AF850332

ENDOCRINOLOGY: DIABETES AND HYPERTENSION

Dr. Kashieca Yap

ALLIED HEALTH PRESS

Endocrinology: Diabetes and Hypertension

Author: **Dr. Kashieca Yap**

Allied Health Press
4164 Lakeshore Road
Burlington ON L7L 1A4
Canada
www.alliedhealthpress.com
Email: orders@arclereducation.com

© 2025 Allied Health Press
ISBN: 978-1-77956-264-7

This book contains information obtained from highly regarded resources. Reprinted material sources are indicated and copyright remains with the original owners. Copyright for images and other graphics remains with the original owners as indicated. A Wide variety of references are listed. Reasonable efforts have been made to publish reliable data. Authors or Editors or Publishers are not responsible for the accuracy of the information in the published chapters or consequences of their use. The publisher assumes no responsibility for any damage or grievance to the persons or property arising out of the use of any materials, instructions, methods or thoughts in the book. The authors or editors and the publisher have attempted to trace the copyright holders of all material reproduced in this publication and apologize to copyright holders if permission has not been obtained. If any copyright holder has not been acknowledged, please write to us so we may rectify.

General Disclaimer:

This book is a summation of information from different sources and encompasses a wide range of medical conditions, the latest therapy methods, principals and techniques that are used in current practice, at the time of publication. This book offers general information with educational purposes, it is not to be applied or relied on for any diagnostic or treatment purposes. Please do not use the data/matter as a substitute for professional diagnosis and treatment. Please consult your healthcare provider or a licensed physician before making any healthcare queries or treatment choices. The medical information and research findings presented in this book are for educational purposes only and should not be used for the treatment of specific individual patients, as individual cases may vary. The author(s), editors(s) and publisher cannot be held accountable and make no guarantees that the information provided in this book will apply to each and individual patient. This book is meant to serve as a basic guideline and other relevant literature sources should be used for more specific information. This text can be a vital resource for students, trainees, and practitioners, covering essential topics. This book encompasses a wide range of medical conditions and the latest therapy options used in current practice. Through the utilization of many different medical studies this book provides the basics of different medical conditions, which can be used as a basic guide from where medical students, trainees and practitioners can extract necessary information. Further, some of the books have graphic images to explain anatomy for medical/educational purposes only. Hence, the book is intended for students or teachers/staff or individuals with a mature outlook looking to learn or enhance their knowledge.

Notice: Registered trademark of products or corporate names are used only for explanation and identification without intent of infringement.

Allied Health Press publishes wide variety of books and eBooks. For more information about Allied Health Press and its products, visit our website at www.alliedhealthpress.com

ABOUT THE AUTHOR

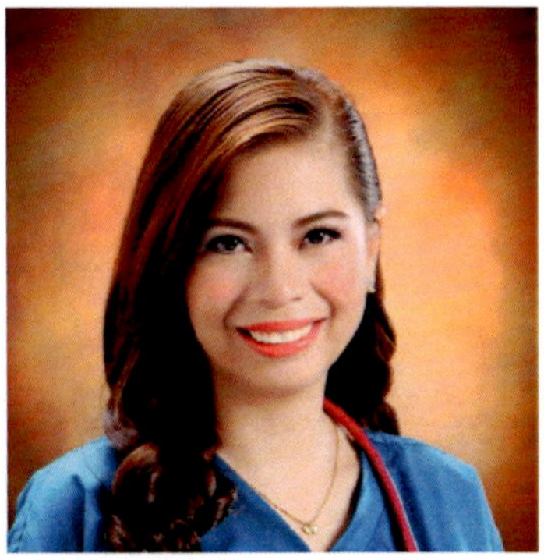

Kashieca Yap, M.D., is a devoted medical doctor and medical writer. She currently works as a general practice physician in a rural town, where she handles adult and pediatric cases, infectious diseases, and chronic medical conditions. Kashieca also lectures on mental health, clinical pharmacology, physiology, and psychiatry and is an enthusiastic researcher and medical writer. She obtained her medical degree from Cebu Doctor's University College of Medicine and further developed her clinical skills at a large public hospital. Alongside her professional endeavors, Kashieca dedicates her time to volunteering at NGOs and medical missions, reaching out to people in geographically isolated areas. Her unwavering passion for medicine and her strong desire to serve people is a testament to her compassion and skill as a healthcare professional.

Word Roots, Prefixes, and Suffixes by Chapter

Chapter 1 Epidemiology of Hypertension in Diabetes

hyper- high or excessive

-osis abnormal condition of a disease Example: hematosis ketosis

-oid resembling

anti- describing something as 'against' or 'opposed to' another

Chapter 2 Hypertension in Chronic Kidney Disease

Anti- opposite, against

Bi two

Calc- relating to calcium

Cyst- prefix denoting a bladder esp. the urinary bladder

Dia- through, throughout

Chapter 3 Diabetes and Hypertension in People with Sleep Apnea

a- Without, lack of Apnea

dys- Bad, difficult, painful Dyspnea

hypo- Under, below, deficient Hypopnea

-pnea Breathing Apnea

Chapter 4 Resistant Hypertension: Etiology, Evaluation and Management

endo- inside

epi- upon

hypo- below

inter- between, among

para- alongside, near

Chapter 5 Diabetes and Cardiovascular Disease

a- absence of, without

bi- two

brady- slow

endo- within, in

epi- on, upon, over

Chapter 6 Hypertension, Diabetes, and the Eye

Tens Derived from the Latin "tendere," meaning to stretch.

Hyper- Means over, above, or excessive.

-ion Indicates a process or condition.

Ophthalm- Derived from the Greek "ophthalmos," meaning eye.

Chapter 7 Endocrine Hypertension in Children

acr/o extremities, height

aden/o gland

adip/o fat

adren/o adrenal glands

endocrin/o endocrine

Chapter 8 Endocrine Hypertension in Pregnant Woman

gravid/o pregnancy

nat/o birth

Culd/o Retrouterine pouch (cul-de-sac)

dys- painful, labored, difficult

Chapter 9 Imaging for Patients with Endocrine Hypertension

angi- blood vessel

ante- describing something as positioned in front of another thing

arteri(o)- of or pertaining to an artery

chrom(ato)- color

Chapter 10 Systematic Approach for the Diagnosis and Management of Endocrine Hypertension

endo- inside

epi- upon

hypo- below

inter- between, among

intra- within

-lysis, -lyso destruction

Table of Contents

LIST OF FIGURES

edema. The conspicuous absence of lipid, bleeding and fibrosis make correct recognition difficult at first glance. (b) Photo of the same eye later that day after PRP was applied. He opted to be initially treated with simultaneous injection of intravitreal steroids

Figure 6.6. Red-free (top) and mid-phase fluorescein angiographic images (bottom) depict microaneurysms—seen as hyper fluorescent spots. A small amount of lipid is seen inferior to the foveola top right image, indicating CSDME. This would be monitored closely, and patient would be advised of the great importance of HTN, BS and lipid control

Figure 6.7. Right (a) and left (b) eye red-free photos depicting moderate NPDR and bilateral CSDME. Lipid is threatening the foveal center (a), and a peri-foveal microaneurysm is causing foveal edema (b). Both eyes display cotton-wool spots indicative of moderate nonproliferative diabetic retinopathy. Patient was treated with focal laser (a) and intravitreal therapy (b), as the microvascular abnormality was judged too close to the fovea to treat safely with laser. Both eyes must be monitored very closely for progression to PDR. PRP laser may be necessary within months, or if patient is judged unreliable to follow-up

Figure 6.8. (a) This is a normal fundus fluorescein mid-phase circulation image of the right eye . The retinal vessels show fluorescence about 1 min after fluorescein intravenous dye injection. (b) Note the healthy (magnified) appearance of the capillary network surrounding the anatomical foveola. The extent of the central black area represents the so-called foveolar avascular zone

Figure 6.9. Red-free photos (top) and late-phase fluorescein angiographic photos (bottom) of the right and left eyes. Diffuse CSDME with circinate lipid exuation is evident

Figure 6.10. Red-free photos (top) and late-circulation fluorescein angiographic images (bottom). Large areas of hypo fluorescence are seen consistent with nonperfusion/ischemia. Neovascularization, which is hyper fluorescent, tends to occur at borders of these areas (so-called watershed zones). Fibrosis is evident in the upper right photo, in a commonly seen con figuration. This is very severe PDR of both eyes (o.u.)

Figure 6.11. (a – f) This 45-year-old long-standing IDDM patient has very severe, flat NVE (a , b) which has invaded the macula in the right eye (a). He recently had PRP at another facility in the o.d. (a , c) and attributes his 20/25 vision to that event. Extensive hyper fluorescent areas represent NVE (d – f). There is a conspicuous absence of NVD and VH, though, and his uncorrected vision is excellent (20/25 R and 20/20 L). He is at high risk of sudden, near simultaneous blindness. His macular disease will be treated with intravitreal therapy (Avastin) R , focal and grid laser L , and aggressive scatter PRP laser (o.u.)

Figure 6.12. Upper images depict SD-OCT (Heidelberg) (left) in a normal macula and its associated topographic thickness map in microns (right). Lower images depict SD-OCT (left) in chronic CSDME and associated topographic thickness map in microns (right). ILM internal limiting membrane, BM Bruch's membrane

Figure 6.13. SD-OCT image (Optovue ™) which depict macular edema of the right eye (a) and a nice foveal contour several months after focal laser of the left (b)

Figure 6.14. This patient had "perfect" vision until occurrence of " floaters" R several days before presentation. He had severe PDR which was occult and unrecognized until she experienced a "sentinel bleed" in the form of VH R (a , c). Aggressive PRP will be applied in an exigent fashion, as further bleeding will necessitate urgent PPV. L will be treated with aggressive PRP (b , d , e). Surgery in this setting is quite treacherous as the risk of intra- and postoperative bleeding is high in the un- or inadequately lasered eye

LIST OF TABLES

PREFACE

Diabetes is a major cardiovascular risk factor worldwide. Heart rate and heart rate variability are crucial predictors of cardiovascular and total morbidity and mortality in diabetic patients. The combination of arterial hypertension and diabetes negatively affects cardiovascular remodeling and outcomes. Thus, determining the optimal blood pressure threshold for initiating antihypertensive therapy and the target blood pressure in diabetic patients remains a topic of debate. A comprehensive cardiac assessment, including 24-hour ECG, ambulatory blood pressure monitoring, and echocardiography, is now available to evaluate cardiac damage in diabetic patients.

A 24-hour ECG can assess heart rate variability, providing valuable information on the autonomic nervous system, which plays a key role in adverse outcomes in diabetic patients. Ambulatory blood pressure monitoring offers data on daytime, nighttime, and 24-hour blood pressure values, as well as circadian blood pressure patterns (dipping and non-dipping), all of which are crucial in diabetic patients.

This book aims to underscore the significance of blood pressure, heart rate, and arterial hypertension in diabetic patients.

The incidence and prevalence of type 2 diabetes are on the rise, with projections indicating a global increase from 171 million in 2000 to 366 million by 2030. The number of adults with hypertension is also expected to increase by 60%, reaching 1.56 billion by 2025. Hypertension affects around 70% of diabetic patients, occurring twice as often in individuals with diabetes compared to those without. The prevalence of concurrent hypertension and diabetes varies among different ethnic, racial, and social groups. Importantly, hypertension significantly raises the risk of vascular complications and chronic kidney disease in diabetic patients. The overlap between hypertension and diabetes also substantially increases the risk of ischemic cerebrovascular disease, retinopathy, and sexual dysfunction. Diabetes mellitus independently increases the risk of coronary artery disease, with a markedly higher risk when hypertension is present.

Endocrine hypertension, accounting for 10% of secondary hypertension cases, can be diagnosed in about 1% of all hypertensive patients. This type of hypertension, primarily due to conditions like primary aldosteronism, hypercortisolism, pheochromocytoma, hyperparathyroidism, and thyroid dysfunctions, involves hormonal mechanisms that affect blood pressure regulation. Pathological mechanisms exacerbated by hormonal excess contribute to the organ damage seen in endocrine hypertension. This condition is often associated with metabolic disorders such as diabetes and dyslipidemia, further elevating cardiovascular risk. Advances in genetic and molecular biology have enhanced our understanding of the hormonal mechanisms and pathophysiological pathways in endocrine hypertension, offering prospects for tailored approaches in the future. This text provides updates on diagnostic and therapeutic strategies for managing endocrine hypertension and its related organ damage.

This comprehensive book aims to provide a thorough understanding of the intricate interplay between diabetes and hypertension within the field of endocrinology. It explains the pathophysiology, epidemiology, diagnosis, and management of these conditions, offering insights into their impact on various organ systems. By exploring the latest research and treatment strategies, the book aims to enhance the knowledge and skills of endocrinologists, diabetologists, cardiologists, nephrologists, and other healthcare professionals involved in the care of patients with diabetes and hypertension. Additionally, it seeks to raise awareness among medical students, researchers, and educators about the growing burden of these diseases and the importance of multidisciplinary approaches in their management. Finally, this book aspires to serve as a valuable resource for advancing clinical practice, research, and education in the field of endocrinology and related disciplines.

Chapter 1

EPIDEMIOLOGY OF HYPERTENSION IN DIABETES

Contents

INTRODUCTION

It is well recognized that having diabetes and hypertension together can compound the negative clinical outcomes associated with both microvascular and macrovascular disease. Therefore, an integrated strategy that combines appropriate glycemic control with optimal blood pressure and lipid control is necessary for effective diabetes management. The pathophysiology of hypertension in diabetes includes immune system abnormalities, detrimental environmental factors, vascular endothelial dysfunction, and increased activation of the renin-angiotensin-aldosterone system. Maladaptive changes in the autonomic nervous system also play a role. Numerous randomized controlled trials have demonstrated that lowering high blood pressure in diabetics reduces morbidity. Because most patients with diabetes are at higher risk of cardiovascular disease (CVD) than those without diabetes, attention must be given to individual risk factors and comorbidities with a goal of less than 130/80 mm Hg. The approach to controlling blood pressure in these patients includes good glycemic control, optimizing weight, encouraging exercise, and reducing harmful environmental factors like exposure to air pollution. It is crucial to choose a therapy carefully and to take pertinent side-effect profiles into account. Drug combinations should be selected after careful consideration of the potential for both positive and negative drug interactions. While combined use of these agents is not advised due to poor renal outcomes, angiotensin-converting enzyme inhibitors and angiotensin receptor blockers remain preferred agents for the initiation of antihypertensive therapy. When starting therapy for glycemic control, consideration should be given to the antihypertensive, renal, and cardiovascular disease-lowering properties of the newer antidiabetic agents, such as SGLT inhibitors and GLP1 receptor agonists (Oparil et al., 2003).

Orientation and Directional Terms

Term	Definition	Illustration
Diabetes	Diabetes is a disease that occurs when your blood glucose, also called blood sugar, is too high. Glucose is your body's main source of energy. Your body can make glucose, but glucose also comes from the food you eat.	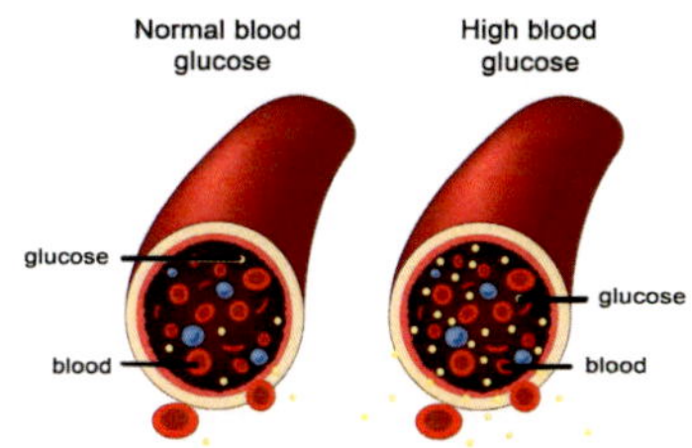
Orthostatic hypotension	Orthostatic hypotension is a drop in blood pressure on standing to a certain extent. It hampers the quality of life and increases the risk of falls, cardiovascular diseases, dementia, depression, and death. Orthostatic hypotension is defined as a sudden drop in blood pressure upon standing from a sitting or supine position.	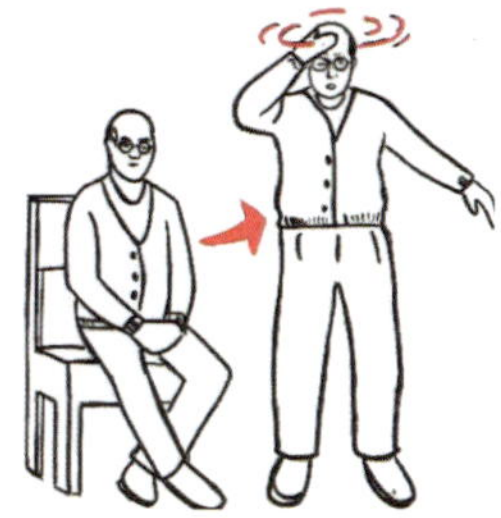
Renin-angiotensin-aldosterone system (RAAS)	The renin-angiotensin-aldosterone system (RAAS), or renin-angiotensin-system (RAS) is a regulator of blood pressure and cardiovascular function. Dysregulated RAAS is implicated in high blood pressure, cardiovascular and kidney conditions, and medications targeting RAAS can improve these conditions.	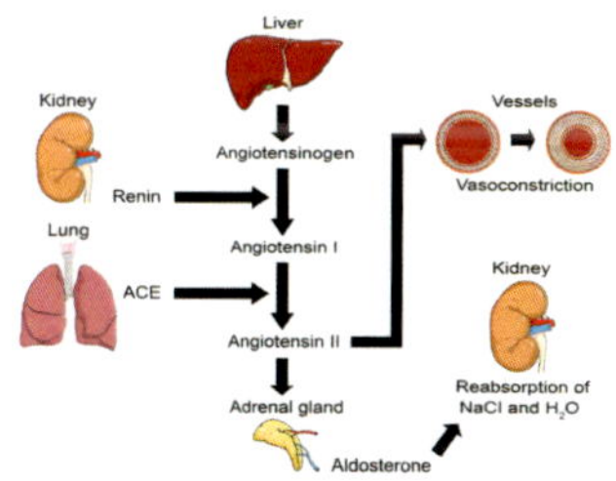
Angiotensin	Angiotensin is a peptide endocrine hormone and an important part of the renin-angiotensin-aldosterone system, an inter-related endocrine system important in volume and blood pressure control. Angiotensinogen, an alpha-globulin, and the peptide prohormone are synthesized primarily by the liver and circulate in plasma.	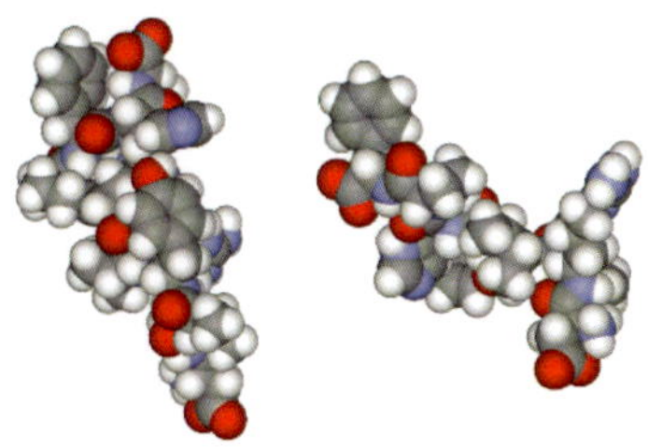
DASH diet	DASH is an acronym for "Dietary Approaches to Stop Hypertension" which is a diet rich in fruits, vegetables, whole grains, and dairy. It limits sugar-sweetened foods and beverages, red meat, and added fats. In addition to its effect on blood pressure, it is designed to be a well-balanced approach to eating for the general public.	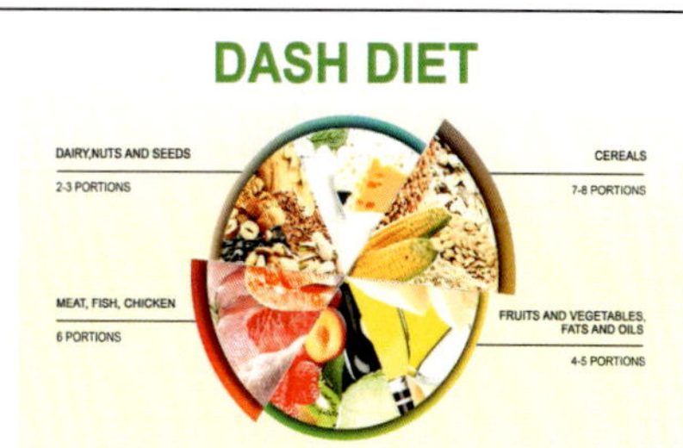

1.1. PATHOPHYSIOLOGY OF HYPERTENSION IN DIABETES

Increased activation of the renin-angiotensin-aldosterone system (RAAS), complex interactions between the autonomic nervous system, a maladaptive immune system, and unfavorable environmental factors are all contributing factors to the pathophysiology of hypertension in diabetes. The following factors have been the focus of therapeutic interventions because they are important players in the pathophysiology of hypertension (see Figure 1.1) (Sowers et al., 2001).

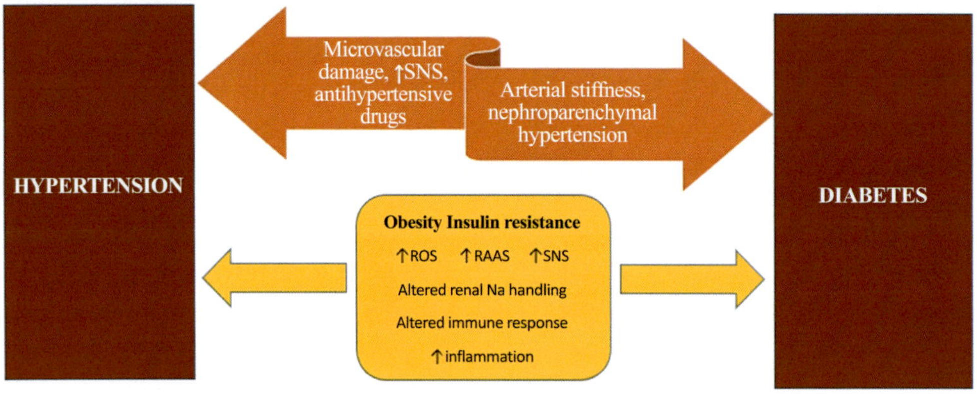

Figure 1.1. *Relationship between hypertension and diabetes.*

Source: https://link.springer.com/article/10.1007/s13410-022-01143-7.

1.1.1. Sedentary Lifestyle, Excessive Caloric Intake, and Insulin Resistance

An increased risk of exacerbating insulin resistance has been linked to adiposity, which can be caused by a sedentary lifestyle and an excessive calorie intake. Insulin resistance has been connected, in turn, to elevated vascular oxidative stress, inflammation, and endothelial dysfunction, which is marked by reduced vascular nitric oxide bioactivity. These factors all contribute to vascular stiffness, which raises blood pressure over time and predisposes to CVD (Figure 1.2) (Oparil et al., 2003).

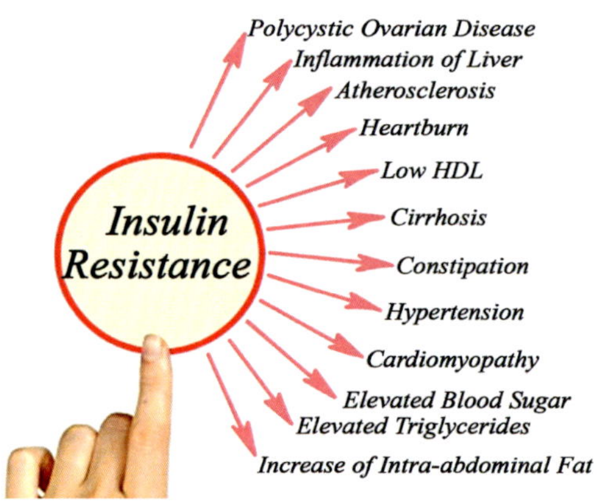

Figure 1.2. *Insulin resistance.*

Source: https://www.nature.com/collections/hhhcddbahe.

1.1.2. Elevated Intravascular Volume

The total sodium content of the body has a strong influence on intravascular volume. The primary extracellular cation in humans is sodium, which has osmotic activity that influences effective arterial blood volume. A positive sodium balance may arise from an imbalance between sodium loss and intake. As a result, the intravascular sodium concentration rises, which increases intravascular volume by encouraging an influx of water along the osmotic gradient. According to the Frank Starling Law, an increase in intravascular volume subsequently causes an increase in venous return to the heart, which increases cardiac output and ultimately raises arterial pressure. Additionally, there is mounting evidence that, in states of obesity and insulin resistance, like those experienced by the majority of T2DM patients, increased activation of sodium inward transport in endothelial cells leads to elevated blood pressure and increased vascular stiffness.

Increasing glomerular filtration and compensatory urinary salt excretion usually lower elevated blood pressure (BP) caused by intravascular volume expansion. Pressure natriuresis is the term used to describe this phenomenon of increased excretion of salt in a state of elevated blood pressure. Unfortunately, secondary changes within the kidney microvasculature and maladaptive changes within the glomerular apparatus itself, which lower glomerular filtration and stimulate sodium reabsorption, mean that this mechanism alone is unable to correct persistently elevated blood pressure. Overt chronic kidney disease (CKD) and end stage renal disease (ESRD), which are both characterized by simultaneous volume overload and persistent hypertension, are the conditions in which these alterations are most noticeable. Restoring normal vascular volume is necessary to control hypertension in CKD/ESRD patients, which can be done with diuretics or dialysis (Van et al., 2013).

1.1.3. Premature Vascular Aging

Variations in the elasticity of the vessel lumen have an impact on how easily blood can pass through arteries. Even slight decreases in lumen diameter have the potential to cause an exponential rise in blood flow resistance. Individuals suffering from hypertension frequently exhibit anatomical and functional alterations that negatively impact the lumen of arterioles and small arteries. Elevated blood pressure can cause vascular remodeling, low-grade inflammation, vascular fibrosis, and stiffening that are associated with hypertension in people with diabetes. Therefore, diabetes patients exhibit accelerated premature vascular aging, which is characterized by increased vascular smooth muscle contraction and resistance, vascular stiffness, and impaired endothelial-mediated relaxation. These maladaptive vascular alterations expedite the detrimental effects of hypertension on vessel integrity in addition to aiding in the development of hypertension.

1.1.4. Autonomic Nervous System Dysregulation

Autonomic nervous system function plays a significant role in BP regulation. Blood pressure is regulated by both the parasympathetic and sympathetic nervous systems. Increased peripheral vascular resistance, heart rate, ventricle contraction force, and fluid retention are all caused by increased sympathetic activity. The sum of these physiological processes leads to an increase in blood pressure. A decrease in parasympathetic outflow also raises heart rate and causes a relative increase in sympathetic hyperactivity, both of which raise blood pressure. Insulin resistance, sleep apnea, and central obesity are associated with dysregulation of these pathways. Resistant hypertension, an activated RAAS, and elevated sympathetic activity are frequently present in conjunction with hypertension linked to these disorders. Moreover, insulin resistance and the risk of type 2 diabetes are also encouraged by sympathetic nervous system activation. T2DM-related autonomic dysfunction may also exacerbate hypertension by contributing to these alterations. Improvements in insulin sensitivity, better glycemic control, and lower blood pressure are linked to renal denervation, which interrupts the central sympathetic outflow, indicating the importance of these pathways in the etiology of hypertension and diabetes.

1.1.5. Renin Angiotensin Aldosterone System (RAAS)

The RAAS pathway is essential for preserving normal blood pressure. The pathophysiology of hypertension is closely associated with RAAS activation due to the elevated levels of plasma aldosterone, which have effects on the kidneys and cardiovascular system. Strong vasoconstrictor angiotensin II directly raises the tone of smooth muscle in the blood vessels. Angiotensin II also increases aldosterone secretion, which encourages the retention of water and salt and raises blood pressure by expanding the volume. Even when there is no increase in angiotensin levels, obesity is linked to higher plasma aldosterone levels. This increase is believed to be partially caused by the expanded adipose tissue's secretion of aldosterone-releasing factors. Since angiotensin converting enzyme (ACE) inhibitors, angiotensin II receptor blockers (ARBs), and increasingly mineralocorticoid receptor antagonists are the mainstays of blood pressure management in people with diabetes, an understanding of the physiology of RAAS is crucial.

The kidney's juxtaglomerular cells secrete the proteolytic enzyme renin. Circulating angiotensinogen is broken down by renin into angiotensin I. Angiotensin I is subsequently changed into angiotensin II by ACE in the lung capillaries. Renin production and release are closely regulated by many interrelated factors, including sodium chloride concentration in the distal tubule of the nephron, renal perfusion pressure, and sympathetic nervous system stimulation of renin-secreting cells.

When there is hypovolemia-induced renal hypoperfusion, RAAS is physiologically activated. Angiotensin II production rises as a result of a series of events triggered by the juxtaglomerular apparatus's release of renin. Following direct vasoconstriction, angiotensin II increases blood pressure by stimulating aldosterone secretion, which causes salt and water retention and restores intravascular volume (Lewington et al., 2002).

Inappropriate RAAS and sympathetic nervous system activation is linked to obesity and insulin resistance. High plasma aldosterone levels have been associated with increased adiposity, which suggests that RAAS may be chronically overactive in obesity. In classical insulin-sensitive tissues, it has been demonstrated that angiotensin II and aldosterone inhibit insulin metabolic signaling. This likely contributes to a decrease in endothelial-mediated vascular relaxation and the emergence of hypertension. Through non-genomic mechanisms like increased serine phosphorylation of insulin receptor substrate 1, decreased phosphatidylinositol 3-kinase engagement and protein kinase B stimulation, decreased insulin metabolic signaling, and impaired nitric oxide-mediated vascular relaxation, angiotensin II and aldosterone may also contribute to insulin resistance. It is becoming more widely known that increased vascular stiffness and related increases in hypertension and CVD are caused by elevated aldosterone in combination with hyperinsulinemia, which is frequently present in obesity and insulin resistance.

1.1.6. Renal Dysfunction

There is a reciprocal relationship between renal dysfunction and hypertension in diabetic individuals. Hypertension is a known risk factor for chronic kidney disease in diabetes, but diabetic nephropathy can also lead to the development of hypertension. This connection is particularly noticeable in type 1 diabetics without prior hypertension. Studies have shown that microalbuminuria often comes before hypertension in this group, and the prevalence of hypertension increases as kidney disease worsens, reaching 90% in type 1 diabetics with end-stage renal disease. The proposed mechanisms for this relationship include volume expansion due to increased renal sodium reabsorption, peripheral vasoconstriction from endothelial dysfunction, dysregulated activation of the RAAS system, upregulation of endothelin, and downregulation of nitric oxide.

1.1.7. Role of Innate and Adaptive Immunity

There is growing evidence that vascular disease and hypertension brought on by angiotensin II and aldosterone are related to both innate immunity and acquired immunity. According to research on animals, T cells and macrophages mediate the oxidative damage linked to these effects, and complete expression of these negative effects is contingent upon intact T cell function. Conversely, T regulatory cells' protective qualities in animal models point to a possible therapeutic role for these cells, though as of right now, these interventions are only possible in a research setting.

1.1.8. Environmental and Socioeconomic Factors

White and Black Americans differ significantly in their rates of hypertension. Despite Black Americans being more aware of and receiving treatment for their hypertension than White Americans, this gap is widening. The recent Covid-19 pandemic has increased this gap, with communities of color experiencing disproportionately high rates of morbidity and mortality. There have been suggestions that the differences in Covid outcomes can be attributed to the same social, economic, and environmental injustices that support obesity, diabetes, and hypertension.

People living in these communities frequently consume low-cost, high-salted, high-calorie foods, which inevitably results in obesity and hypertension. In addition, a lack of secure outdoor areas deters physical activity, and targeted advertising promotes unhealthy choices like smoking.

A study of Black and White Americans residing in long-term integrated neighborhoods provides additional evidence for these effects. Although the odds ratio for hypertension was higher in Blacks in the sample population, it was found to be about 30% lower in the Exploring Health Disparities in Integrated Communities-South Western Baltimore (EHDIC-SWB) study when compared to NHANES data. The authors came to the conclusion that a significant amount of the racial differences in people with diabetes and hypertension could be explained by social and environmental exposure (UK Prospective Diabetes Study (UKPDS) Group, 1998).

1.2. BLOOD PRESSURE MEASUREMENT AND MONITORING

Precise blood pressure measurement is essential for diagnosing and successfully treating hypertension. The majority of the time, blood pressure is measured in a doctor's office using either the oscillometric approach used in automated devices or the auscultatory method of listening to Korotkoff sounds. Because oscillometric devices are more convenient to use and reduce inter-observer variability in manual measurements, the auscultatory method has mostly been replaced by them. But it is crucial to keep in mind that, if certain measures are ignored, even automated measurements may turn out to be inaccurate. After the patient has rested for three to five minutes, measurements should be taken while they are seated or lying down, ideally with an empty bladder. No exertion, exercise, eating, smoking, or stressful situations for at least half an hour before taking a blood pressure reading. In a span of two weeks, three readings will be optimal. To guarantee accurate readings, the device should be calibrated on a regular basis.

An incorrect cuff size is a common cause of reading errors. It is advised that the cuff bladder's width be roughly half of the arm circumference and that its length match the patient's arm circumference as measured at the midpoint of the olecranon and acromion processes. Because obesity is becoming more common, using cuffs that are too small can lead to an overestimation of blood pressure. Even with all these safety measures, there can still be a lot of variation in one reading from another, which is why the American Heart Association (AHA) advises getting at least two readings every clinic visit. (Muntner et al., 2019)

A fully automated non-invasive procedure called ambulatory blood pressure monitoring (ABPM) involves placing a blood pressure cuff on the non-dominant arm and taking readings every 15 to 30 minutes for a full day. ABPM has a better prognostic value for target organ damage and cardiovascular outcomes than in-office blood pressure monitoring. The main benefit of ABPM over office monitoring, which depends on individual measurements, is its comprehensiveness. Different blood pressure patterns that cannot be identified with office measurements alone, such as sustained, white-coat, masked, and nocturnal hypertension, as well as non-dipping or reverse-dipping patterns, can be detected. These patterns need to be treated very differently because they are linked to different cardiovascular outcomes. When ABPM readings are consistently normal but office measurements are in the hypertensive range, the condition is known as "white-coat hypertension."

This phenomenon is linked to low cardiovascular risk and is not a sign that antihypertensive medication is necessary. It is ascribed to the influence of an observer during the measurement. However, it should be noted that people with white coats are more likely to experience persistent hypertension and should thus undergo routine monitoring. Conversely, "masked hypertension" describes a state in which ABPM readings fall into the hypertensive range, despite office measurements being normal.

This phenomenon is linked to elevated cardiovascular risk, similar to what is observed in cases of long-term hypertension. Crucially, masked hypertension is more prevalent in patients with diabetes and obesity. Aggressive antihypertensive therapy is thought to benefit these patients, but no randomized controlled trials have been conducted to support this theory.

Normal blood pressure readings follow a physiologic circadian rhythm, with a drop of over 10% during the night compared to daytime readings. Patients with a non-dipping pattern are those whose blood pressure decreases by less than 10%. This non-dipping pattern has been linked to cardiovascular autonomic neuropathy and is more common in diabetics. Its role in the development of diabetic complications is less clear. Due to its effects on renal hemodynamics, blood flow distribution, and circulating plasma volume, hyperglycemia itself can affect the typical nocturnal dip.

1.3. BLOOD PRESSURE TARGET IN PATIENTS WITH DIABETES

It is impossible to overstate the significance of strict blood pressure management in preventing diabetes-related morbidity. There is growing evidence to support this for both microvascular and macrovascular complications. According to the United Kingdom Prospective Diabetes Study (UKPDS), lowering blood pressure (target blood pressure <150/85 mm Hg) was associated with 44%, 32%, and 34% lower risks of stroke, diabetes-related deaths, and retinopathy, respectively. Systolic blood pressure reduction was found to have a linear relationship with unfavorable outcomes at as low as 120 mm Hg.

A decrease in diastolic blood pressure was associated with a decrease in CVD, according to the Hypertension on Target (HOT) trial. Interestingly, though, this benefit was limited to patients with diabetes, indicating that a different, possibly more aggressive blood pressure target should be set for this population subgroup.

The first study specifically designed to address blood pressure control in subjects with diabetes was the Action in Diabetes and Vascular Disease: Preterax and Diamicron MR Controlled Evaluation (ADVANCE) trial. Impressive results were obtained, with a mean achieved blood pressure of 134/74 mm Hg as opposed to 140/76 mm Hg, indicating a significant reduction in microvascular events, cardiovascular deaths, and all-cause mortality with aggressive reduction in both systolic and diastolic blood pressure.

For patients with diabetes, major medical societies such as the American Diabetes Association (ADA) recommend a target blood pressure of less than 130/80 mm Hg. The Normotensive Appropriate Blood Pressure Control in Diabetes (ABCD) trial was the first to look for support for this recommendation. The intensive treatment group's mean blood pressure of 128/75 mm Hg was below the 130 mm Hg systolic target, despite no specific blood pressure target being pursued. Comparing the creatinine clearance (primary outcome) and cardiovascular events over a five-year follow-up period to the placebo group revealed no discernible differences (mean blood pressure 137/81). There were notable improvements in the acute treatment group's albuminuria, stroke risk, and retinopathy progression.

The Action to Control Cardiovascular Risk in Diabetes (ACCORD) blood pressure trial cast doubt on the idea of aiming for a systolic blood pressure of less than 130 mm Hg. A systolic target of less than 120 mm Hg (intensive therapy) was compared to a systolic target of less than 140 mm Hg (standard therapy) in this sizable randomized control trial. There was no discernible difference between the two groups in terms of the combined CVD outcomes (heart attack, stroke, and cardiovascular death) with over 4500 patients and a mean follow-up of 4 years and 7 months. Significantly, there was a 40% decrease in the risk of stroke, which is comparable to the ABCD trial's findings (Suh et al., 2009).

The Systolic Blood Pressure Intervention Trial (SPRINT) was the most recent large-scale randomized control trial that looked at a lower systolic blood pressure goal. In this study, the benefits of treatment were compared between groups receiving intensive treatment (whose systolic blood pressure target was less than 120 mm Hg) and standard treatment (whose target was less than 140 mm Hg). At one year, the standard treatment group's mean systolic blood pressure was 136.2 mm Hg, while the intensive treatment group's was 121.4 mm Hg. The intensive treatment group exhibited significantly lower rates of cardiovascular events, both fatal and nonfatal, as well as death from all causes, according to the results. With a hazard ratio of 1.88 (P<0.001), serious adverse events that were either definitely or possibly related to the intervention occurred statistically more frequently in the group receiving intensive treatment. 9361 participants with a median follow-up of 3.26 years were included in this study; however, patients with diabetes were not included. Because of its study design, the SPRINT trial cannot be directly applied to the diabetic population, but it does support a lower goal.

The ACCORD trial may not have had enough power to demonstrate a statistically significant difference for the primary endpoint, according to some experts. The same primary endpoint from the SPRINT trial was examined in a recent pooled analysis that combined data from the ACCORD and SPRINT trials. In addition to myocardial infarction, stroke, and CVD death, the primary endpoint was different from the ACCORD trial in that it also included unstable angina and acute decompensated heart failure.

Table 1.1. *Key Outcome Studies and Results*

Outcome Study	**Intervention**	**Results**
United Kingdom Prospective Diabetes Study (UKPDS)	Blood pressure reduction (< 150/85 mmHg)	44% risk reduction in stroke 32% risk reduction in diabetes related deaths 34% risk of retinopathy
Hypertension On Target Trial (HOT)	Lower diastolic blood pressure	Reduction in CVD
Action in Diabetes and Vascular Disease: Preterax and Diamicron MR Controlled Evaluation trial (ADVANCE)	Reduced systolic and diastolic blood pressure (134/74mmHg vs 140/76mmHg)	Reduction in microvascular events, cardiovascular deaths, and all-cause mortality
Normotensive Appropriate Blood Pressure Control in Diabetes Trial (ABCD)	Intensive blood pressure control (128/75mmHg vs 137/81mmHg)	Reduction in progression of retinopathy, albuminuria, and absolute risk of stroke No difference in creatinine clearance or cardiovascular events
ACCORD Study Group Trial	Intensive blood pressure control (Systolic target <120mmHg vs <140mmHg)	40% risk reduction for stroke No difference for combined CVD outcomes (heart attack, stroke, and cardiovascular death)
Systolic Blood Pressure Intervention Trial (SPRINT)	Intensive blood pressure control (Systolic target <120mmHg vs <140mmHg) Achieved mean blood pressure 121.4mmHg vs 136.2mmHg	Reduced rates of fatal and nonfatal cardiovascular evens and death Increased adverse events related to intensive group

Source: https://www.ncbi.nlm.nih.gov/books/NBK279027/.

Both patients with and without diabetes showed a significant positive effect from the intensive treatment group, according to the final analysis. This implies that patients with type 2 diabetes may not benefit differently from aggressive blood pressure lowering (to less than 130/80 mm Hg). It should be mentioned that blood pressure was measured in the SPRINT and ACCORD trials under very controlled circumstances, which should have resulted in lower readings than in traditional clinic settings. This finding begs the question of whether similar cardiovascular benefits could be obtained in real-world situations by using more lenient targets (Brown et al., 2000).

Numerous excellent randomized controlled trials have demonstrated that treating elevated blood pressure in diabetics reduces morbidity. It seems that patients with type 2 diabetes are especially vulnerable to the harmful effects of hypertension on the development and course of cardiovascular disease. When deciding on lower treatment targets for patients with diabetes who have hypertension, consideration needs to be given to co-morbidities, patient preferences, and individual risk factors. For example, a young person who would benefit from a reduction in stroke risk and retinopathy progression without experiencing the unfavorable side effects of hypotension, syncope, and hyperkalemia—symptoms that are more frequently experienced by the elderly and those with multiple co-morbidities—might be better off having a lower blood pressure target (Table 1.1).

1.4. THE RELATIONSHIP BETWEEN HYPERGYCEMIA AND HYPERTENSION IN DIABETIC PATIENTS

1.4.1. Hyperglycemia elevates Blood Pressure

The volume of exchangeable sodium in vivo that is higher in diabetic patients than in non-diabetics due to hyperglycemia is the main cause of hypertension in these patients. In a study, the volume of exchangeable sodium in patients with type 1 diabetes was found to be between 2800 and 3000 mEq per 1.73 m^2, which is roughly 10% higher than in non-diabetics. Patients with overt albuminuria had a significantly higher volume of exchangeable sodium than patients with normoalbuminuria or microalbuminuria. However, the study purportedly did not discover any variations in the amount of circulating plasma between individuals with diabetes and those without it. Moreover, there was a positive correlation between the mean blood pressure and the volume of exchangeable sodium in diabetic patients. The primary cause of this is thought to be elevated sodium glucose co-transporter (SGLT) 2 levels, which increase glucose and sodium (Na) reabsorption. It is possible for the glomerular filtration rate (GFR) to rise, or for hyperfiltration to become apparent. Such an excess of bodily fluid volume is not related to the renin-angiotensin (RA) system. Put another way, the majority of diabetics frequently exhibit normal or slightly low plasma renin activity and aldosterone concentration values. Additionally, the blood test results indicate a high level of inactive renin and a decrease in the conversion to active type. However, advances in molecular biology are progressively yielding new information and discoveries. Examples include the pathophysiological significance of prorenin and (pro)renin receptors, the mechanism by which high salt intake activates mineralocorticoid receptors inside the kidneys, and the local intrarenal acceleration of tissue RA systems.

1.4.2. Diabetes is a salt-sensitive Hypertension

Patients with diabetes are thought to have high glomerular blood pressure, a flatter pressure-diuresis curve, and salt-sensitive hypertension. The reabsorption of sodium from the renal tubules is accelerated by hyperinsulinemia brought on by insulin resistance. Consuming too much salt prevents the nocturnal blood pressure from falling, or, to put it another way, the patient's nocturnal blood pressure is raised above normal to expel extra sodium, preventing them from falling asleep. Reducing salt intake has been shown to improve vascular endothelial cell functions and insulin resistance. Numerous clinical results support this claim, even in patients with diabetes and impaired glucose tolerance (Blonde et al., 2015).

1.4.3. Blood Pressure Drops with Improvement of Hyperglycemia

Blood pressure is known to decrease as hyperglycemia improves after educational hospitalization and the start of hypoglycemic medication. It has been reported that pioglitazone and metformin, which reduce insulin resistance, have mild hypotensive effects. Some newer hypoglycemic medications, however, have hypotensive properties that are superior to these medications. Daily doses of 1.2–1.8 mg of liraglutide, for example, have been shown to produce hypotensive effects of 2.7–6.6 mmHg in SBP when used in conjunction with GLP-1 receptor agonists. DPP-4 inhibitors, which block the action of dipeptidyl peptidase (DPP)-4, are said to exhibit some hypotensive effects, albeit to a lesser extent than GLP-1 receptor agonists. There is debate because the exact mechanism by which GLP-1 and GLP-1 receptor agonists lower blood pressure has not been fully determined. It appears, however, that these medications also directly inhibit natrium-hydrogen exchanger 3 (NHE3) in the proximal tubules, preventing the reabsorption of sodium and glucose and promoting natriuretic activity in addition to the previously mentioned vasodilating effects. Since DPP-4 binds to NHE3, NHE3 activity is inhibited when DPP-4 inhibitors act from the luminal side, leading to natriuresis. On the other hand, SGLT2 inhibitors prevent sodium and glucose from being reabsorbed in the proximal tubules, which results in natriuresis. As a result, both blood pressure and body weight decrease. A 16- to 24-week administration of these drugs decreased diastolic blood pressure (DBP) by 1.1–2.7 mmHg and SBP by 2.6–5.6 mmHg in a phase II or III clinical study carried out in Japan, as indicated in Table 1.2. According to a meta-analysis conducted in the US and Europe, SBP decreased by 3.77 mmHg (95% confidence interval [CI]: −4.65 to −2.90) and DBP decreased by 1.75 mmHg (95% confidence interval [CI]: −2.27 to −1.23) in 21 placebo-controlled studies. The EMPA-REG BP study, in which 825 type 2 diabetic patients with hypertension received empagliflozin for 12 weeks, has just released its results.

Table 1.2. *Effects of SGLT2 Inhibitors on HbA1C, Body Weight (BW) and Systolic, and Diastolic Blood Pressure (SBP and DBP)*

	ipriglralfozin 50 m	**dapagliflozin 5 mg**	**dapagliflozin 10 mg**	**luseogliflozin 2.5 mg**	**tofogliflozin 20 mg**	**canagliflozin 100 mg**	**empagliflozin 10 mg**	**empagliflozin 25 mg**
Periods	16w	24w	24w	24w	24w	24w	24w	24w
ΔHbA1C	−1.24	−0.4	−0.45	−0.75	−0.77	−1.03	−0.74	−0.85
ΔBW	−1.47	−1.29	−1.38	−1.77	−1.87	−3	−1.93	−2.15
ΔSBP	−3.1	−2.8	−2.7	−5.6	−4.4	−5.16	−2.6	−3.4
ΔDBP	−1.1	NA	NA	−2.5	−2.7	−2.61	−0.6	−1.5

Source: *Katayama, S., Hatano, M. & Issiki, M. Clinical features and therapeutic perspectives on hypertension in diabetics. Hypertens Res 41, 213–229 (2018). https://doi.org/10.1038/s41440-017-0001-5.*

Table 1.3. *Recent Cardiovascular Outcome Studies Using SGLT2 Inhibitor or GLP-1 Receptor Agonist*

	Subjects	*n*	Duration	3P-MACE	CV death	All-cause mortality	Non-fatal MI	Non-fatal stroke	Hospitalization due to HF	Nephropathy$^{\#}$	Retinopathy
EMPA-REG	CVD history(+)	7020	3.1 yr	0.86^{***}	0.62***	0.68^{***}	0.87	1.24	0.65^{**}	0.61^{***}	
LEADER	High risk of CVD	9340	3.8 yr	0.87^{**}	0.78^{**}	0.85^{*}	0.88	0.89	0.87	0.78^{**}	1.15
SUSTAIN-6	CVD history (+)	3297	2 yr	0.74^{***}	0.98	1.05	0.74	0.61*	1.11	0.64^{**}	1.76*

Source: *Katayama, S., Hatano, M. & Issiki, M. Clinical features and therapeutic perspectives on hypertension in diabetics. Hypertens Res 41, 213–229 (2018). https://doi.org/10.1038/s41440-017-0001-5.*

According to the findings, the group receiving empagliflozin experienced a drop in daytime SBP of roughly 10 mmHg in comparison to the placebo group. The 24-hour mean SBP of the empagliflozin group was 3.44 mmHg lower than that of the placebo group following the administration of 10 mg/day and 4.16 mmHg lower following the administration of 25 mg/day. At that time, the mean 24-hour DBP reduction level was 1.36 and 1.72 mmHg, respectively. We still remember the startling outcomes of the empagliflozin-using EMPA-REG OUTCOME study. In this secondary prevention study, 10, 25, or 10 mg/day of empagliflozin were administered to 7028 type 2 diabetic patients with a history of CVD. After that, they were monitored for a mean of 3½ years. As indicated in Table 1.3, the groups receiving empagliflozin experienced HRs of p in contrast to the placebo group.

1.5. MANAGEMENT OF BLOOD PRESSURE IN PATIENTS WITH DIABETES

Particularly in individuals with diabetes, hypertension is a significant risk factor for cardiovascular morbidity and mortality. Individuals with normal blood pressure (BP) are not as likely to develop diabetes as those with hypertension, who have a two to three times higher risk. Individuals with type 2 diabetes are two to four times more likely than non-diabetic individuals to die from cardiovascular (CV) causes. Diabetes and hypertension together have a catastrophic effect on the CV system. Blood pressure control is especially helpful for diabetic patients, but only about 30% of these patients achieve the current blood pressure target (Smits et al., 2016).

Compared to age-matched subjects without type 2 diabetes, patients with the disease have a roughly two-fold higher incidence of hypertension. In people with diabetes, blood pressure readings greater than 130/80 mmHg are considered high.

Recent studies have shown strong correlations between age and body mass index (BMI) with the prevalence of diabetes mellitus and hypertension. The highest rates of diabetes (50%) and hypertension (72.6%) were found in patients over 60 years old and those with a BMI over 50. In the NHANES survey from 1999-2004, the simultaneous prevalence of hypertension and diabetes in the US population was only 2% in the 30-54 age group, but increased to 12.4% in the 65-74 age group.

1.5.1. BP Characteristics in Patients with Diabetes Mellitus

Individuals with diabetes experience higher baseline heart rates and less reduction in nocturnal blood pressure due to autonomic neuropathy, as well as more isolated systolic hypertension than their non-diabetic counterparts. Furthermore, people with diabetes have increased blood pressure variability, a higher risk of orthostatic hypotension, and a higher resistance to treatment for their hypertension.

Due to their poor response to treatment and relatively low target blood pressure, these patients pose significant challenges to blood pressure control.

1.5.2. BP and Target Organ Damage in Diabetes Mellitus

Diabetes mellitus is the primary cause of end-stage renal disease (ESRD), blindness, and nontraumatic amputations in western nations. It is also linked to an increased risk of cardiovascular disease. Patients who have both hypertension and diabetes are far more likely to have coronary heart disease (CHD) than those who only have one of the two conditions. The incidence of CHD during a 4-year period in the Prospective Cardiovascular Munster (PROCAM) trial was 6 per 1,000 in individuals without hypertension, diabetes, or hyperlipidemia, 14 or 15 per 1,000 in individuals with hypertension or diabetes, respectively, and as high as 48 per 1,000 in patients who had both hypertension and diabetes.

Compared to what would be predicted with either hypertension or diabetes mellitus alone, the coexistence of diabetes and hypertension causes a more severe cardiomyopathy. It was demonstrated that the prevalence of left ventricular hypertrophy was only 32% in patients with a comparable level of hypertension without diabetes, compared to 72% in patients with both diabetes and hypertension.

In all age groups, hypertension—primarily systolic—has a strong and direct correlation with stroke. Patients with hypertension who also have diabetes have a stroke risk that is more than doubled. Patients with diabetes and hypertension have a 44% lower risk of stroke when their blood pressure is lowered.

Diabetes mellitus is a primary cause of end-stage renal disease. A well-established risk factor for ESRD, hypertension is responsible for 27% of all ESRD cases in the US and 33.4% of ESRD cases among African Americans. In diabetic patients, blood pressure control can delay the development of renal disease. Diabetic retinopathy can be brought on by diabetes mellitus, and its onset is sped up by hypertension.

1.5.3. What Should be the Target BP in Diabetes Mellitus?

Reducing blood pressure in diabetic patients to less than 130/80 mmHg is advised by current guidelines. Numerous studies have demonstrated the advantages of strict blood pressure control in patients with type 2 diabetes. Evidence from the Hypertension Optimal Treatment study showed that lowering blood pressure to the lowest target level (diastolic blood pressure ≤80 mmHg) in patients with both type 2 diabetes and hypertension reduced major CV events by 51% when compared to the group whose target was ≤90 mmHg. The UK Prospective Diabetes Study results (UKPDS 38) corroborated these conclusions. In that study, patients with type 2 diabetes who were hypertensive and had tight control over their blood pressure (average of 144/82 mmHg in the "tight" control group vs. 154/87 mmHg in the "less tight" control group) were linked to a 44% decrease in the risk of stroke events and a 37% decrease in microvascular-related endpoints. An additional examination of the UKPDS revealed that, without a threshold, every 10 mmHg drop in systolic blood pressure was linked to a 12% decrease in the risk of any type 2 diabetes-related complication. Intense blood pressure control was linked to improvements in secondary outcomes in the Appropriate Blood Pressure Control in Diabetes (ABCD) trial, but it had no effect on the primary endpoint.

The Joint National Committee (JNC) and the American Diabetes Association both suggested a target blood pressure (BP) based on these data. <130/80 mmHg for patients with diabetes and <125/75 mmHg for those with proteinuria. However, a meticulous review of the literature and results from recent publications cast doubt on the validity of these current recommendations. In the Action in Diabetes and Vascular disease, preterAx and diamicorN MR Controlled Evaluation (ADVANCE) trial, active treatment (BP = 136/73 mmHg) reduced the relative risk of a major macrovascular or microvascular event by 9% as compared to the placebo treatment (BP = 140/73 mmHg). The authors stated that the study treatment was not affected by the initial BP levels. However, the mean initial BP of the population studied was 145/81 mmHg and 7,655 (68.5%) patients had a history of current antihypertensive treatment. Analysis of subgroups revealed that, in patients with no history of hypertension, active treatment did not reduce the rate of occurrence of CV events. It is noteworthy that the systolic BP achieved in this trial was > 130 mm Hg, or 136 mm Hg. The systolic blood pressure attained in other studies demonstrating the advantages of lowering blood pressure stayed above 130 mmHg (Mistry et al., 2008).

Six thousand and four hundred diabetes patients participated in the International Verapamil SR-Trandolapril (INVEST) study, and they were split into three groups based on the mean systolic blood pressure that was attained. The authors assessed the impact of a very low systolic blood pressure of less than 115 mmHg. The primary outcome rate during the INVEST follow-up was 19% in the "not-controlled" group, 12% in the "usual" group, and 13% in the "tight control" group, respectively (P < 0.001 for the not-controlled group vs. the other teams). When comparing the tight control group to the usual control group, the rate of all-cause mortality was significantly higher (11% vs. 10.2%; P is equal to 0.035). In comparison to usual control, tight control was linked to a higher death rate during the extended follow-up (adjusted hazard ratio 1.15 (95% confidence interval 1.01–1.32); P = 0.04). A lower systolic blood pressure of less than 115 mmHg was linked to a higher mortality risk. This study has several limitations: it only included patients with CHD and divided patients into groups based on blood pressure achieved. It also represents an observational analysis of a randomized control study (Maliha et al., 2015).

In individuals with type 2 diabetes who are at high risk for major CV events, the ACCORD BP trial examined whether therapy aimed at normal systolic blood pressure (<120 mmHg) lowers the incidence of such events. Diabetic patients were randomized to receive either standard therapy, which aimed for a systolic blood pressure of less than 140 mmHg, or intensive therapy, which targeted a BP of less than 120 mmHg. The primary endpoint rate was the same in both groups, despite a 14.2 mmHg difference in systolic blood pressure. Significant adverse events related to antihypertensive medication, such as hypotension, bradycardia, hyperkalemia, and renal deterioration, were more common in the intensive therapy group (3.3%) than in the standard therapy group (1.3%) (P < 0.001). However, intensive therapy was linked to a lower rate of stroke—a predetermined secondary outcome—than standard therapy. It has been demonstrated that strict blood pressure control did not slow the rate at which diabetic retinopathy progresses in a recent extra analysis of the ACCORD trial. The findings of these recent studies indicate that, even in patients with diabetes, there may be little to no benefit to aggressively lowering blood pressure. In fact, the patient may even be in danger if their blood pressure is lowered too much. The recommended target blood pressure for patients with diabetes is 135/85 mmHg, as the previously mentioned target of less than 130/80 has not been substantiated by new data. In some diabetic patients who also have proteinuria, lower blood pressure may be appropriate; however, this should be recorded in prospective trials.

1.5.4. How to Achieve Target BP

1.5.4.1. Nonpharmacologic Therapy

Nonpharmacologic treatment for hypertension, diabetes, and possibly both of these conditions can be beneficial. Examples of this include weight loss, a low-sodium diet, and regular exercise. Still, no credible research indicates that losing weight in and of itself will lower blood pressure over time.

The Swedish Obese Subjects (SOS) study evaluated changes in CV risk factors in surgically treated subjects over 2- and 10-year follow-up periods, and compared the results with those of matched control subjects who received conventional treatment. Following two years, there was a 0% increase in body weight in the control group and a 23.4% decrease in the surgery group ($P < 0.001$); ten years later, there was a 1.6% increase in the control group and a 16.1% decrease in the surgery group ($P < 0.001$). After two and ten years, the surgically treated group's incidence rates of diabetes were significantly lower than those of the control group, while there was no difference in the incidence of hypertension between the groups. Systolic blood pressure had increased by 0.5 mmHg in the control group and decreased by 4.4 mmHg in the surgery group at the 2-year follow-up ($P < 0.001$). However, at the 10-year follow-up, there was no significant difference in the change in systolic blood pressure between the groups. Thus, there are still some questions about whether weight loss has long-term antihypertensive effects. Nonetheless, this approach ought to be supported going forward, as it might improve lipid profile and glycemia.

According to the Dietary Approaches to Stop Hypertension (DASH) trial, individuals without diabetes can reduce their blood pressure by following a healthy diet. This diet might provide diabetic patients with an extra nutritional strategy for managing their hypertension. The goals of lifestyle therapy include cutting back on sodium to less than 1,500 mg per day, getting rid of extra weight, consuming more fruits and vegetables (8–10 servings per day) and low-fat dairy products (2-4 servings per day), avoiding binge drinking, and engaging in physical activity. For patients with diabetes whose blood pressure is 130–139/80–89 mmHg, a three- to six-month initial trial of nonpharmacologic therapy may be appropriate. However, medication therapy should be started in addition to nonpharmacologic therapy when the blood pressure is ≥140/90 mmHg (Zinman et al., 2015).

1.5.4.2. Drug Therapy

1. Renin Angiotensin Aldosterone System Blockers

Angiotensin-converting enzyme (ACE) inhibitors and angiotensin receptor blockers (ARBs) are two examples of renin-angiotensin-aldosterone system (RAAS) blockers that are now the mainstay of treatment for patients with diabetes and hypertension. ACE inhibitors decrease the morbidity and mortality associated with CV disease in high-risk diabetic patients. Studies have demonstrated the positive impact of both drug classes on surrogate endpoints, including the reduction of microalbuminuria, the deceleration of the progression from microalbuminuria to macroalbuminuria, and the deceleration of the decline in renal function. Although RAAS blockers have a theoretical advantage over other antihypertensive medications, there isn't any conclusive proof that they work better in these patients. However, because diabetic patients have a higher risk of cardiovascular disease, they are preferred for these patients (Neal et al., 2013).

Direct renin inhibitors, like aliskiren, block the effects of renin and cause a decrease in plasma renin activity, in contrast to ACE inhibitors and ARBs, which reactively induce an increase in plasma renin activity. However, before aliskiren can be recommended for patients with both diabetes and hypertension, more findings from long-term studies are needed.

Patients with diabetes who have bilateral renal artery stenosis or renal failure, as well as those with hyporeninemic hypoaldosteronism, are more likely to experience hyperkalemia and renal deterioration when RAAS blockers are taken. Close monitoring of kidney functions and electrolytes is necessary soon after drug initiation because these side effects typically manifest shortly after drug initiation. It is crucial to remember that, following the start of RAAS blocker therapy, a slight rise in creatinine (up to 20%–25%) is considered to be "nephroprotective." Unpredictable factors like dehydration, concurrent drug use (such as nonsteroidal anti-inflammatory drugs) and intravenous contrast can cause hyperkalemia and deterioration in renal function. Crucially, a dose of an ACE inhibitor that was previously well tolerated in a particular patient may no longer be appropriate as the illness and renal failure worsen. When using any RAAS blocker as monotherapy, blood pressure is typically not sufficiently controlled in patients with diabetes and hypertension. Just 9% of the diabetes patients in the Losartan Intervention for Endpoint Reduction in Hypertension study (LIFE) continued on losartan monotherapy. It is true that in these patients, monotherapy with any drug class hardly ever results in the desired blood pressure; instead, two or more prescriptions must be written together (Imai et al., 2011).

2. Combinations of RAAS blockers

Better than either of them alone, combination therapy combining ACE inhibitors and ARBs can block the RAAS. This combination may work in concert to reduce microalbuminuria, but it has little to no additive effect on blood pressure. The Ongoing Telmisartan Alone and in Combination with Ramipril Global End-point Trial (ONTARGET), a recent large clinical study, revealed that, in high-risk patients, telmisartan, an ARB, plus ramipril, an ACE inhibitor, was more effective in lowering blood pressure than ramipril alone. However, it did not lower the primary endpoints and was linked to an increased risk of hypotension, syncope, and renal failure. For this reason, patients with diabetes and hypertension should not receive combination therapy involving an ACE inhibitor and an ARB. The combination treatment of aliskiren and losartan, an ARB, was successful in lowering albuminuria and preserving renal function, in contrast to combination therapy involving an ACE inhibitor and an ARB. To validate the effectiveness of this combination therapy involving aliskiren and ARB in lowering CV endpoints, more research is required.

3. Calcium Channel Antagonists

Calcium channel blockers are effective at lowering blood pressure and have been shown to be just as beneficial in patients with diabetes and hypertension as traditional therapy. Non-dihydropyridine calcium antagonists like verapamil and diltiazem appear to be more effective in reducing proteinuria compared to dihydropyridines and are almost as effective as ACE inhibitors. Most long-term studies on the benefits of calcium antagonists in treating hypertension have used the dihydropyridine amlodipine. In patients with diabetes and hypertension, calcium antagonists have been shown to have similar effects on coronary heart disease, less impact on reducing the risk of heart failure, and a slightly greater reduction in the risk of stroke compared to conventional therapy. They have also shown similar benefits to RAAS blockers in reducing the risk of stroke, coronary heart disease, and overall mortality. In the ASCOT trial, amlodipine-based treatment proved more effective in reducing cardiovascular events compared to atenolol-based therapy. Calcium antagonists are effective at lowering blood pressure and reducing variability regardless of other health conditions, medications, diet, or lifestyle factors. They are well tolerated and have neutral effects on metabolism.

4. β-Blockers

In general, patients with diabetes and hypertension should not receive β-blockers as their first line of treatment; however, in some cases, they may be helpful as an adjunct. β-blockers have a positive effect on both diabetes and concomitant heart failure, as both conditions are known to increase sympathetic activity. Law et al. conducted a meta-analysis recently which demonstrated that in patients with a history of CHD, β-blockers have a unique effect in preventing recurrent CHD events while lowering blood pressure. Results from patients who were randomly assigned to receive an ACE inhibitor or a β-blocker in the UKPDS trial were comparable. However, neither of the two medication classes was found to significantly lower the risk of CHD in a study (Ruggenenti et al., 2011). Because of their adverse effect on endocrine metabolism, β-blockers are not thought to be the best medication for use in patients who also have hypertension and diabetes. It has been demonstrated that β-blockers worsen insulin resistance, raise triglycerides, lower HDL cholesterol, cause systemic weight gain, and conceal hypoglycemia. It has never been demonstrated that β-blockers as a class lower the risk of heart attacks and strokes in patients with mild hypertension. In the ASCOT trial, both in the overall group and in a subset of patients with diabetes, an atenolol-based regimen prevented fewer CV events than an amlodipine-based regimen.

Generally speaking, only patients with diabetes for whom there are indications for this drug class should be able to take β-blockers. These indications include tachycardia or sympathetic excess symptoms, the existence of congestive heart failure, or the requirement for an additional medication for uncontrolled hypertension (Tillin et al.,.2011).

5. Diuretics

The antihypertensive medication arsenal has included and continues to include thiazide diuretics. Chlorthalidone was found to be more effective in preventing stroke in black patients than doxazosin mesylate, an α-blocker, and lisinopril, an ACE inhibitor, in the Antihypertensive and Lipid-Lowering Treatment to Prevent Heart Attack Trial (ALLHAT). Chlorthalidone has been demonstrated to be equally effective as both an ACE inhibitor and a calcium antagonist in lowering CV-related morbidity and mortality in 13,100 diabetic patients who took part in the ALLHAT. The effectiveness of diuretics in lowering CV-related morbidity and mortality in the elderly has been demonstrated by many placebo-controlled trials. In the Systolic Hypertension in the Elderly Program (SHEP), chlorthalidone decreased the rate of major CV events by 32%, the rate of all-cause mortality by 13%, and the rate of total stroke by 36% among elderly patients (over 60) with isolated systolic hypertension. Chthalidone had the same positive effects on patients with and without diabetes.

Indapamide, a thiazide-like diuretic, decreased the risk of stroke, congestive heart failure, and all-cause mortality in very elderly hypertensive patients participating in the recent Hypertension in the Very Elderly Trial (HYVET). Thus, it seems that the use of chlorthalidone or indapamide should continue to be an option, at least for older patients.

Diuretics, however, have a well-established history of adversely affecting endocrine metabolism, including insulin resistance and electrolyte balance. Although loop diuretics may not be as diabetogenic as thiazides, there is not enough justification for using them in diabetic patients unless there is an elevated creatinine level.

Hyponatremia, which seems to be especially common in older women, may be brought on by thiazides. Patients can avoid this side effect by taking a low to medium dose of a diuretic and being advised to consume fewer fluids. Gout and hyperuricemia are frequent clinical problems in diabetic patients. Thiazide diuretics raise uric acid levels, and in patients who are vulnerable, their careless use may result in a gout attack. Over the course of a few years of follow-up, there was no increase in cardiovascular morbidity or mortality due to the adverse effects of diuretics on glucose metabolism. Recent results from the SHEP study's 15-year follow-up revealed that thiazide's diabetogenic effect had no effect on cardiovascular morbidity or mortality. The long-term safety of diuretics is still unknown, as is the case with most medication classes used to treat hypertension. Consequently, diuretics should only be used in small doses and in conjunction with other medications like ACE inhibitors and ARBs in patients who have both diabetes and hypertension.

6. Aldosterone antagonists

In certain patients, aldosterone antagonists like eplerenone and spironolactone can be very beneficial. It has been demonstrated that these medications lessen surrogate endpoints like left ventricular hypertrophy and microproteinuria as well as target organ disease. In diabetic nephropathy, spironolactone provides more renoprotection when added to a regimen that includes maximal ACE inhibition as opposed to adding losartan, an ARB. Spironolactone is especially useful for patients with aldosterone breakthrough and hypertension whose serum potassium level is low (<4 mmol/l). Compared to spironolactone, eplerenone appears to have a less severe side-effect profile because it does not appear to induce gynecomastia. Nevertheless, these medications should only be used sparingly and in small doses because patients with diabetes and hypertension are more likely to develop hyperkalemia (hyporeninemic hypoaldosteronism, renal impairment, and/or ACE inhibitor/ARB treatment). Potassium and creatinine will also need to be closely watched.

7. α-Blockers

It has been demonstrated that α-Blockers improve metabolic and endocrine parameters. The ALLHAT trial has shown that chlorthalidone is more effective than alpha-blockers in preventing congestive heart failure and CHD, even in spite of these apparent positive surrogate endpoint effects of the former. Drugs classified as α-blockers should no longer be used as the first line of treatment for simple hypertension. Nonetheless, they might be helpful in patients exhibiting prostatism symptoms and as a third or fourth step of therapy (Benavente et al., 2013).

1.5.4.3. Combination Therapy

Reaching blood pressure targets with monotherapy is extremely challenging, and most patients need a combination of two or three medications to reach their goals. A blocker of the RAAS, either an ACE inhibitor or an ARB, represents the cornerstone of the antihypertensive arsenal for patients with diabetes plus hypertension, so the key question should be which combination is preferable. The American Diabetes Association recommends a low dosage of a thiazide diuretic as a second step. The combination therapy involving an ACE inhibitor, benazepril, and hydrochlorothiazide was found to be less effective in lowering the risk of the predefined primary endpoints than the combination therapy involving benazepril and amlodipine, according to the recent Avoiding cardiovascular Events through combination Therapy in Patients Living with Systolic Hypertension (ACCOMPLISH) trial. Furthermore, compared to benazepril plus hydrochlorothiazide, combination therapy involving benazepril plus amlodipine significantly slowed the advancement of nephropathy. Combination therapy with benazepril plus amlodipine was found to be more effective than benazepril plus hydrochlorothiazide in reducing the rate of primary endpoints in 6,946 diabetes patients included in the ACCOMPLISH trial (hazard ratio: 0.79%, 95% confidence interval: 0.68–0.92, P = 0.003). We propose that, unless there is a clear indication for diuretics, such as a history of congestive heart failure, a calcium antagonist should be prescribed in addition to a RAAS blocker in light of the results of the ACCOMPLISH trial. Triple therapy is often necessary for many patients and consists of a calcium antagonist, a RAAS blocker, and a low-dose thiazide diuretic. Patients with congestive heart failure or rapid heartbeat can benefit from using β-blockers. When a patient has low serum potassium (<4 mmol/l), aldosterone antagonists should be taken into consideration. A thiazide diuretic should be continued, and serum potassium levels should be checked often, particularly in patients with chronic renal failure, to prevent hyperkalemia. α-blockers and/or anti-adrenergic agents are additional add-on therapies for patients receiving quadruple drug therapy. Combination therapy involving an ACE inhibitor and an ARB is not advised, as was previously stated. However, the addition of the renin inhibitor aliskiren should be taken into consideration for patients with microalbuminuria or diabetic nephropathy who do not respond to a combination therapy that includes a maximal dose of a RAAS blocker (Figure 1.3).

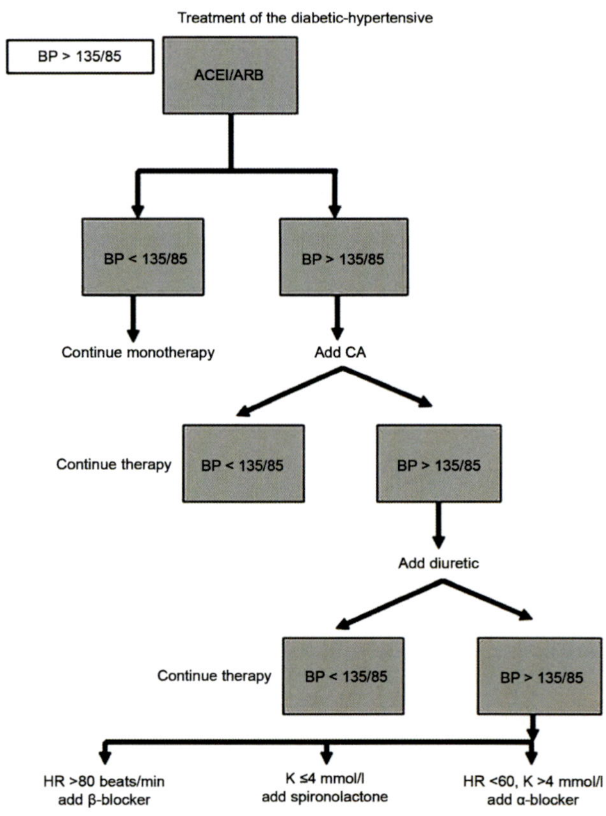

Figure 1.3. *Treatment of diabetic-hypersensitive.*

Source: https://academic.oup.com/ajh/article/24/8/863/226345.

Fixed-dose combinations of medications may be useful to reduce the number of medications taken and increase compliance.

1.5.4.4. Resistant Hypertension

Compared to patients with hypertension alone, those with diabetes are more resistant to antihypertensive medication. Additionally, patients with diabetes plus hypertension typically have lower rates of blood pressure control because the target blood pressure in individuals with both conditions at the same time is lower than in individuals with hypertension alone. About 75% of patients in the ACCOMPLISH trial met the blood pressure target, compared to only ~45% of patients with diabetes. To rule out a white-coat effect, 24-hour ABPM should be carried out when resistant hypertension is suspected. Treatable secondary causes like renal artery stenosis, primary hyperaldosteronism, pheochromocytoma, sleep apnea, and drug-induced hypertension should be ruled out if 24-hour ambulatory blood pressure monitoring confirms the diagnosis of resistant hypertension. Weight loss, sodium restriction, and regular exercise should be promoted after secondary causes have been ruled out. When necessary, we advise stepping up the dose of the diuretic and, if needed, adding an aldosterone antagonist to the treatment plan.

1.5.4.5. Very Elderly Patients

Elderly people frequently have both diabetes and hypertension, and their rate of cardiovascular events is higher. The most recent HYVET study demonstrated that very old patients can benefit from blood pressure reduction; however, the proportion of patients with diabetes in this study was very small (<7%). In patients 75 years of age and older, perindopril-indapamide administration safely lowers blood pressure and lowers the risk of major adverse clinical outcomes, according to a recent analysis of the ADVANCE trial results broken down by age. Furthermore, patients ≥75 years of age saw a higher absolute benefit than those <65. It is evident that treating elderly patients with both diabetes and hypertension necessitates greater caution when choosing medications because these patients are more likely to experience adverse events and orthostatic hypotension. Lower dosages, closer titration of treatment, and patient monitoring with standing blood pressure measurements are all preferred (Palacio et al., 2014).

1.5.4.6. Adjunct Therapy: Glycemic and Lipid Level Regulation

Examining the event rates of diabetes patients in randomized trial cohorts makes it more evident that statins are effective in lowering the frequency of adverse events in this high-risk group. Compared to a placebo, simvastatin has been demonstrated to reduce the rate of CHD in this group by approximately 50%. 2,838 diabetic patients with a baseline mean low-density lipoprotein (LDL) of 118 mg/dl were randomly assigned to receive atorvastatin or a placebo in the CARDS study. Following a median follow-up of approximately 4 years, the primary endpoint was reduced by 37%. There was a 27% decrease in overall mortality and a 48% decrease in the frequency of strokes. The early termination of the study was due to the established benefits of atorvastatin therapy for patients diagnosed with type 2 diabetes.

According to the most recent American Diabetes Association guidelines, all patients with type 2 diabetes who are older than 40 and have one or more cardiovascular disease risk factors, such as hypertension, should receive lipid-lowering therapy regardless of their baseline levels of low-density lipoprotein cholesterol. If the low-risk patient's LDL cholesterol is more than 100 mg/dl, a statin should be prescribed. The main objective is LDL <100 mg/dl in people without overt CV disease, while LDL <70 mg/dl in people with overt CV disease.

In type 2 diabetes, maintaining glucose control is crucial primarily to avoid microvascular complications. Compared to insulin and sulphonylurea therapy, glucose control with metformin therapy appears to reduce the risk of diabetes-related endpoints in patients with the disease and is linked to less weight gain and hypoglycemic events. For this reason, metformin is regarded as the preferred first-line pharmacological treatment for individuals with type 2 diabetes. Achieving hemoglobin A_{1c} (HbA_{1c}) <7% is the aim of glycemic control.

1.6. EPIDEMIOLOGY OF HYPERTENSION ASSOCIATED WITH DIABETES MELLITUS

Clinical consensus suggests that hypertension is more common in diabetic patients than in the general population. When two common but arbitrary conditions are studied in conjunction, numerous methodological issues arise that must be addressed to validate this association using epidemiological methods. The pathogenesis of diabetic macrovascular and microvascular disease has been linked to hypertension; therefore, one crucial question that remains unanswered is whether treating hypertension will lessen the burden of death and morbidity on diabetic patients.

1.6.1. Frequency of Hypertension among Diabetic Patients

Several studies have tried to show a link between hypertension and diabetes mellitus, but challenges in methodology have made it hard to interpret the results. Past studies typically used a case-control approach, comparing the blood pressure of diabetic patients to non-diabetic controls. However, these studies often lacked clear definitions of the diabetic group's characteristics, such as age, obesity levels, kidney disease, diabetes type, and treatment methods, which could affect blood pressure. The same lack of clarity was found in the non-diabetic control groups, which were often made up of hospital patients, visitors, or medical staff (Schrader et al., 2005).

Numerous factors, such as the time of day, room temperature, amount of rest before BP measurement, history of cigarette smoking, posture, stress, and medication, are known to affect an individual's arterial blood pressure level. Another issue is observer variation, which can be reduced with proper observer training and the application of blind or random-zero sphygmomanometers. It is important to consider the arm girth and use the proper cuff size. It is evident from these methodological considerations that measurements in cases and controls in any BP study should be performed by the same observers using appropriate quality control in standardized settings. However, these requirements have not been met in many sizable, frequently cited studies on diabetics, making it challenging to interpret their findings. Within the Freedman et al. study. Hamilton et al.'s study provided control data on 1100 diabetic patients. of blood pressure in a randomized outpatient group, and it is evident that the study conditions for the cases and controls were different. With the exception of the age range of 70 to 79 years, the prevalence of hypertension (defined as diastolic blood pressure >100 mm Hg) was not significantly higher in diabetic patients in either gender. In their diabetic group, malignant hypertension was absent and severe hypertension (diastolic blood pressure > 125 mm Hg) was uncommon. Keen, among others. The control data from Hamilton et al. were also utilized in their clinical study involving 735 diabetics. and discovered that there were no systematic blood pressure differences between the diabetics and the controls; however, the diastolic blood pressure scores were higher for the diabetics under the age of forty.

These two studies did not categorize patients based on the type of diabetes. However, patients with juvenile onset insulin-dependent diabetes (IDD) were the subjects of two studies. When Moss examined the systolic blood pressure of 889 non-diabetics and 123 diabetic children between the ages of 8 and 20, she discovered that the diabetics' blood pressure was considerably higher than the non-diabetics. A second study, conducted in 1964 at the Joslin Clinic with 900 IDD patients, used control data from the Framingham Study and the U. S. Overview of High Blood Pressure. Compared to controls, patients with IDD had a higher prevalence of hypertension, which is defined as systolic blood pressure of at least 160 mm Hg or diastolic blood pressure of at least 95 mm Hg, especially in female subjects. There was no consistent correlation found in either of these two studies between the length of diabetes and hypertension.

Gerber et al. emphasized the importance of the population source when studying the potential link between hypertension and diabetes. They found that hypertension and diabetes were more commonly found together in a hospital clinic population (6.0%) compared to a work-site population (1.9%). This discrepancy is known as Berkson's paradox, which warns against concluding disease co-occurrence based solely on hospital populations. To address methodological challenges in clinic-based studies, Pell and D'Alonzo examined the blood pressure of 662 diabetic employees compared to an equal number of nondiabetic employees from the DuPont Company. They discovered that hypertension was 54% more prevalent in diabetic individuals, even before the diabetes diagnosis, and increased across all body weight categories. This suggests that studying blood pressure in diabetic patients identified through population surveys may offer a more accurate representation of disease associations.

Garcia et al. stated from the Framingham Study that diabetics' mean systolic blood pressure increased, with female subjects experiencing this effect more than male subjects; however, the degree of obesity was not taken into account. Even after adjusting for age and degree of obesity, people with newly diagnosed and borderline diabetes in both sexes had systolic blood pressure that was significantly higher in the Bedford Survey than in people without the condition. The Whitehall Study of male civil servants in London produced similar findings, however, the mean blood pressure of those with pre-existing diabetes was not raised. Diabetes patients' systolic blood pressure was higher than controls' in a population survey conducted in Maryland, USA; however, obesity was not taken into account. When age and obesity were taken into account, the mean blood pressure of older adults in California between the ages of 50 and 79 was found to be lowest in non-diabetics, intermediate in those with recently discovered disease, and highest in those with a history of diabetes. Nevertheless, the differences were only statistically significant for the female subjects, and their magnitude was small.

In conclusion, there appears to be some evidence linking diabetes to a higher incidence of systolic hypertension, especially in older age groups. However, the evidence linking diabetes to diastolic hypertension is less compelling. The finding that young people with IDD have higher systolic blood pressure may have significant prognostic implications; therefore, this finding needs to be confirmed by carefully planned studies that consider the methodological issues raised (Masakane et al., 2017).

1.6.2. Possible Mechanisms for the Relationship between Hypertension and Diabetes

Several studies in non-diabetic populations found statistically significant relationships between blood pressure and different glycemia measurements. This association appeared to be stronger in people with higher heart rates and to be unaffected by age, level of obesity, or heart rate. There have been attempts to explain this correlation in terms of the impact of humoral or neutral sympathetic pathways on the regulation of blood pressure and blood glucose. Though heart rate is thought to be an indicator of sympathetic activity, there is still a relationship between these two variables after adjusting for it, so this is unlikely to be a full explanation. Drury reviewed additional potential pathogenic mechanisms for the correlation between diabetes and hypertension. These include anomalies related to the renin-angiotensin system, insulin and renal sodium metabolism, and catecholamines. Because measuring the biochemical variables in a large number of subjects presents methodological challenges, it is difficult to confirm such hypotheses through epidemiological studies. Seldom can endocrine disorders like thyrotoxicosis, pheochromocytoma, Cushing's syndrome, acromegaly, and primary hyperaldosteronism cause secondary hypertension or diabetes. Diabetes does not appear to be associated with an increased risk of renal artery stenosis.

1.6.3. Hypertension and Mortality in Patients with Diabetes

The etiology of diabetic macrovascular and microvascular disease is unclear, but both cohort and insurance studies showed that elevation of both systolic and diastolic blood pressure increases mortality among individuals with diabetes. Individuals with diabetes and those with glucose intolerance are more likely to die from coronary heart disease (CHD) and stroke in developed nations. The relative significance of cardiovascular risk factors identified for normoglycemic populations is still unknown for these hyperglycemic groups.

In a subsequent study involving 371 diabetics and 742 controls, Dupree and Meyer discovered that individuals with diabetes and a systolic blood pressure of 160 mm Hg or higher were four times more likely to experience mortality compared to normotensive controls. For those with lower blood pressure levels, the risk of mortality increased by 1.5 times. Additionally, in a 10-year follow-up of individuals with borderline diabetes from the Bedford Survey, systolic blood pressure was identified as a significant predictor of coronary heart disease mortality, even after accounting for age and obesity.

There was no difference in the association between cardiovascular disease frequency and risk factors, such as blood pressure, over a 20-year duration (the Framingham Study) between individuals with and without diabetes. The Whitehall Study contradicted this, showing that systolic and diastolic pressures were more consistently associated with CHD mortality in patients with diabetes and glucose intolerance than were cholesterol, obesity, and cigarette smoking. Subjects with glucose intolerance had higher relative risks of dying from coronary heart disease (CHD) than subjects with normoglycemia when subjects were randomly split into hypertensive and normotensive groups. Only when systolic blood pressure was used was the relative risk higher for the diabetic group. Cohort studies and analyses of national death statistics revealed a higher risk of stroke death in people with diabetes. In the Whitehall Study, men with diabetes and glucose intolerance also had higher rates of stroke mortality; systolic blood pressure and age played significant roles in this increased risk. Measured cardiovascular risk factors were unable to account for a significant portion of the excess mortality risk in both CHD and stroke mortality.

In individuals diagnosed with diabetes before the age of 31, renal disease plays a significant role in mortality, accounting for 31% of all deaths. Those with persistent proteinuria have three to four times higher mortality rates compared to those without proteinuria. Keen et al. found a strong correlation between blood pressure levels and microalbumin excretion rate in diabetics, which can predict the development of clinical renal disease. Studies have also shown that hypertension is common in young individuals with type I diabetes and diabetic nephropathy, potentially worsening renal disease progression. Mogensen and Parving et al. suggested that antihypertensive treatment could slow down the decline in renal function in patients with diabetic nephropathy (Gregg et al., 2014).

1.6.4. Geographical Variation in Frequency of Hypertension among Diabetics

The majority of the previously discussed clinic- and population-based studies on diabetes and hypertension were conducted in developed societies. The World Health Organization (WHO) Multinational Study of Vascular Disease in Diabetics has provided additional data on the prevalence of hypertension in a range of diabetic populations. In all, 6695 men and women with diabetes, ages 35 to 54, from 14 centers took part in the prevalence investigation. A random sample of patients with diabetes, stratified by age, sex, and length of diabetes, was taken from each center. Arterial blood pressure was measured as part of the standard examination procedures. About 34% of the patients had hypertension (systolic blood pressure above 160 mm Hg, diastolic blood pressure above 95 mm Hg, or receiving hypertension treatment); this percentage was slightly higher in women (36.0%) than in men (31.8%). Men's and women's hypertension frequencies were highest in Berlin (GDR) and Moscow, while women's frequencies were lowest in London and Arizona. There was no correlation between these discrepancies and the centers' varying levels of obesity.

A Closer Look

The Impact of Hypertension on Microvascular Disorders

It is common knowledge that people with diabetes, especially those with type 1 diabetes, experience elevated blood pressure, hypertension, and the advancement of diabetic nephropathy. Conversely, hypertension frequently coexists with type 2 diabetes in patients. Even if blood pressure was normal at first, it frequently increases as diabetic nephropathy progresses, leading to hypertension. In any case, the development of hypertension as a complication accelerates the course of diabetic nephropathy in the patient. Thus, it is possible to say that the development of diabetic nephropathy and the deterioration of renal function are mutually reinforcing factors in hypertension.

Despite only studying a 1% diabetic population, the Multiple Risk Factor Intervention Trial looked into the connection between blood pressure and end-stage renal failure. According to the trial, if an optimal blood pressure of less than 120/80 mmHg was used as the reference, the risk of developing end-stage renal failure increased by 1.9 in the case of high-normal blood pressure (130–139 mmHg/85–89 mmHg), by 3.1 in the case of mild hypertension (140–159 mmHg/90–99 mmHg), and by 11.2 in the case of severe hypertension. The five stages of diabetic nephropathy are generally recognized as follows: dialysis, end-stage renal failure, overt albuminuria, normoalbuminuria, and microalbuminuria. The United Kingdom Prospective Diabetes Study (UKPDS) revealed that approximately 25% of patients experienced microalbuminuria after a ten-year follow-up. According to the study, the annual rates of progression from normoalbuminuria to microalbuminuria, overt albuminuria to end-stage renal failure and renal replacement therapy, such as dialysis, were 2%, 2.8%, and 2.3%, respectively, for the various stages of diabetic nephropathy. As a result, albuminuria is a sign of diabetic nephropathy advancement. Additionally, many studies have shown that albuminuria is a predictor of cardiovascular disease. The UKPDS also reported that the death rate from cardiovascular disease increased significantly as albuminuria increased with each stage of diabetic nephropathy.

The onset and progression of diabetic nephropathy (urinary albumin (Alb)/creatinine (Cr) exceeding 300 mg/g·Cr on two consecutive occasions) in a Japanese study on the prevention of the onset of vascular complications in diabetes and the suppression of its progression (Japan Diabetes Complications Study: JDCS), which involved 1,558 type 2 diabetics whose urinary Alb/Cr was either normal (<30 mg/g·Cr) or low-microalbuminuria (30 to <150 mg/g·Cr). Up to eight years later, the rate of nephropathy onset was only 6.67/1000 person years.

Summary

- The coexistence of diabetes and hypertension is known to have a multiplicative effect on adverse clinical outcomes with respect to both microvascular and macrovascular disease.
- The pathophysiology of hypertension in diabetes involves maladaptive changes in the autonomic nervous system, vascular endothelial dysfunction, and enhanced activation of the renin-angiotensin-aldosterone system, immune function alterations, and harmful environmental factors.
- Insulin resistance has been linked in turn to an increased vascular oxidative stress, inflammation, and endothelial dysfunction characterized by diminished vascular nitric oxide bioactivity, all of which promote vascular stiffness resulting in a persistent elevation of blood pressure and the promotion of CVD.
- Increased blood pressure (BP) from intravascular volume expansion is typically corrected by a rise in glomerular filtration and compensatory urinary salt excretion.
- The autonomic nervous system is an important determinant of BP. Both the sympathetic and the parasympathetic systems are involved in the regulation of BP.
- There is emerging evidence that innate immunity and acquired immunity are involved in angiotensin II and aldosterone-induced hypertension and vascular disease.
- Ambulatory blood pressure monitoring (ABPM) is a fully-automated non-invasive modality that involves placement of a blood pressure cuff on the non-dominant arm with measurements every 15 to 30 minutes over the course of a 24-hour period.
- The Hypertension on Target (HOT) trial showed a reduction in CVD with a lowering of diastolic blood pressure. Interestingly however, this benefit was only seen in patients with diabetes, suggesting the need for establishing a different and perhaps more aggressive blood pressure target in this population subgroup.
- Patients with T2DM appear to be particularly susceptible to the deleterious effects of hypertension in the initiation and progression of CVD. In the treatment of hypertension in patients with diabetes attention must be paid to individual risk factors, co-morbidities, and patient preferences when considering lower treatment targets.
- Several factors are known to influence the level of arterial BP in an individual, including time of day, room temperature, period of rest preceding BP measurement, prior cigarette smoking, posture, stress, and medication.
- Hypertension is a powerful risk factor for cardiovascular morbidity and mortality, particularly in patients with diabetes. Patients with hypertension are at two to three times higher risk of developing diabetes than patients with normal blood pressure (BP).
- Patients with diabetes have more isolated systolic hypertension and, because of autonomic neuropathy, they experience less reduction in nocturnal BP and higher baseline heart rates than their counterparts who do not have diabetes.
- Diabetes mellitus is associated with a high risk for CV disease and is the leading cause of end-stage renal disease (ESRD), blindness, and nontraumatic amputations in western countries.

- Nonpharmacologic therapy such as weight loss, low-sodium diet and regular exercise has beneficial effects in patients with hypertension, those with diabetes, and possibly also in those who have both these disorders.
- Blockers of the renin–angiotensin–aldosterone system (RAAS). Blockers of RAAS, either angiotensin-converting enzyme (ACE) inhibitors or angiotensin receptor blockers (ARBs), have become the cornerstone of the management of patients with hypertension plus diabetes.
- Patients who have diabetes alongside hypertension are more resistant to antihypertensive treatment than those with hypertension alone.

References

1. Benavente, O. R., Coffey, C. S., Conwit, R., et al. (2013). Blood-pressure targets in patients with recent lacunar stroke: The SPS3 randomised trial. *Lancet, 382*(9891), 507–515. https://doi.org/10.1016/S0140-6736(13)60852-1.
2. Blonde, L., Pencek, R., & MacConell, L. (2015). Association among weight change, glycemic control, and markers of cardiovascular risk with exenatide once weekly: A pooled analysis of patients with type 2 diabetes. *Cardiovascular Diabetology, 14*, 12.
3. Brown, M. J., Castaigne, A., de Leeuw, P. W., Mancia, G., Palmer, C. R., Rosenthal, T., & Ruilope, L. M. (2000). Influence of diabetes and type of hypertension on response to antihypertensive treatment. *Hypertension, 35*(4), 1038–1042.
4. Gregg, E. W., Yanfeng, L., Wang, J., Burrows, N. R., Ali, M. K., Rolka, D., Williams, D. E., & Geiss, L. (2014). Changes in diabetes-related complications in the United States, 1990–2010. *New England Journal of Medicine, 370*(16), 1514–1523.
5. Imai, E., Chan, J. C., Ito, S., et al. (2011). Effects of olmesartan on renal and cardiovascular outcomes in type 2 diabetes with overt nephropathy: A multicenter, randomized, placebo-controlled study. *Diabetologia, 54*(11), 2978–2986.
6. Lewington, S., Clarke, R., Qizilbash, N., Peto, R., & Collins, R. (2002). Age-specific relevance of usual blood pressure to vascular mortality: A meta-analysis of individual data for one million adults in 61 prospective studies. *Lancet, 360*(9349), 1903–1913.
7. Maliha, G., & Townsend, R. R. (2015). SGLT2 inhibitors: Their potential reduction in blood pressure. *Journal of the American Society of Hypertension, 9*(1), 48–53.
8. Masakane, I., Taniguchi, M., Nakai, S., Tsuchida, K., Goto, S., Wada, A., Ogata, S., Hasegawa, T., Hamano, T., Hanafusa, N., Mizuguchi, J., & Nakamoto, H. (2017). An overview of regular dialysis treatment in Japan (as of 31 December 2015). *Therapeutic Apheresis and Dialysis, 50*(1), 1–62.
9. Mistry, G. C., Maes, A. L., Lasseter, K. C., Davies, M. J., Gottesdiener, K. M., Wagner, J. A., & Herman, G. A. (2008). Effect of sitagliptin, a dipeptidyl peptidase-4 inhibitor, on blood pressure in nondiabetic patients with mild to moderate hypertension. *Journal of Clinical Pharmacology, 48*(5), 592–598.
10. Muntner, P., Shimbo, D., Carey, R. M., Charleston, J. B., Gaillard, T., Misra, S., Myers, M. G., Ogedegbe, G., Schwartz, J. E., Townsend, R. R., Urbina, E. M., Viera, A. J., White, W. B., &

Wright, J. T., Jr. (2019). Measurement of blood pressure in humans: A scientific statement from the American Heart Association. *Hypertension, 73*(5), e35–e66.

11. Neal, B., Perkovic, V., Zeeuw, D., Mahaffey, K. W., Fulcher, G., Stein, P., Desai, M., Shaw, W., Jiang, J., Vercruysse, F., et al. (2013). Rationale, design, and baseline characteristics of the canagliflozin cardiovascular assessment study (CANVAS)—A randomized placebo-controlled trial. *American Heart Journal, 166*(2), 217–223.
12. Oparil, S., Zaman, M. A., & Calhoun, D. A. (2003). Pathogenesis of hypertension. *Annals of Internal Medicine, 139*(9), 761–776.
13. Palacio, S., McClure, L. A., Benavente, O. R., et al. (2014). Lacunar strokes in patients with diabetes mellitus: Risk factors, infarct location, and prognosis: The secondary prevention of small subcortical strokes study. *Stroke, 45*(9), 2689–2694.
14. Ruggenenti, P., Fassi, A., Ilieva, A. P., et al. (2011). Effects of verapamil added-on trandolapril therapy in hypertensive type 2 diabetes patients with microalbuminuria: The BENEDICT-B randomized trial. *Journal of Hypertension, 29*(2), 207–216.
15. Schrader, J., Lüders, S., Kulschewski, A., et al. (2005). Morbidity and mortality after stroke, eprosartan compared with nitrendipine for secondary prevention: Principal results of a prospective randomized controlled study (MOSES). *Stroke, 36*(6), 1218–1226.
16. Smits, M. M., Muskiet, M. H., Tonneijck, L., Hoekstra, T., Kramer, M. H., Diamant, M., & van Raalte, D. H. (2016). Exenatide acutely increases heart rate in parallel with augmented sympathetic nervous system activation in healthy overweight males. *British Journal of Clinical Pharmacology, 81*(4), 613–620.
17. Sowers, J. R., Epstein, M., & Frohlich, E. D. (2001). Diabetes, hypertension, and cardiovascular disease: An update. *Hypertension, 37*(4), 1053–1059.
18. Suh, D. C., Kim, C. M., Choi, I. S., Plauschinat, C. A., & Barone, J. A. (2009). Trends in blood pressure control and treatment among type 2 diabetes with comorbid hypertension in the United States: 1988–2004. *Journal of Hypertension, 27*(10), 1908–1916.
19. Tillin, T., Orchard, T., Malm, A., et al. (2011). The role of antihypertensive therapy in reducing vascular complications of type 2 diabetes: Findings from the DIabetic REtinopathy Candesartan Trials-Protect 2 study. *Journal of Hypertension, 29*(7), 1457–1462.
20. UK Prospective Diabetes Study (UKPDS) Group. (1998). Effect of intensive blood-glucose control with metformin on complications in overweight patients with type 2 diabetes (UKPDS 34). *Lancet, 352*(9131), 854–865.
21. Van Buren, P. N., & Toto, R. D. (2013). The pathogenesis and management of hypertension in diabetic kidney disease. *Medical Clinics of North America, 97*(1), 31–51.
22. Zinman, B., Wanner, C., Lachin, J. M., Fitchett, D., Bluhmki, E., Hantel, S., Mattheus, M., Devins, T., Johansen, O. E., Woerle, H. J., et al. (2015). Empagliflozin, cardiovascular outcomes, and mortality in type 2 diabetes. *New England Journal of Medicine, 373*(22), 2117–2128.

Chapter

2

HYPERTENSION IN CHRONIC KIDNEY DISEASE

Contents

INTRODUCTION

The primary cause of the current global disease burden is hypertension, a public health concern. Heart disease, stroke, and kidney failure have this as their primary modifiable risk factor. Both CKD and uncontrolled hypertension can result from chronic kidney disease (CKD), which is also a common cause of hypertension. There is a higher chance of unfavorable outcomes related to the heart and brain when hypertension and chronic kidney disease interact. This is especially important when resistant hypertension, which is frequently observed in CKD patients, is present (Agarwal et al., 2006).

There are several factors that contribute to the multifactorial pathophysiology of hypertension associated with chronic kidney disease (CKD). These pathogenic mechanisms include changes in the activity of the renin-angiotensin-aldosterone system, increased sympathetic nervous system, and sodium dysregulation. Standardized blood pressure (BP) measurement is crucial for determining the hypertension diagnosis and treatment in chronic kidney disease (CKD). A second way to evaluate the diurnal variation in blood pressure that CKD patients frequently experience is through the use of ambulatory blood pressure monitoring. Despite new guidelines and data from clinical trials, the ideal blood pressure target for treating hypertension in the general population and in people with chronic kidney disease (CKD) is still up for debate.

Patients with CKD-associated hypertension may find medical therapy demanding and complex. In the case of treatment-resistant hypertension, further assessment by a hypertension specialist might be necessary to rule out pseudo-resistance and manageable secondary causes. A crucial part of managing hypertension in patients with chronic kidney disease (CKD) is treating the condition with a mix of antihypertensive medications, including selecting the right diuretic based on the estimated glomerular filtration rate. Non-pharmacological methods, such as dietary salt restriction, should be incorporated into the management of hypertension in patients with chronic kidney disease (CKD) in addition to drug treatment (Agarwal et al., 2016).

Orientation and Directional Terms

Term	Definition	Illustration
Angiotensin-converting enzyme (ACE) inhibitors	ACE inhibitors reduce the production of the hormone "angiotensin." This allows the blood vessels to relax and dilate, thereby lowering blood pressure.	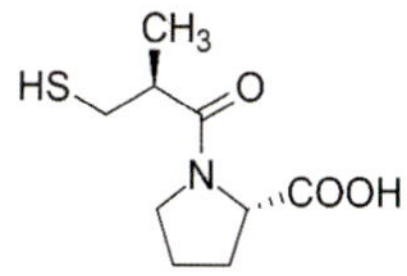
Beta-blockers	These medications cause the following effects on the heart, which help to lower blood pressure: • reducing heart rate • reducing the heart's workload • reducing the heart's output of blood	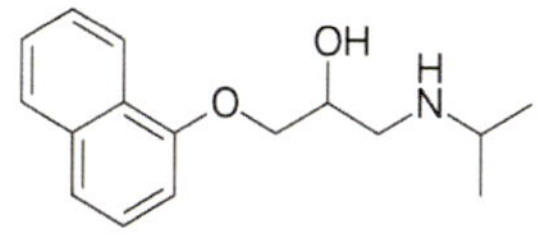
Diuretics	These medications help the body remove excess sodium and water, which reduces blood volume and helps manage blood pressure.	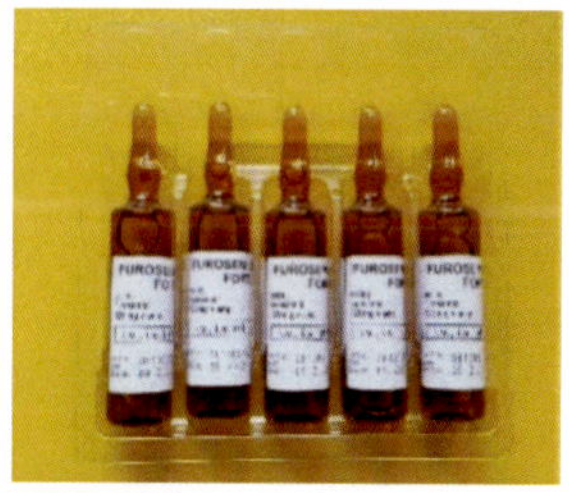
Blood pressure	Blood pressure is the pressure of blood pushing against the walls of your arteries. Arteries carry blood from your heart to other parts of your body. Your blood pressure normally rises and falls throughout the day.	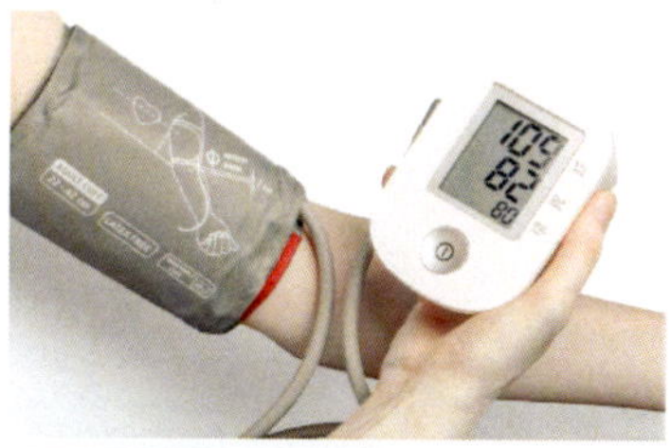
α-Blockers	Alpha-blockers are a type of blood pressure medicine. Alpha-blockers lower blood pressure by keeping a hormone called norepinephrine from tightening the muscles in the walls of smaller arteries and veins. As a result, the blood vessels remain open and relaxed. This improves blood flow and lowers blood pressure.	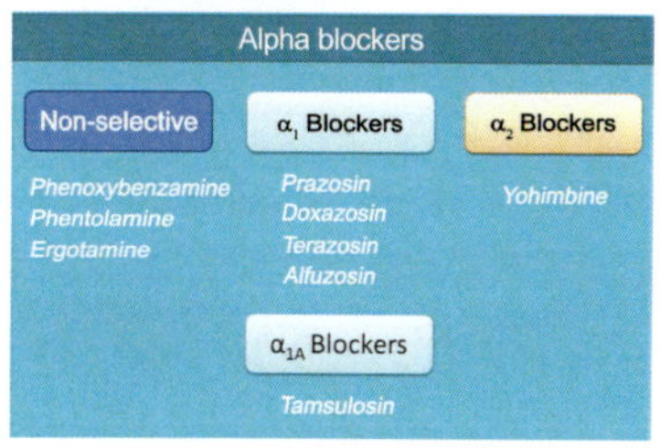

2.1. PATHOGENESIS OF HYPERTENSION IN CHRONIC KIDNEY DISEASE (CKD)

Several mechanisms influence the management of chronic kidney disease (CKD) by contributing to the development of hypertension. (Fig. 2.1). Increased sympathetic tone in patients with chronic kidney disease (CKD) is a result of afferent signals produced by functionally declining kidneys. The renin-angiotensin-aldosterone system (RAAS), which encourages salt and water retention, is upregulated when eGFR decreases. This is made worse by BP's heightened sensitivity to salt. Advanced chronic kidney disease (CKD) is characterized by endothelial dysfunction (eGFR < 30 mL/min/1.73 m^2), and a strong correlation has been found between it and hypertension. Along the whole spectrum of CKD, increased arterial stiffness is also observed (Townsend et al., 2010) and is a separate risk factor for CVD events. It is also linked to the development of hypertension. After hypertension sets in, many variables, such as elevated oxidative metabolism and the ensuing relative renal hypoxia, may accelerate the advancement of blood pressure and CKD (Figure 2.1). (Fine et al., 2008).

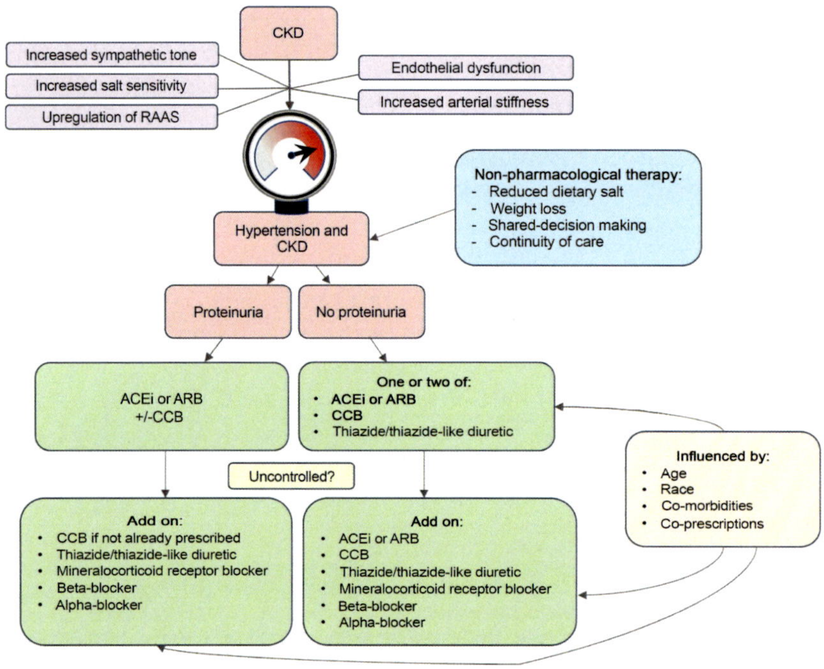

Figure 2.1. *Pathogenesis and management flow-chart of hypertension in chronic kidney disease. ACEi angiotensin converting enzyme inhibitor, ARB angiotensin II receptor antagonist (blocker), CCB calcium channel antagonist (blocker), CKD chronic kidney disease, RAAS renin–angiotensin–aldosterone system.*

Source: Pugh D, Gallacher PJ, Dhaun N. Management of Hypertension in Chronic Kidney Disease. Drugs. 2019 Mar;79(4):365-379. doi: 10.1007/s40265-019-1064-1. Erratum in: Drugs. 2020 Sep;80(13):1381. PMID: 30758803; PMCID: PMC6422950.

In terms of health, there is a 10–20% nocturnal drop in blood pressure. This is regulated by multiple elements, such as changes in autonomic function throughout the day, excretion of salt, and the RAAS (Fabbian et al. 2013). An elevated risk of CVD morbidity and mortality as well as the advancement of CKD is linked to dysregulation of these systems in CKD, which results in non-dipping or even rising nocturnal blood pressure.

2.2. DIAGNOSIS AND CLASSIFICATION OF HYPERTENSION IN CHRONIC KIDNEY DISEASE

To confirm the diagnosis of hypertension and modify antihypertensive medication, the 2017 American Heart Association/American College of Cardiology (AHA/ACC) guideline emphasizes that assessment and management of hypertension should be based on standardized methods of blood pressure (BP) measurement. It also suggests using home or ambulatory BP monitoring (ABPM) (Table 2.1) (Aronow et al., 2017).

Table 2.1. *Definitions of Normal and Abnormal BP Based on the 2017 AHA/ACC Guideline in Patients With CKD*

BP Classification[a]	**Office BP**	**Daytime ABPM or Home BP**
Normal or elevated BP	<130/80 mm Hg	<130/80 mm Hg
Sustained hypertension	≥130/80 mm Hg	≥130/80 mm Hg
White coat hypertension	≥130/80 mm Hg	<130/80 mm Hg
Masked hypertension	<130/80 mm Hg	≥130/80 mm Hg
Difficult-to-Control BP	**Definition**	
Resistant hypertension	Receiving ≥3 antihypertensive agents, 1 of which is a diuretic, without adequate BP control	
Refractory hypertension	Receiving ≥3 antihypertensive agents, 1 of which is a thiazide-type diuretic and another of which is spironolactone, without adequate BP control	

Abbreviations: ABPM, ambulatory blood pressure monitoring; AHA/ACC, American Heart Association/American College of Cardiology; BP, blood pressure; CKD, chronic kidney disease.

aAs recommended by the 2017 ACC/AHA guidelines.

Source: *Whelton et al. J Am Coll Cardiol. 2018;71(19):2199-2269.*

Similarly, the 2018 European Society of Hypertension/European Society of Cardiology (ESH/ESC) guideline acknowledges the limited diagnostic accuracy of blood pressure recordings obtained during a single office visit and suggests two approaches for diagnosing hypertension: either blood pressure measurement should be done repeatedly in the office or blood pressure should be monitored outside of the office. Table 2.2 provides an overview of BP measurement methods and diagnostic thresholds in accordance with American and European guidelines.

Table 2.2. *Techniques of BP Measurement*

Parameter	**Routine office BP**	**Unattended automated office BP**	**Home BP**	**Ambulatory BP**
Description	Manual or automated oscillometric measurements without specification of seated rest and with an observer in the room	Multiple automated oscillometric measurements after a 5-minute seated and without observer in the room	BP recordings obtained twice daily by the patients themselves at home typically with a validated oscillometric device	Automated BP measurements typically 3 times/ hour during daytime and 2 times/hour during nighttime
Monitoring schedule	Office visit	Office visit	At least 3 and preferably 7 days	24-Hour recording on a usual day
White-coat effect	Yes	Reduced vs. routine recordings	No	No
Assessment of nighttime BP/ nocturnal dipping	No	No	No	Yes
Association with target-organ damage	Poor	Moderate	Moderate	Strong
Association with cardiovascular and kidney outcomes	Poor	Few outcome data	Superior to routine office BP	Strong
Need for patient training	No	No	Yes	Yes
Availability in daily clinical practice	Yes	Limited	Yes	Limited
Diagnostic threshold according to the 2017 AHA/ACC guideline[	≤130/80 mm Hg	≤130/80 mm Hg	≤130/80 mm Hg	24-Hour: ≤125/75 mm Hg Daytime: ≤130/80 mm Hg Nighttime: ≤110/65 mm Hg
Diagnostic threshold according to the 2018 ESH/ESC guideline	≤140/90 mm Hg	≤135/85 mm Hg	≤135/85 mm Hg	24-Hour: ≤130/80 mm Hg Daytime: ≤135/85 mm Hg Nighttime: ≤120/70 mm Hg

Abbreviations: AHA/ACC, American Heart Association/American College of Cardiology; BP, blood pressure; ESH/ESC, European Society of Hypertension/European Society of Cardiology.

:

2.2.1. Office BP Monitoring

The Systolic Blood Pressure Intervention Trial (SPRINT) was a groundbreaking study that had to be ended early due to the significant heart-protective benefits of intensive blood pressure lowering. The trial involved 9,361 participants with systolic blood pressure (SBP) over 130 mm Hg and high cardiovascular risk. Participants were either placed in an intensive group aiming for an SBP under 120 mm Hg or a standard group aiming for an SBP under 140 mm Hg. The study protocol required participants to rest for 5 minutes in a quiet room before having three blood pressure measurements taken at 1-minute intervals using a research-grade technique, with no observer present at most sites.

The Ambulatory Blood Pressure SPRINT Ancillary Study (Drawz et al., 2017), 897 SPRINT participants had ABPM three weeks after the follow-up visit after 27 months. The correlation between research-grade office SBP and daytime ambulatory SBP was only moderate (Spearman coefficient: 0.56). Research-grade office SBP underestimated daytime ambulatory SBP by −6.8 mm Hg with wide 95% confidence intervals (−32.7 to 19.3 mm Hg) in the intensive treatment arm. The mean difference between research-grade office and daytime ambulatory SBP in the standard-treatment arm was –3 mm Hg, but the 95% limits of agreement were again wide (–3 mm Hg to 24 mm Hg).

The same research-grade technique used in SPRINT was used to measure blood pressure in 275 patients with chronic kidney disease (CKD) whose office blood pressure was within the normotensive range (<140/90 mm Hg). The results were compared to a single automated office blood pressure measurement taken on the same day in the presence of an observer and without any restrictions on seated rest. There was poor agreement between measurements and a significant mean difference between research-grade and routine office SBP (mean difference: −12.7 mm Hg; 95% limits of agreement: −46.1 to 20.7). The research-grade office SBP underestimated daytime ambulatory SBP by −7.9 mm Hg (95% limits of agreement: −33.2 to 17.4 mm Hg), in contrast to the popular belief that office BP is usually higher than daytime ambulatory BP. On the other hand, regular office SBP readings overestimated daytime ambulatory SBP by 4.8 mm Hg (with 95% limits of agreement ranging from -26.9 to 36.5 mm Hg). While SBP was linked to echocardiographically confirmed left ventricular hypertrophy regardless of how it was measured, the correlation was stronger with ambulatory and research-grade measurements than with routine office BP readings.

When combined, these diagnostic-test studies show that there are large 95% limits of agreement, meaning that neither routine nor research-grade office blood pressure measurements can consistently replace ABPM in individual patients. Standardized methods, however, lessen the bias present in regular office blood pressure readings.

2.2.2. Identification of BP Phenotypes with the Use of Out-of-office BP Monitoring

The utilization of remote blood pressure monitoring in combination with in-office measurements allows for the differentiation of white-coat and masked hypertension phenotypes, which aids in the categorization of hypertension severity (Figure 2.2). The International Database of Ambulatory BP in Renal Patients (I-DARE) collaborative group provided an estimate of the prevalence of BP phenotypes among 7,518 patients with CKD. 1,868 patients (25%) had controlled hypertension (CH), 1,488 patients (20%) had white-coat effect (WCE), 1,239 patients (16%) had masked uncontrolled hypertension (MUCH), and 2,923 patients (39%) had sustained uncontrolled hypertension (SUCH), based on a threshold of <140/90 mm

Hg for office BP and <130/80 mm Hg for 24-hour ambulatory BP (Drawz PE et al., 2017). Four factors were linked to increased risk of MUCH and SUCH: male gender, diabetes, using at least four antihypertensive drugs, and moderate-to-severe proteinuria (Agarwal, 2017).

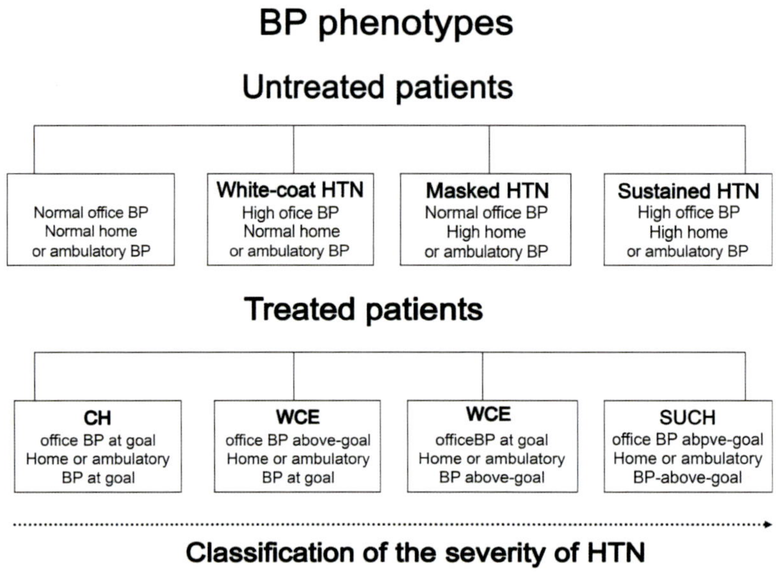

Figure 2.2. *BP phenotypes identified with concomitant use of office and out-of-office BP monitoring in treated and untreated subjects. Abbreviations: BP, blood pressure; CH, controlled hypertension; HTN, hypertension; MUCH, masked uncontrolled hypertension; SUCH, sustained uncontrolled hypertension; WCE, white-coat effect.*

Source: Panagiotis I Georgianos, Rajiv Agarwal, Hypertension in Chronic Kidney Disease (CKD): Diagnosis, Classification, and Therapeutic Targets, American Journal of Hypertension, Volume 34, Issue 4, April 2021, Pages 318–326, https://doi.org/10.1093/ajh/hpaa209.

The prevalence of different blood pressure phenotypes varies significantly depending on how blood pressure is measured and how hypertension is defined. In a study of 333 veterans with stage 2-4 chronic kidney disease who had controlled blood pressure in the doctor's office (<140/90 mm Hg), the prevalence of masked uncontrolled hypertension (MUCH) changed depending on the criteria used. For example, MUCH was found in 26.7% of participants when defined as daytime ambulatory blood pressure ≥135/85 mm Hg, and 32.8% when defined as 24-hour ambulatory blood pressure ≥130/80 mm Hg. However, the prevalence increased to 56.1% when either daytime blood pressure ≥135/85 mm Hg or nighttime blood pressure ≥120/70 mm Hg were considered. When home blood pressure monitoring was used (≥135/85 mm Hg), the prevalence of MUCH was 50.8%. This highlights the importance of considering both daytime and nighttime blood pressure measurements when diagnosing MUCH, as nocturnal hypertension is common in the chronic kidney disease population. In fact, nighttime blood pressure elevation was the only abnormality found in nearly half of the patients in this study.

It is reasonably reproducible to diagnose MUCH. In this study (Agarwal et al., 2016), office and out-of-office blood pressure readings were repeated four weeks apart to evaluate the reproducibility of MUCH diagnosis. 2016,]. When ABPM was used, there was a 75%–78% agreement in MUCH detection (k coefficient: 0.44–0.51), but only a 63%–65% agreement (k coefficient: 0.25) when home blood pressure records were used. The prevalence of MUCH increased with increases in office SBP, rising from 2% and 17% in the 90–110 and 110–119 mm Hg subgroups to 34% and 66% in the 120–129 and 130–139 mm Hg subgroups, respectively. Research-grade office SBP is a strong predictor of MUCH. As a result, if office blood pressure falls within the prehypertensive range, ABPM should be used to confirm the diagnosis of MUCH. Remarkably, office SBP was not found to be superior to home SBP in the diagnosis of MUCH, as confirmed by ABPM. Taking home blood pressure recordings without the same level of care, like waiting five minutes to sit still before taking the reading, could be one of the causes (Ahmed et al., 2010).

There is a well-established belief that the staging of chronic kidney disease and the severity of hypertension are related. However, the body of evidence is increasingly pointing to proteinuria as the factor more closely associated with the severity of hypertension rather than the estimated glomerular filtration rate (eGFR). Regardless of the method used to measure blood pressure—routine office, standardized office, home, or 24-hour ambulatory—the log of the urinary protein-to-creatinine ratio (UPCR) showed the strongest association with SBP in a cross-sectional analysis of 232 veterans with CKD that sought to investigate the relationship of 17 risk factors for hypertension with SBP. The association between UPCR and hypertension, however, was stronger when hypertension was measured using out-of-office blood pressure readings as opposed to office readings. In contrast, eGFR was not found to be a significant factor in determining SBP independently by any method. A study involving 336 veterans with or without CKD found a correlation between proteinuria and eGFR with the average level of 24-hour ambulatory SBP. However, when both factors were considered together in the same regression model, it was discovered that proteinuria, not eGFR, was the primary determinant of hypertension severity. Additionally, compared to the stage of CKD, increases in proteinuria had a greater impact on disrupting circadian variation and the average level of 24-hour ambulatory SBP (Alencar de Pihno et al., 2019).

In patients with chronic kidney disease (CKD), there is a gradual increase in left ventricular mass index, aortic pulse wave velocity, and log of UPCR as hypertension severity progresses from mild (CH) to moderate (MUCH) and severe (SUCH). However, after considering factors such as age, sex, race, other cardiovascular risks, and treatment, the connection between left ventricular mass index and pulse wave velocity with blood pressure classification weakens, while the link between proteinuria and the seriousness of hypertension remains. If this relationship is indeed causal, renal mechanisms may play a more significant role than cardiovascular damage in MUCH or SUCH.

Increases in 24-hour, daytime, and nighttime ambulatory blood pressure are strongly linked to a higher risk of unfavorable outcomes related to the kidneys and cardiovascular system among patients with chronic kidney disease (CKD); office blood pressure measurements by themselves, however, do not provide predictive information. Cardiorenal risk stratification is made easier by classifying the severity of hypertension and concurrently assessing office and ambulatory blood pressure. For instance, 489 hypertensive CKD patients were categorized into 4 phenotypes in a prospective cohort study based on their achievement of office (<140/90 mm Hg) and ambulatory (<135/85 during the day and <120/70 at night) blood pressure control. During a 5.2-year follow-up, individuals with WCE did not show an increased risk of cardiovascular morbidity and mortality compared to those with CH (hazard ratio: 1.55; 95% confidence interval: 0.75–3.19). However, those with MUCH (HR: 3.17; 95% CI: 1.50–6.69) and SUCH (HR: 2.83; 95% CI: 1.50–5.34) had an increased risk. When compared to CH, the risk of end-stage kidney disease (ESKD) or death was not higher in WCE (HR: 1.24; 95% CI: 0.67–2.27), but was elevated in MUCH (HR: 3.59; 95% CI: 2.05–6.27) and SUCH (HR: 2.96; 95% CI: 1.83–4.78) [Minutolo R. et al., 2014]. These findings remained significant even after adjusting for various risk factors. Therefore, while WCE indicates a lower-risk phenotype, the cardiorenal risk associated with MUCH is comparable to or even higher than that of SUCH.

2.3. MEASUREMENT OF BLOOD PRESSURE (BP) IN CKD

Accurate blood pressure measurements are necessary for the successful management of hypertension. In reality, blood pressure readings from clinics or offices are frequently used to guide hypertension treatment. Due to white-coat hypertension, diurnal variations in blood pressure, and a lack of repeat measurements, these could be erroneous. As a result, the clinical problem may not be precisely defined by this BP snapshot. There are several recognized forms of hypertension, and they are linked to differing levels of cardiovascular disease risk (Table 2.3). More accurate techniques for measuring blood pressure should be employed to detect these and adjust treatment accordingly (Appel et al., 2010).

Table 2.3. *Association of Hypertension Phenotype with All-Cause Mortality*

BP Phenotype	**Description**[a]	**All-cause Mortality Hazard Ratio (95% CI)**
Normotension	Normal clinic BP, normal 24-h ABPM	Reference
White-coat hypertension	High clinic BP, normal 24-h ABPM	1.79 (1.38–2.32)
Sustained hypertension	High clinic BP, high 24-h ABPM	1.80 (1.41–2.31)
Masked hypertension	Normal clinic BP, high 24-h ABPM	2.83 (2.12–3.79)

Values represent patients on treatment and without chronic kidney disease.

ABPM ambulatory blood pressure monitoring, BP blood pressure, CI confidence interval

aNormal clinic BP defined as < 140/90 mmHg. Normal 24-h BP defined as < 130/80 mmHg

Source: Pugh D, Gallacher PJ, Dhaun N. Management of Hypertension in Chronic Kidney Disease. Drugs. 2019 Mar;79(4):365-379. doi: 10.1007/s40265-019-1064-1. Erratum in: Drugs. 2020 Sep;80(13):1381. PMID: 30758803; PMCID: PMC6422950.

In patients with chronic kidney disease (CKD), 24-hour ambulatory blood pressure monitoring (ABPM) is a more reliable indicator of CVD events and a more accurate representation of BP phenotype. The 24-hour ABPM makes it possible to evaluate the BP's daily variation as well. An alternate, less resource-intensive tactic is home blood pressure monitoring. Compared to those who do not, those who get home readings show better overall blood pressure control. The 2017 American College of Cardiology (ACC) guidelines support out-of-office blood pressure measurement to confirm the diagnosis of hypertension and for titrating blood pressure-lowering medication in all patients, which is in line with current hypertension guidelines. Use only validated home blood pressure monitors to guarantee accuracy. The expected relationship between clinic and out-of-clinic blood pressure measurements is also described in the ACC guidelines. It is suggested that a blood pressure measurement at the clinic of 140/90 mmHg roughly corresponds to a home blood pressure value of 135/85 mmHg and to daytime and nighttime ABPM values of 135/85 and 120/70 mmHg, respectively (Brenner et al., 2001).

2.4. GOALS OF BP REDUCTION AND CONSENSUS TARGETS

As more research comes to light, the ideal blood pressure targets for treating CKD hypertension have changed (Figure 2.3) (Kotchen, 2011). The randomized SPRINT trial was terminated in September 2015 before it could be completed, as the interim analysis revealed that the group assigned to an intensive systolic blood pressure goal of less than 120 mm Hg had a 25% lower risk of cardiovascular disease and a 27% lower risk of all-cause mortality when compared to the standard group assigned to systolic blood pressure of less than 140 mm Hg.

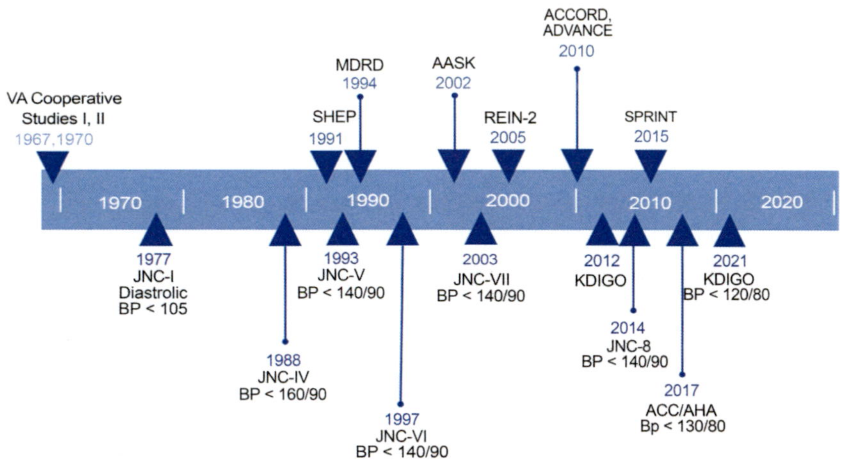

Figure 2.3. *United States blood pressure guidelines for chronic kidney disease (CKD) hypertension targets over time. Above timeline: Hypertension trials with CKD participants from 1960 to 2018 (not all inclusive). Below timeline: Guidelines and hypertension treatment targets from 1960 to 2021. CKD: chronic kidney disease; AASK: African American study of kidney disease and hypertension; ACCORD: Action to control cardiovascular risk in diabetes; ADVANCE: The action in diabetes and vascular disease: preterax and diamicron controlled evaluation trial; HTN: hypertension; KDIGO: Kidney disease improving global outcomes; MDRD: Modification of diet in renal disease; REIN-2: Blood-pressure control for renoprotection in patients with non-diabetic chronic renal disease; SPRINT: Systolic blood pressure intervention trial; SHEP: Systolic hypertension in the elderly program; VA: Veterans affairs.*

Source: Chang A et al. Blood Pressure Goals in Patients with CKD. CJASN Jan 2019, 14 (1) 161–169.

Recent recommendations from the clinical practice guidelines for Kidney Disease Improving Global Outcomes (KDIGO) in 2021 have favored more intensive treatment up to an SBP of less than

120 mm Hg. Subgroup analysis testing the two BP targets (SBP < 120 vs. SBP < 140 mm Hg) among 2,600 CKD patients in SPRINT led to this recommendation. After a median follow-up of 3.3 years in the intensive arm, the results showed lower composite cardiovascular outcome (HR 0.81; 95% CI, 0.63-1.05) and lower mortality (HR 0.72; 95% CI, 0.53-0.99). Fortunately, there was only one instance of a more marked decline in the estimated glomerular filtration rate (eGFR) in the intensive group during the first six months (-0.47 vs. -0.32 mL/min/1.73 m^2/year; P <.05) and no other significant kidney outcomes, such as the development of end-stage kidney disease (ESKD) or a reduction of more than 50% in eGFR. 03), ascribed to an immediate hemodynamically mediated reduction in the renal blood flow, without experiencing any additional noteworthy alterations throughout the rest of the investigation (Cheung et al., 2017).

The SPRINT trial's primary outcome heterogeneity set it apart from the three earlier trials comparing BP targets in CKD. Instead of cardiovascular outcomes, kidney outcomes (ESKD and reduced eGFR) were the primary outcomes in the Modification of Diet in Renal Disease (MDRD) trial, the African American Study of Kidney Disease and Hypertension (AASK) trial, and the Blood-Pressure Control for Renoprotection in Patients with Non-diabetic Chronic Renal Disease (REIN-2) trial (Klahr et al., 1994; Greene et al., 2002; Ruggenenti et al., 2005). Due to the low number of cardiovascular and mortality events in these studies, data synthesis for evidence-based practice guidelines is difficult. Malhotra and colleagues conducted a meta-analysis. subsequently looked at mortality in CKD subgroups, including these three trials, and found that the intensive blood pressure control group had a lower death rate (HR 0.86; 95% confidence interval, 0.76-0.97; P = .01). All four studies' intense blood pressure targets, however, did not prove to be helpful in lowering kidney outcomes. Considered collectively, an intensive blood pressure target appears suitable for lowering cardiovascular complications, especially considering the increased cardiovascular risk associated with chronic kidney disease.

By identifying two distinct BP phenotypes in hypertensive CKD patients—masked uncontrolled hypertension, or MUCH—and white coat hypertension, or WCH—the 24-hour ABPM can assist in ensuring BP targets are met. MUCH is wildly underappreciated; it is defined as normal blood pressure in the clinic but uncontrolled blood pressure outside the office. Patients with clinically normotensive chronic kidney disease (CKD) who are uncontrolled outside of the office may be at higher risk for cardiovascular disease (CVD) and experience a faster decline in kidney function. Patients with WCH account for up to 30% of patients with clinically uncontrolled hypertensive CKD. They have uncontrolled blood pressure in the clinic but normal blood pressure outside of the office. Under- and overtreatment, respectively, have resulted from the diagnostic failure of these two phenotypes (Parati G, Stergiou G, O'Brien E, et al., 2014). Ku et al. revealed a U-shaped relationship between the clinic and ambulatory SBP difference and increased mortality but no ESKD risk, demonstrating the clinical significance of these conditions among 610 participants in the AASK trial. It is unknown, though, if this trial can be applied to all hypertensive CKD patients. If it turns out that ABPM-based treatment strategies slow target organ damage and lower future CV events, the ongoing 4-year prospective randomized MASked-unconTrolled hypERtension (MASTER) management based on office BP or on ambulatory blood pressure measurement study may help resolve this uncertainty (Casas et al., 2005).

2.5. MANAGEMENT OF HYPERTENSION IN CHRONIC KIDNEY DISEASE

For the majority of patients with CKD and HTN, agents that not only lower blood pressure but also decrease proteinuria are advised as first-line therapy; data suggest that reducing proteinuria may have major long-term benefits in terms of cardiovascular and renal outcomes. HTN and CKD may be treated with a variety of antihypertensive drug classes. For this patient population, agents that target the renin-angiotensin-aldosterone system (RAAS), such as angiotensin receptor blockers (ARBs) or angiotensin-converting enzyme (ACE) inhibitors, are typically recommended as first-line antihypertensive therapy (Cushman et al., 2010).

2.5.1. BP Control for Renal Protection

The first randomized trial to examine the impact of standard (target mean arterial pressure [MAP] 107 mmHg) versus intensive (target MAP 92 mmHg) blood pressure control on the rate of eGFR decline in a US population with chronic kidney disease (CKD) (eGFR 13–55 mL/min/1.73 m^2). was the Modification of Diet in Renal Disease (MDRD) study. When compared to standard BP control, intensive blood pressure management did slow the rate of eGFR decline in patients with baseline proteinuria greater than 1 g/day. Nevertheless, individuals without proteinuria did not experience this benefit. These findings were confirmed in a non-diabetic African American population in 2002 by AASK (African American Study of Kidney Disease and Hypertension), with a GFR of 20–65 mL/min/1.73 m^2. In this study, 1094 patients were randomly assigned to receive either intensive (MAP 97 mmHg) or standard (MAP 102–107 mmHg) blood pressure control for a minimum of three years. Once more, only patients with baseline proteinuria greater than 1 g/day showed that severe blood pressure control could slow the progression of CKD (Appel et al., 2010). The purpose of the REIN-2 (Ramipril Efficacy in Nephropathy-2) study was to determine if standard blood pressure control with an ACE inhibitor alone was inferior to intensive blood pressure control with the addition of a dihydropyridine calcium channel antagonist (blocker) (CCB) to those already established on an ACE inhibitor. People with CKD and baseline proteinuria greater than 1 g/day were included in the study. Although BP was lowered with the addition of a CCB, renoprotection was not improved (Ruggenenti et al., 2005).

2.5.2. BP Control for Cardiovascular Protection

In patients with type 2 diabetes mellitus and normal renal function (serum creatinine < 133 μmol/L), the ACCORD (Action to Control Cardiovascular Risk in Diabetes) study compared the effects of intensive (target systolic BP < 120 mmHg) versus standard (target systolic BP < 140 mmHg) blood pressure control on cardiovascular outcomes (myocardial infarction [MI], stroke, or death from CVD) (Cushman et al., 2010). The risk of dying from CVD did not differ significantly between the intensive and standard treatment groups, despite a sustained difference in attained blood pressure. Intensive blood pressure control did, however, result in a lower risk of stroke.

The systolic blood pressure target was compared in the 2015 publication of SPRINT (Systolic Blood Pressure Intervention Trial). < 140 mmHg with a more intensive systolic goal of < 120 mmHg in 9361 non-diabetic patients at elevated CVD risk (defined as the presence of CVD, CKD, age > 75 years, or a 10-year risk of CVD of at least 15%. A statistically significant decrease in the primary outcome, which is a composite of MI, acute coronary syndrome, stroke, heart failure, or death from CVD, was shown by the intensive treatment group. There was also a noteworthy decrease in the secondary outcome of death from all causes. The trial was terminated early after three of its planned five-year duration due to the large effect size. Severe blood pressure control decreased all-cause death in individuals with chronic kidney disease (CKD; n = 2666; mean GFR 47.9 mL/min/1.73 m^2), with an effect size comparable to that of the cohort as a whole. On renal outcomes, such as the rate of eGFR decline, this had no effect. Sadly, individuals with eGFR. < 20 mL/min/1.73 m^2 and/or proteinuria > 1 g/day were not allowed to participate in SPRINT, nor were people with diabetes, which can cause up to 45% of CKD in developed nations. However, SPRINT indicates that CKD patients who receive intensive blood pressure control have lower CVD morbidity and mortality. Notably, despite no change in the rate of CKD progression, extended follow-up data from the AASK and MDRD studies now available also point to a long-term survival benefit from intensive blood pressure lowering (Drawz et al., 2017).

It should be mentioned that any trial's outcome could be significantly impacted by the BP measurement technique chosen. After five minutes of distraction-free sitting in a quiet room, participants in SPRINT had their blood pressure measured. Because our clinic's blood pressure is probably higher, SPRINT blood pressure may not be directly comparable to it. This could be the cause of the beneficial findings for such a low target BP. Notably, those receiving intensive treatment had a higher chance of suffering from acute kidney injury (AKI). Furthermore, intensive treatment increased the risk of developing chronic kidney disease (CKD) during the study in individuals with normal renal function at baseline. An examination conducted by Zhang and colleagues. (Zhang et al., 2018) that examined kidney damage biomarkers in this cohort to determine whether these changes reflect true renal injury. They discovered that the severe blood pressure reduction employed in SPRINT was linked to a drop in kidney damage indicators, such as ACR, anti-chitinase-3-like protein 1, and uromodulin. This suggests that benign modifications to renal blood flow, as opposed to pathological processes, could be the cause of the observed changes in eGFR.

The best blood pressure target for chronic kidney disease (CKD) is not well-established based on the evidence currently available. As a result, rules differ. The outcomes of SPRINT served as the foundation for a more stringent BP target in the 2017 ACC guidelines. Nevertheless, this more thorough approach has not been incorporated into the 2018 ESC/ESH guidelines. This could be seen as the Americans giving cardiovascular protection a higher priority than renoprotection, and the Europeans doing the opposite. Analyzing the available data makes it possible to comprehend the reasoning behind these choices, providing a foundation for developing individualized treatment programs that account for co-morbidities, CVD risk, the rate at which expected eGFR declines, and other patient characteristics. A person's blood pressure objectives may alter as they get older or have more severe illnesses. Consequently, it is important to view BP management in CKD as a dynamic process (Fabbian et al., 2013).

2.5.3. Achieving BP Targets

Reaching blood pressure goals is difficult. Despite receiving intensive care, which included monthly medication reviews, SPRINT showed that more than 50% of patients in the intensive treatment group were unable to reach the desired systolic blood pressure. Findings indicate that achieving blood pressure goals may be even more difficult for people with CKD than for people with hypertension in general. The majority of CKD patients do not achieve target blood pressure (BP) even when treated with multiple antihypertensive agents and non-pharmacological interventions (Georgianos and Agarwal, 2019).

2.5.4. Non-Pharmacological Treatment

In the context of CKD, there are several non-pharmacological treatments for hypertension. A Slagman et al. study discovered that lowering dietary sodium intake to a target of <50 mmol/day (~3 g/day of salt) reduced systolic blood pressure by an additional ~10 mmHg in individuals who were already on RAAS blockade. It has also been shown that restricting to a target of less than 100 mmol/day (~ 6 g/day of salt) reduces proteinuria by approximately 25%, an effect that cannot be explained by lowering blood pressure alone. Some people's blood pressure is not significantly affected by the effects of dietary sodium. On the other hand, BP becomes more sensitive to dietary sodium load as GFR decreases. In real life, restricting one's sodium intake can be challenging. Measurements of urinary sodium by Slagman et al. showed that, even with frequent counseling sessions, the group aiming for less than 50 mmol/day had an average daily sodium intake of 106 mmol. The daily intake for individuals without dietary restrictions was 186 mmol. Recognizing individual dietary preferences and establishing reasonable targets (less than 100 milligrams of sodium per day) while working with a dietitian can increase the chances of making significant and long-lasting dietary modifications (Greenland and Peterson, 2017).

Losing weight can slow the progression of CKD and is effective in lowering blood pressure and proteinuria. A mean weight reduction of approximately 4% can reduce proteinuria by approximately 30 % in overweight patients (body mass index [BMI] > 27 kg/m^2) with CKD and proteinuria (> 1 g/24 h). In CKD, the advantages of a multidisciplinary approach have also been shown. Santschi and colleagues' systematic review demonstrates that after community pharmacists were introduced, hypertensive patients' achievement of blood pressure goals improved. Specialized nursing care significantly enhanced the management of CVD risk factors, including blood pressure, at one and two years in patients with stage 3–4 chronic kidney disease (CKD), according to the MASTERPLAN (Multifactorial Approach and Superior Treatment Efficacy in Renal Patients with the Aid of Nurse Practitioners) study carried out in the Netherlands (Gritter et al., 2022).

2.5.5. Pharmacological Treatment

Antihypertensive drugs are typically needed in addition to non-pharmacological therapies for chronic kidney disease (CKD), despite their advantages. Certain pharmaceutical treatments have additional renoprotective and/or cardioprotective effects in addition to their direct BP-lowering effects, which may occur independently of these effects. As a result, the medication of choice should take the patient's need for risk reduction into account. A combination drug therapy is often required to meet blood pressure targets, so polypharmacy risks must also be taken into account.

2.5.5.1. Renin–Angiotensin–Aldosterone System Blockade

Patients with chronic kidney disease (CKD) benefit greatly from the cardioprotective and renoprotective effects of angiotensin II receptor antagonists (ARBs) and ACE inhibitors. RAAS blockade can lower systolic blood pressure in individuals with CKD and hypertension by about 20 mmHg. This is comparable to the BP reduction that diuretics and CCBs provide. Crucially, though, these medications provide a BP-independent decrease in proteinuria in both non-diabetic and diabetic CKD patients, and as a result, they are widely recognized as the initial line of treatment for hypertension in these patients.

Recently, there has been doubt about the superior renoprotective effect of RAAS blockade in patients with non-proteinuric CKD. According to a systematic review conducted by Casas and colleagues, the better renal outcomes linked to RAAS blockade are most likely the result of a BP-lowering effect alone. If another antihypertensive were to reduce blood pressure in the same way, this effect might be replicated. Consequently, CCBs and thiazide or thiazide-like diuretics should be taken into consideration as alternative first-line options in this population, even though ACE inhibitors may be used as first-line agents in those with hypertension and non-proteinuric CKD (Jennings and Taber, 2008).

Chronic ACE inhibition can cause angiotensin II reactivation in up to 50% of patients, which blunts the effects of RAAS blockade. Thus, it has been postulated that cardiovascular and renal outcomes could be enhanced by adding an ARB to those already known to inhibit ACE. This question was intended to be addressed in patients at high risk of CVD by the ONTARGET. 25,620 patients were followed up for a median of 56 months after being randomly assigned to receive combination therapy consisting of both agents, ACE inhibitors, or ARB. Combination therapy was linked to a higher rate of side effects but did not significantly lower the primary outcome of dying from heart failure, stroke, MI, or CVD (Kasiske et al., 2004).

The Veterans Affairs Nephropathy in Diabetes (VA NEPHRON-D) study looked at renal outcomes in a group of CKD patients who were diabetic. Once more, combination treatment involving an ACE inhibitor and an ARB increased adverse events but did not significantly lower the primary endpoint of CKD progression, ESRD, or death. For patients with CKD, combination therapy utilizing both an ACE inhibitor and an ARB is no longer recommended. Notably, participants in these trials had a high risk of developing renal vascular disease, which is characterized by a partially dependent GFR on a functional RAAS. Double angiotensin blockade reduces proteinuria more than monotherapy does in patients with conditions like immunoglobulin A (IgA) nephropathy, the primary glomerular cause of end-stage renal disease (ESRD) in the United States. Compared to VA NEPHRON-D and ONTARGET patients, these patients are younger and have a lower cardiovascular risk. It is currently unknown whether this translates into a larger benefit for the kidneys and cardiovascular system (Knoll et al., 2016).

Possible side effects of RAAS blockade include the emergence of AKI and hyperkalemia. Following the start of RAAS blockade, a decrease in intraglomerular pressure frequently results in an increase in serum creatinine. Losartan or placebo was administered to 1513 patients with diabetic nephropathy, which is defined as proteinuria exceeding 0.5 g/day or serum creatinine between 115 and 265 μmol/L, as part of the RENAAL (Reduction in End Points in Noninsulin-Dependent Diabetes Mellitus with the Angiotensin II Antagonist Losartan) study. During the first three months of treatment, the losartan group's eGFR decreased more (-2.3 vs. -1.6 mL/min/1.73 m^2).

It is unclear what this brief decline in eGFR means. ARB or ACE inhibitor-induced initial eGFR decline has been associated with unfavorable cardiorenal outcomes, according to observational data from the primary care context in the United Kingdom. On the other hand, regardless of the initial rate of decline, RENAAL patients randomly assigned to losartan had a slower rate of eGFR decline compared with placebo after a mean follow-up period of 3.4 years. According to current guidelines, after starting RAAS blockade, a rise in serum creatinine of up to 30% with subsequent stabilization should be accepted as this is likely to confer longer-term renoprotection (Ku et al., 2019). The use of RAAS blockade in patients with advanced chronic kidney disease (eGFR < 30 mL/min/1.73 m2) is also unclear because most large randomized trials have not included this population. An observational study conducted by Ahmed and colleagues. [El Kossi M, El Nahas AM, Kamath NS, Ahmed AK. 2010] showed that stopping RAAS blockade significantly increased eGFR in a cohort of UK patients with advanced CKD, sometimes delaying the initiation of renal replacement therapy. Consequently, the STOP-ACEi national multicenter randomized trial of ACE inhibitor/ARB withdrawal in advanced chronic kidney disease has commenced. For patients with advanced chronic kidney disease (CKD), the decision about starting or continuing RAAS blockade is still up for debate until trial results are available (Lambers et al., 2012).

2.5.5.2. Diuretics

Up to 50% of patients with CKD experience volume overload, which is frequently subclinical and a separate risk factor for CVD. Diuretic therapy has been demonstrated to improve arterial stiffness and left ventricular mass index in patients with chronic kidney disease (CKD) and can lessen volume expansion. Diuretics have antihypertensive and cardioprotective properties, which is why they are commonly used in combination medication therapy for chronic kidney disease (CKD) (Lewis et al., 2021).

First-line therapy for non-proteinuric chronic kidney disease (CKD) may involve monotherapy with a thiazide (e.g., bendroflumethiazide) or thiazide-like diuretic (e.g., indapamide). A diuretic treatment may also restore the natural nocturnal drop in blood pressure that is associated with chronic kidney disease. Because the tubular mechanism of action of loop diuretics (like furosemide) depends first on glomerular filtration, higher doses of these medications are frequently needed in patients with lower eGFRs. Nevertheless, loop diuretics are valuable medications. Given how potent a loop and thiazide diuretic combination is, caution should be exercised to prevent fluid depletion. Patients with polycystic kidney disease should generally avoid using diuretics because of the accelerated growth of cysts and loss of excretory function that comes with using them.

In patients with CKD, mineralocorticoid receptor antagonists (blockers) like spironolactone effectively lower blood pressure; however, they also increase the risk of hyperkalemia. Since these medications have been shown to enhance diastolic and systolic function in early chronic kidney disease (CKD), patients who also have concurrent left ventricular dysfunction may find special benefit from them. It is not clear if this effect results from BP lowering on its own. To address this, a randomized trial called SPIRO-CKD [Spironolactone in Chronic Kidney Disease] has been finished, comparing spironolactone with the thiazide-like diuretic chlorthalidone in patients with stage 3 CKD. The results are being awaited. When used as a fourth-line add-on therapy for hypertensive patients without CKD, spironolactone lowers blood pressure more effectively than bisoprolol or doxazosin (Li et al., 2006).

2.5.5.3. Calcium Channel Antagonists (Blockers)

In CKD, dihydropyridine and non-dihydropyridine CCBs are both helpful in controlling hypertension. In non-proteinuric CKD, dihydropyridine CCBs (like amlodipine) can be used alone or in combination as first-line treatment. Their impact is less effective in proteinuric CKD than RAAS blockade. However, adding a dihydropyridine CCB to patients with established RAAS blockade who have proteinuria improves blood pressure control without making proteinuria worse. The recently revised ESC/ESH guidelines, which support combination therapy with an ACE inhibitor and CCB as first-line therapy in patients with proteinuria, reflect this. Non-dihydropyridine CCBs, like verapamil, are just as good at controlling blood pressure as dihydropyridine CCBs, but they have a greater impact on reducing proteinuria (Mayer et al., 2018).

To reduce CVD mortality in people with hypertension who are also at high risk of developing CVD (defined as having diabetes, left ventricular hypertrophy, peripheral arterial disease, CKD, or a history of CVD), combination therapy with amlodipine and an ACE inhibitor was compared to hydrochlorothiazide and an ACE inhibitor in the ACCOMPLISH (Avoiding Cardiovascular Events through Combination Therapy in Patients Living with Systolic Hypertension) trial. A doubling of baseline serum creatinine or reaching ESRD was the predetermined endpoint of CKD progression in this multicenter, double-blind, randomized trial. Because amlodipine and ACE inhibitors were more effective at reducing CVD mortality, the trial was stopped early.

Notably, regardless of achieved blood pressure levels, the amlodipine group also had a noticeably lower risk of CKD progression. This shows that in this at-risk group, adding amlodipine to ACE inhibitor therapy has a greater renoprotective effect than adding a thiazide diuretic. Despite being well tolerated overall, CCBs have the potential to exacerbate peripheral edema, which can be especially problematic for people with chronic kidney disease (McMohan et al., 2021).

2.5.5.4. β-Blockers

As β-adrenoceptor antagonists, β-blockers effectively lower blood pressure in patients with chronic kidney disease (CKD) by affecting the dysregulated sympathetic nervous system. These medications have well-established cardioprotective properties, making CKD patients especially benefit from them. β-blockers have also been shown in animal studies to exhibit renoprotective effects, such as a decrease in the progression of interstitial fibrosis after renal injury. In patients with chronic kidney disease (CKD), observational and prospective studies have shown that β-blocker therapy improves survival when compared to placebo. In spite of this, people with CKD use β-blockers less frequently than people without it (Minutolo et al., 2014).

Concerns about reduced renal excretion, systemic accumulation, and glycaemic control may account for some of the underuse observed in CKD patients. Despite the possible risks associated with specific β-blocker classes, these medications are safe to use in all stages of renal impairment. Hepatically excreted β-blockers and those with additional vasodilatory properties (like carvedilol) may be especially useful in cases where dosage adjustments are necessary. Comparing β-blockers directly to ACE inhibitors has revealed that they provide less effective renoprotection. However, the AASK study did show that CKD patients treated with metoprolol had lower rates of ESRD and death compared to those treated with amlodipine. Thus, β-Blockers should be regarded as beneficial supplements for patients with established RAAS blockade, especially when overt CVD coexists (Parati et al., 2014).

2.5.5.5. α-Blockers

In combination therapy, peripherally acting α-blockers (α-adrenoceptor antagonists) like doxazosin are frequently utilized to manage hypertension in patients with chronic kidney disease. This could be the result of both positive effects on glycaemic control and a pharmacokinetic profile that is unaffected by decreasing eGFR. Numerous investigations have exhibited their effectiveness as supplemental treatment for hypertension in individuals with chronic kidney disease. As other agents are more effective in reducing the incidence of CVD, α-Blockers should not be the first choice for first-line therapy.

2.5.5.6. Chronotherapy

The hypothesis is that evening dosing could reverse the non-dipping nocturnal blood pressure observed in chronic kidney disease (CKD) since the timing of antihypertensive medications can affect the diurnal variation of blood pressure. In a study conducted by Hermida and colleagues, participants were randomly assigned to take one or more antihypertensives at night or to take all antihypertensive medication upon waking. This allowed the researchers to examine the effects of nocturnal antihypertensive dosing in 661 patients with CKD. Compared to the group that took all of their medications in the morning, the nocturnal dosing group had significantly better blood pressure control and a lower incidence of CVD death, MI, and stroke after a median follow-up period of 5.4 years. Thus, chronotherapy would seem to be one of the easier ways to help people with CKD and hypertension get better results (Picard et al., 2020).

2.5.5.7. Adherence

Treatment adherence is no more superior in patients with CKD than in those without, despite the dangers of CKD developing into ESRD and patients needing dialysis and/or transplantation. As CKD worsens, adherence gets better, but when patients begin dialysis, it gets worse once more.

Table 2.4. *Commonly Prescribed Antihypertensive Drugs, Usual Drug Doses, Precautions and Side Effects*

Drug Class and Druga	**Usual Dose**	**Common Side Effects**	**Potential Contraindications**	**Additional Considerations**
ACEIs				
Lisinopril PerindoprilRamipril Trandolapril	10–40 mg/day2–8 mg/day5–10 mg/day0.5–4 mg/day	Cough; angioedema; hyperkalemia; leucopenia; anemia	Hyperkalemia; pregnancy; bilateral renal artery stenosis	First-line antihypertensive agents in patients with severely increased albuminuria
ARBs				
CandesartanIrbesartan Losartan Olmesartan Telmisartan Valsartan	8–32 mg/day75–300 mg/day50–100 mg/day10–40 mg/day40–80 mg/day80–320 mg/day	Cough (less commonly than with ACEIs); angioedema; hyperkalemia; anemia	Hyperkalemia; pregnancy; bilateral renal artery stenosis	First-line antihypertensive agents in patients with severely increased albuminuria
Dihydropyridine CCBs				
Amlodipine Felodipine Manidipine	5–10 mg/day5–10 mg/day10–20 mg/day	Lower-extremity edema; gingival; hypertrophy		Worsening of albuminuria

Non-dihydropyridine CCBs				
Verapamil Diltiazem	180–360 mg/day180–360 mg/day	Constipation; gingival hyperplasia	2nd or 3rd degree heart block	Reduction in albuminuria; increase the levels of calcineurin and mTOR inhibitors; drug interactions (i.e., β-blockers, statins)
Thiazide or thiazide-like diuretics				
Hydrochlorothiazide Chlorthalidone Metonazole	12.5–25 mg/day12.5 mg/day2.5 mg/day	Hyperuricemia; hypercalcemia; hyponatremia; hypokalemia; hyperglycemia	Hyponatremia; hypokalemia; hypercalcemia; volume depletion	The thiazide-like diuretic chlorthalidone is effective in lowering BP in patients with stage 4 CKD and poorly controlled hypertension
Loop diuretics				
Furosemide Torsemide	40–80 mg/day20 mg/day	Hearing loss; hypokalemia; hypocalcemia; hyponatremia	Volume depletion	Torsemide has better bioavailability and longer elimination half-life as compared with furosemide
Steroidal MRAs				
Spironolactone Eplerenone	25–50 mg/day50–100 mg/day	Hyperkalemia; metabolic acidosis; gynecomastia	Hyperkalemia	Spironolactone is useful in resistant hypertension as fourth-line therapy
β-adrenergic receptor blockers				
Atenolol Bisoprolol Carvedilol Metoprolol Nebivolol	25–100 mg/day2.5–10 mg/day12.5–25 mg twice daily50–100 mg twice daily2.5–10 mg/day	Bradycardia; hyperkalemia; fatigue; depression; sexual dysfunction	Bradycardia; asthma; chronic obstructive pulmonary disease; 2nd or 3rd degree heart block	β-blockers are recommended for the management of hypertension in patients with specific cardiovascular indication for their use

[a]This is a list of selected medications from each antihypertensive drug category; the use of antihypertensive agents may differ from country to country.

mTOR: mammalian target of rapamycin.

Source: *Panagiotis I Georgianos, Rajiv Agarwal, Hypertension in chronic kidney disease—treatment standard 2023, Nephrology Dialysis Transplantation, Volume 38, Issue 12, December 2023, Pages 2694–2703, https://doi.org/10.1093/ndt/gfad118.*

Research looking into CKD patients' reasons for non-compliance emphasizes the value of communication and the perceived efficacy of the relevant therapies. Adverse effects, drug interactions, and pill burden are also significant factors. Hence, wherever feasible, antihypertensive regimens should be made simpler while taking into account the number, timing, and type of interventions. Continuity of care may also be important; therefore, whenever feasible, try to arrange for patients to see the same doctor for each visit. This has been shown to improve results (Table 2.4) (Rahman et al., 2020).

2.5.6. Managing Hypertension in the Context of Hemodialysis

Blood pressure and the consequences of CVD in patients receiving hemodialysis have a complicated relationship. Lower blood pressure does not always correspond to better survival in this cohort, unlike in the general population and in people with pre-dialysis chronic kidney disease. There is not enough data to set BP targets for this group. In a study conducted over three years, 125,928 hemodialysis patients were categorized into various pre-dialysis systolic blood pressure categories. The patients with a pre-dialysis systolic blood pressure of less than 120 mmHg had the highest mortality rate. Higher pre-dialysis blood pressure was protective; individuals with pre-dialysis systolic blood pressure between 160 and 180 mmHg had the lowest mortality. Although this "inverse epidemiology" has been shown before, little is still known about it. Adverse clinical results may also be predicted by changes in blood pressure during hemodialysis. Intradialytic hypertension has been linked to higher 30-day mortality and hospitalization rates, according to retrospective data (Santschi et al., 2011). It is controversial how best to take blood pressure readings from patients receiving hemodialysis. Changes in fluid and electrolyte levels can cause large differences in pre- and post-dialytic blood pressure. Mayer and associates used 24-hour ABPM administered right before a dialysis session to investigate the association between mortality and systolic blood pressure in a cohort receiving home hemodialysis. A U-shaped relationship between 24-hour systolic ABMP and all-cause mortality was observed during the 3-year follow-up period, indicating a higher risk of death for individuals with either very low or very high blood pressure. An analysis of subgroups showed a linear relationship between people with and without CVD. A lower blood pressure was linked to a higher death risk in patients with CVD. For those without CVD, the opposite was true, which explains the overall U-shaped curve. This highlights the necessity of individualized blood pressure treatment regimens that take co-morbidities into account for patients receiving hemodialysis. For a long time, patients have had access to CVD risk calculators that estimate their personal risk of experiencing CVD events. Not only do innovative risk calculators like QRISK®3 now incorporate individuals with chronic kidney disease (CKD), but many risk calculators specifically intended for the hemodialysis population have also been created and verified (Slagman et al., 2011).

In patients receiving hemodialysis, sodium and water overload may be the main causes of hypertension. However, despite intensive ultrafiltration, hypertension frequently endures. There are few data that support the use of all antihypertensive classes. Utilizing β-blockers is especially appealing since they lessen arterial stiffness and left ventricular hypertrophy, two conditions that are accelerated in end-stage renal disease (ESRD), as well as some of the arrhythmogenic effects of dialysis. The selection of β-blockers is still controversial, partly because different patients clear drugs to varying degrees during dialysis.

2.5.7. Managing Hypertension Following Kidney Transplantation

There is not any randomized clinical trials investigating the most effective ways to treat hypertension after kidney transplantation, similar to hemodialysis. Several factors can lead to the development of hypertension, which is common following transplantation. After a kidney transplant, over 90% of recipients who are on an immunosuppressive regimen based on calcineurin inhibitors (CNI) will develop hypertension. Uncontrolled blood pressure is also more common. At one year, less than half of patients manage a systolic blood pressure of less than 140 mmHg. As the primary cause of death after kidney transplantation, higher blood pressure is linked to worse graft outcomes and increased risk of cardiovascular disease (CVD). A retrospective analysis of 1666 kidney transplant recipients showed that for every 10 mmHg increase in systolic blood pressure, there was an approximately 5% increased risk of graft failure and death (Kasiske et al., 2004). For the majority of patients, broader cardioprotection—which includes antiplatelet medication and lipid-lowering—is probably advantageous.

The selection of an antihypertensive medication is contingent upon multiple factors, such as the duration since transplantation, concurrent medications involving immunosuppression, and co-morbidities. Because there is a chance that serum creatinine will temporarily increase during this vulnerable period, RAAS blockade has historically been avoided in the early post-transplant period. Nevertheless, early RAAS blockade (within 12 weeks post-transplant) appears to improve left ventricular hypertrophy and proteinuria at 1 year without lowering eGFR, according to a systematic review by Jennings and Taber. Given the elevated risk of cardiovascular disease (CVD) in this population, these drugs—whether started early or not—are thought to be crucial after kidney transplantation. On the other hand, post-transplant renoprotection is still unknown. An investigation by Knoll et al. examined the impact of ramipril versus placebo in 212 transplant recipients who had proteinuria at least three months after the transplant in an effort to allay this uncertainty. Ramipril did not significantly reduce the doubling of serum creatinine, ESRD, or death after a 48-month follow-up period. This group's low rates of ACE inhibitor use—as few as 30% of patients with diabetes and/or CVD receiving RAAS blockade six months after transplant—reflect this uncertainty (Thompson et al., 2015).

Afferent arteriolar vasoconstriction is brought on by CNIs like tacrolimus, which are the cornerstone of post-transplant immunosuppression therapy. Dihydropyridine CCBs have the potential to induce afferent arteriolar vasodilatation in patients receiving CNIs, which may explain some of the evidence supporting their potential benefit in this setting. Because non-dihydropyridine CCBs disrupt CNI metabolism, it is necessary to closely monitor drug levels.

A Closer Look

Mechanism of Hypertensive Kidney Disease

Arteriolosclerosis, a condition in which the walls of small arteries and arterioles thicken and narrow due to the accumulation of hyaline (a pink, amorphous, homogenous material) in the kidneys as a result of benign arterial hypertension, is the result. Tubular atrophy, interstitial fibrosis, glomerular alterations (smaller glomeruli with varying degrees of hyalinization, from mild to sclerosis of glomeruli), and scarring surrounding the glomeruli (periglomerular fibrosis) are the results of the ensuing insufficient blood flow. Kidney failure will develop in later stages. The tubules of functional nephrons are dilated and frequently have hyaline casts in the tubule opening. Blood and protein in the urine is a common side effect of glomerular damage brought on by hypertensive nephropathy (Whelton et al., 2018).

Renal failure linked to a history of hypertension is known as hypertensive nephropathy. This chronic illness poses a significant risk for the progression of end-stage kidney disease (ESKD). Though the link between chronic kidney disease and hypertension is well established, the underlying mechanism is still unknown. The glomerulus, a network of dense capillaries that facilitates kidney filtration, is the focus of the two proposed mechanisms of hemolytic nephropathy's pathophysiology. One theory attributes the primary cause of HN to glomerular ischemia, while the other places the pathogenesis of HN at the intersection of glomerular hypertension and glomerular hyperfiltration.

Glomerular Ischemia

Long-term high blood pressure can harm the endothelium, also referred to as the blood vessel lining. Plaques accumulate as a result, and they have the potential to lodge in the renal arteries, resulting in stenosis and ischemic kidney disease. This results in insufficient blood flow to the kidney supplied by the constricted renal artery, which in turn reduces the size of the kidneys. Additional effects include thickening of the intima, the blood vessel's innermost layer, and arterial stiffening, which is the result of a slow breakdown of elastic fibers.

Glomerular Hypertension and Glomerular Hyperfiltration

Prolonged glomerular hypertension, and consequently glomerular hyperfiltration, is an alternative mechanism of hypertensive nephropathy. These don't always have to happen at the same time. The theory goes that glomerular sclerosis brought on by hypertension eventually leads to decreased kidney function. The preglomerular arterioles, which are the unaffected nephrons, vasodilate as a compensatory mechanism to boost blood flow to the kidney perfusion and glomerular filtration across undamaged glomeruli (Wright et al., 2015).

Summary

- Many mechanisms contribute to the development of hypertension in CKD and these influence its management. An increase in sympathetic tone, brought about by afferent signals generated by functionally declining kidneys, contributes to the development of hypertension in CKD. As eGFR declines there is an upregulation of the renin–angiotensin–aldosterone system (RAAS) which promotes salt and water retention.
- The application of out-of-office BP monitoring in conjunction with measurements obtained in the office enables the identification of phenotypes of white-coat and masked hypertension, facilitating the classification of the severity of hypertension.
- For the management of hypertension to be effective, accurate BP measurements are essential. In practice, the treatment of hypertension is often based on clinic or office BP recordings. These may be inaccurate due to a lack of repeat measurements, diurnal variation in BP and white-coat hypertension.
- A 24-Hour ambulatory BP monitoring (ABPM) provides a more accurate depiction of BP phenotype and is a better predictor of CVD events in those with CKD than clinic readings. 24-Hour ABPM also allows assessment of the diurnal variation in BP. Home BP monitoring is an alternative strategy that is less resource-intensive.
- Several classes of antihypertensive agents may have a role in the treatment of CKD and HTN. Agents that target the renin-angiotensin-aldosterone system (RAAS), such as angiotensin-converting enzyme (ACE) inhibitors or angiotensin receptor blockers (ARBs), are generally considered first-line antihypertensive therapy for this patient population.
- Acknowledging personal dietary preferences and setting realistic goals (< 100 mmol/day of sodium) under the supervision of a dietitian may improve the likelihood of achieving meaningful and sustained dietary changes.
- Despite the benefits of non-pharmacological interventions in CKD, antihypertensive medications are usually also required. As well as direct BP-lowering effects, certain pharmacological therapies provide additional renoprotective and/or cardioprotective action, which may be independent of their BP-lowering effects. The choice of drug should therefore consider the balance of risk reduction required by the individual. Combination drug therapy is frequently needed to achieve BP targets, and thus the risks of polypharmacy need also be considered.
- ACE inhibitors and angiotensin II receptor antagonists (blockers) (ARBs) have both cardioprotective and renoprotective properties and are therefore of particular value in patients with CKD. RAAS blockade can reduce systolic BP by ~ 20 mmHg in patients with hypertension and CKD.
- Volume overload, often subclinical, affects up to 50% of people with CKD and is an independent risk factor for CVD. Diuretic therapy can reduce volume expansion and has been shown to improve left ventricular mass index and arterial stiffness in those with CKD. Thus, diuretics are frequently used as part of combination drug therapy in CKD and offer antihypertensive and cardioprotective effects.

- Both dihydropyridine and non-dihydropyridine CCBs are useful in the management of hypertension in CKD. Dihydropyridine CCBs (such as amlodipine) can be used as first-line therapy in non-proteinuric CKD, either alone or in combination.
- β-Blockers (β-adrenoceptor antagonists) effectively reduce BP in CKD due to their effect on the dysregulated sympathetic nervous system. The cardioprotective benefits of these drugs are well-established and therefore they are particularly advantageous in those with CKD.
- Peripherally acting α-blockers (α-adrenoceptor antagonists; such as doxazosin) are commonly used as part of combination therapy for the management of hypertension in CKD. This may be due to a pharmacokinetic profile that is undisturbed by declining eGFR in addition to favorable effects on glycaemic control.

References

1. Agarwal, R. (2017). Implications of blood pressure measurement technique for implementation of Systolic Blood Pressure Intervention Trial (SPRINT). *Journal of the American Heart Association, 6*(2), e004536. https://doi.org/10.1161/JAHA.116.004536.
2. Agarwal, R., & Andersen, M. J. (2006). Blood pressure recordings within and outside the clinic and cardiovascular events in chronic kidney disease. *American Journal of Nephrology, 26*(5), 503–510. https://doi.org/10.1159/000097366.
3. Agarwal, R., Pappas, M. K., & Sinha, A. D. (2016). Masked uncontrolled hypertension in CKD. *Journal of the American Society of Nephrology, 27*(4), 924–932.
4. Ahmed, A. K., Kamath, N. S., El Kossi, M., & El Nahas, A. M. (2010). The impact of stopping inhibitors of the renin-angiotensin system in patients with advanced chronic kidney disease. *Nephrology Dialysis Transplantation, 25*(12), 3977–3982.
5. Alencar de Pihno, N., Levin, A., Fukagawa, M., et al. (2019). Considerable international variation exists in blood pressure control and antihypertensive prescription patterns in chronic kidney disease. *Kidney International, 96*(4), 983–994. https://doi.org/10.1016/j.kint.2019.04.032.
6. Appel, L. J., Wright, J. T., Jr, Greene, T., Agodoa, L. Y., Astor, B. C., Bakris, G. L., et al. (2010). Intensive blood-pressure control in hypertensive chronic kidney disease. *New England Journal of Medicine, 363*(10), 918–929.
7. Brenner, B. M., Cooper, M. E., de Zeeuw, D., et al. (2001). Effects of losartan on renal and cardiovascular outcomes in patients with type 2 diabetes and nephropathy. *New England Journal of Medicine, 345*(12), 861–869. https://doi.org/10.1056/NEJMoa011161.
8. Casas, J. P., Chua, W., Loukogeorgakis, S., Vallance, P., Smeeth, L., Hingorani, A. D., et al. (2005). Effect of inhibitors of the renin-angiotensin system and other antihypertensive drugs on renal outcomes: Systematic review and meta-analysis. *Lancet, 366*(9502), 2026–2033.
9. Cheung, A. K., Rahman, M., Reboussin, D. M., et al. (2017). Effects of intensive BP control in CKD. *Journal of the American Society of Nephrology, 28*(9), 2812–2823. https://doi.org/10.1681/ASN.2017020148.
10. Cushman, W. C., Evans, G. W., Byington, R. P., Goff, D. C., Jr, Grimm, R. H., Jr, Cutler, J. A., et al. (2010). Effects of intensive blood-pressure control in type 2 diabetes mellitus. *New England Journal of Medicine, 362*(17), 1575–1585.

11. Drawz, P. E., Pajewski, N. M., Bates, J. T., Bello, N. A., Cushman, W. C., Dwyer, J. P., et al. (2017). Effect of intensive versus standard clinic-based hypertension management on ambulatory blood pressure: Results from the SPRINT (Systolic Blood Pressure Intervention Trial) ambulatory blood pressure study. *Hypertension, 69*(1), 42–50.

12. Fabbian, F., Smolensky, M. H., Tiseo, R., Pala, M., Manfredini, R., & Portaluppi, F. (2013). Dipper and non-dipper blood pressure 24-hour patterns: Circadian rhythm-dependent physiologic and pathophysiologic mechanisms. *Chronobiology International, 30*(1–2), 17–30.

13. Fine, L. G., & Norman, J. T. (2008). Chronic hypoxia as a mechanism of progression of chronic kidney diseases: From hypothesis to novel therapeutics. *Kidney International, 74*(7), 867–872.

14. Georgianos, P. I., & Agarwal, R. (2019). Review: Automated office BP measures are similar to awake ambulatory BP and lower than other office BP measures. *Annals of Internal Medicine, 170*(12), JC69. https://doi.org/10.7326/ACPJ201906180-069.

15. Greenland, P., & Peterson, E. (2017). The new 2017 ACC/AHA guidelines "up the pressure" on diagnosis and treatment of hypertension. *JAMA, 318*(21), 2083–2084. https://doi.org/10.1001/jama.2017.18605.

16. Gritter, M., Wouda, R. D., Yeung, S. M. H., et al. (2022). Effects of short-term potassium chloride supplementation in patients with CKD. *Journal of the American Society of Nephrology, 33*(9), 1779–1789. https://doi.org/10.1681/ASN.2022020147.

17. Jennings, D. L., & Taber, D. J. (2008). Use of renin-angiotensin-aldosterone system inhibitors within the first eight to twelve weeks after renal transplantation. *Annals of Pharmacotherapy, 42*(1), 116–120.

18. Kasiske, B. L., Anjum, S., Shah, R., Skogen, J., Kandaswamy, C., Danielson, B., et al. (2004). Hypertension after kidney transplantation. *American Journal of Kidney Diseases, 43*(6), 1071–1081.

19. KDIGO 2021 Clinical Practice Guideline for the Management of Blood Pressure in Chronic Kidney Disease. (2021). *Kidney International, 99*(3), S1–S87. https://doi.org/10.1016/j.kint.2020.11.003.

20. Klahr, S., Levey, A. S., Beck, G. J., et al. (1994). The effects of dietary protein restriction and blood-pressure control on the progression of chronic renal disease. Modification of Diet in Renal Disease Study Group. *New England Journal of Medicine, 330*(13), 877–884. https://doi.org/10.1056/NEJM199403313301301.

21. Knoll, G. A., Fergusson, D., Chassé, M., Hébert, P., Wells, G., Tibbles, L. A., et al. (2016). Ramipril versus placebo in kidney transplant patients with proteinuria: A multicenter, double-blind, randomized controlled trial. *Lancet Diabetes & Endocrinology, 4*(4), 318–326.

22. Kotchen, T. A. (2011). Historical trends and milestones in hypertension research: A model of the process of translational research. *Hypertension, 58*(4), 522–538. https://doi.org/10.1161/HYPERTENSIONAHA.111.177766.

23. Ku, E., Hsu, R. K., Tuot, D. S., et al. (2019). Magnitude of the difference between clinic and ambulatory blood pressures and risk of adverse outcomes in patients with chronic kidney disease. *Journal of the American Heart Association, 8*(9), e011013. https://doi.org/10.1161/JAHA.118.011013.

24. Ku, E., Lee, B. J., Wei, J., et al. (2019). Hypertension in CKD: Core curriculum 2019. *American Journal of Kidney Diseases, 74*(1), 120–131. https://doi.org/10.1053/j.ajkd.2018.12.044.

25. Lambers Heerspink, H. J., Holtkamp, F. A., Parving, H. H., et al. (2012). Moderation of dietary sodium potentiates the renal and cardiovascular protective effects of angiotensin receptor blockers. *Kidney International, 82*(3), 330–337. https://doi.org/10.1038/ki.2012.74.

26. Lewis, C. E., Fine, L. J., Beddhu, S., et al. (2021). Final report of a trial of intensive versus standard blood-pressure control. *New England Journal of Medicine, 384*(20), 1921–1930.

27. Li, Z., Lacson, E., Jr., Lowrie, E. G., Ofsthun, N. J., Kuhlmann, M. K., Lazarus, J. M., et al. (2006). The epidemiology of systolic blood pressure and death risk in hemodialysis patients. *American Journal of Kidney Diseases, 48*(4), 606–615.

28. Mayer, C. C., Matschkal, J., Sarafidis, P. A., Hagmair, S., Lorenz, G., Angermann, S., et al. (2018). Association of ambulatory blood pressure with all-cause and cardiovascular mortality in hemodialysis patients: Effects of heart failure and atrial fibrillation. *Journal of the American Society of Nephrology, 29*(10), 2409–2417.

29. McMahon, E. J., Campbell, K. L., Bauer, J. D., et al. (2021). Altered dietary salt intake for people with chronic kidney disease. *Cochrane Database of Systematic Reviews, 6*, CD010070.

30. Minutolo, R., Gabbai, F. B., Agarwal, R., Chiodini, P., Borrelli, S., Bellizzi, V., et al. (2014). Assessment of achieved clinic and ambulatory blood pressure recordings and outcomes during treatment in hypertensive patients with CKD: A multicenter prospective cohort study. *American Journal of Kidney Diseases, 64*(5), 744–752.

31. Neal, B., Wu, Y., Feng, X., et al. (2021). Effect of salt substitution on cardiovascular events and death. *New England Journal of Medicine, 385*(12), 1067–1077. https://doi.org/10.1056/NEJMoa2105675.

32. Parati, G., Stergiou, G., O'Brien, E., et al. (2014). European Society of Hypertension practice guidelines for ambulatory blood pressure monitoring. *Journal of Hypertension, 32*(7), 1359–1366. https://doi.org/10.1097/HJH.0000000000000221.

33. Picard, K., Barreto Silva, M. I., Mager, D., et al. (2020). Dietary potassium intake and risk of chronic kidney disease progression in predialysis patients with chronic kidney disease: A systematic review. *Advances in Nutrition, 11*(5), 1002–1015. https://doi.org/10.1093/advances/nmaa027.

34. Rahman, M., Wang, X., Bundy, J. D., et al. (2020). Prognostic significance of ambulatory BP monitoring in CKD: A report from the Chronic Renal Insufficiency Cohort (CRIC) study. *Journal of the American Society of Nephrology, 31*(11), 2609–2621. https://doi.org/10.1681/ASN.2020030236.

35. Ruggenenti, P., Perna, A., Loriga, G., et al. (2005). Blood-pressure control for renoprotection in patients with non-diabetic chronic renal disease (REIN-2): Multicenter, randomized controlled trial. *Lancet, 365*(9463), 939–946. https://doi.org/10.1016/S0140-6736(05)71082-5.

36. Santschi, V., Chiolero, A., Burnand, B., Colosimo, A. L., & Paradis, G. (2011). Impact of pharmacist care in the management of cardiovascular disease risk factors: A systematic review and meta-analysis of randomized trials. *Archives of Internal Medicine, 171*(16), 1441–1453.

37. Slagman, M. C., Waanders, F., Hemmelder, M. H., Woittiez, A. J., Janssen, W. M., Lambers Heerspink, H. J., et al. (2011). Moderate dietary sodium restriction added to angiotensin-

converting enzyme inhibition compared with dual blockade in lowering proteinuria and blood pressure: Randomized controlled trial. *BMJ, 343*, d4366.

38. Thompson, S., James, M., Wiebe, N., et al. (2015). Cause of death in patients with reduced kidney function. *Journal of the American Society of Nephrology, 26*(10), 2504–2511. https://doi.org/10.1681/ASN.2014070714.

39. Townsend, R. R., Wimmer, N. J., Chirinos, J. A., Parsa, A., Weir, M., Perumal, K., et al. (2010). Aortic PWV in chronic kidney disease: A CRIC ancillary study. *American Journal of Hypertension, 23*(3), 282–289.

40. Whelton, P. K., Carey, R. M., Aronow, W. S., et al. (2018). 2017 ACC/AHA/AAPA/ABC/ACPM/AGS/APhA/ASH/ASPC/NMA/PCNA guideline for the prevention, detection, evaluation, and management of high blood pressure in adults: A report of the American College of Cardiology/American Heart Association Task Force on Clinical Practice Guidelines. *Journal of the American College of Cardiology, 71*(19), e127–e248. https://doi.org/10.1016/j.jacc.2017.11.006.

41. Williams, B., Mancia, G., Spiering, W., et al. (2018). 2018 ESC/ESH guidelines for the management of arterial hypertension. *European Heart Journal, 39*(33), 3021–3104. https://doi.org/10.1093/eurheartj/ehy339.

42. Wright, J. T., Jr., Bakris, G., Greene, T., et al. (2002). Effect of blood pressure lowering and antihypertensive drug class on progression of hypertensive kidney disease: Results from the AASK trial. *JAMA, 288*(19), 2421–2431. https://doi.org/10.1001/jama.288.19.2421.

43. Wright, J. T., Williamson, J. D., Whelton, P. K., et al. (2015). A randomized trial of intensive versus standard blood-pressure control. *New England Journal of Medicine, 373*(22), 2103–2116.

44. Zhang, W. R., Craven, T. E., Malhotra, R., Cheung, A. K., Chonchol, M., Drawz, P., et al. (2018). Kidney damage biomarkers and incident chronic kidney disease during blood pressure reduction: A case-control study. *Annals of Internal Medicine, 169*(9), 610–618.

Chapter

DIABETES AND HYPERTENSION IN PEOPLE WITH SLEEP APNEA

3

Contents

INTRODUCTION

Breathing ceases while you sleep due to a condition called sleep apnea. The Greek word for "breathless" is where the word "apnea" originates. Breathing ceases while you sleep, which results in sleep apnea. Either your airway becomes blocked (obstructive sleep apnea) or your brain miscontrols the breathing (central apnea) and this results. The subsequent shortage of oxygen triggers a survival response that arouses you just enough to allow you to start breathing again. That reflex keeps you alive, but it throws off your sleep schedule. This keeps you from getting a good night's sleep and may have other negative effects, such as stressing your heart, which may be fatal. Problems focusing, making decisions, recalling details, or managing your conduct can result from this. Severe health issues are also associated with sleep apnea. Breathing repeatedly stops and starts while you sleep, a common symptom of sleep apnea. This may make it so that your body doesn't get enough oxygen. If someone tells you that you gasp or snore while you sleep, or if you suffer other symptoms of poor quality sleep, like excessive daytime sleepiness, you might want to discuss sleep apnea with your healthcare provider (Sankri-Tarbichi, 2012).

There are two types of sleep apnea.

- Obstructive sleep apnea happens when your upper airway becomes blocked many times while you sleep, reducing or completely stopping airflow. This is the most common type of sleep apnea. Anything that could narrow your airway such as obesity, large tonsils, or changes in your hormone levels can increase your risk for obstructive sleep apnea.
- Central sleep apnea happens when your brain does not send the signals needed to breathe. Health conditions that affect how your brain controls your airway and chest muscles can cause central sleep apnea.

A sleep study may be recommended by your physician to diagnose sleep apnea. Common treatments for sleep apnea include breathing devices like continuous positive air pressure (CPAP) machines and lifestyle modifications. Surgery might be suggested to address the underlying cause of your sleep apnea if these therapies prove ineffective.

Orientation and Directional Terms:

Term	Definition	Illustration
Hypoxaemia	Hypoxemia is low levels of oxygen in your blood. It causes symptoms like headache, difficulty breathing, rapid heart rate and bluish skin.	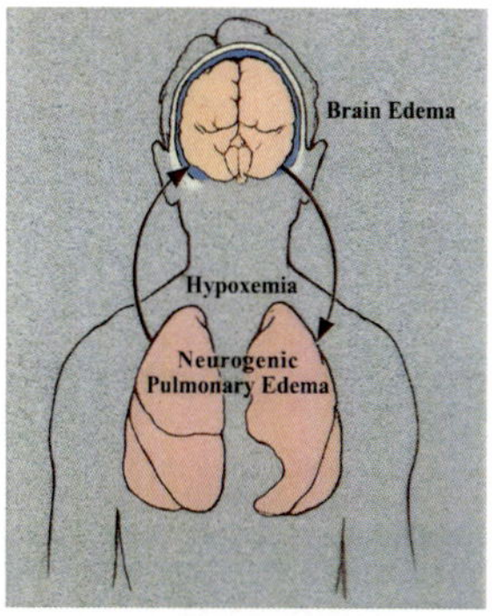
Hypercapnia	Hypercapnia is a buildup of carbon dioxide in your bloodstream. It affects people who have chronic obstructive pulmonary disease (COPD).	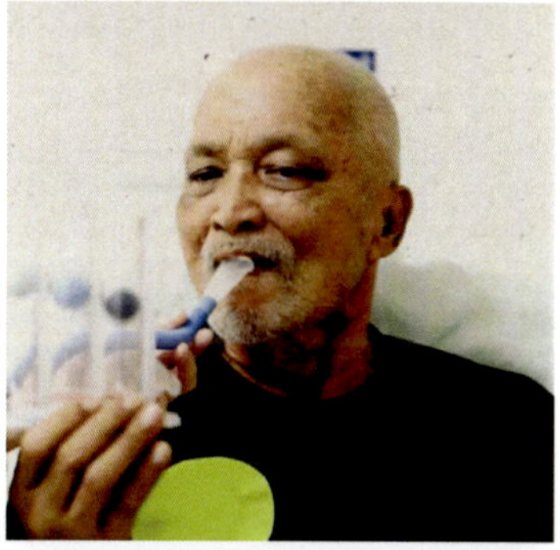
Hypertension	Hypertension, also known as high blood pressure, is a long-term medical condition in which the blood pressure in the arteries is persistently elevated.	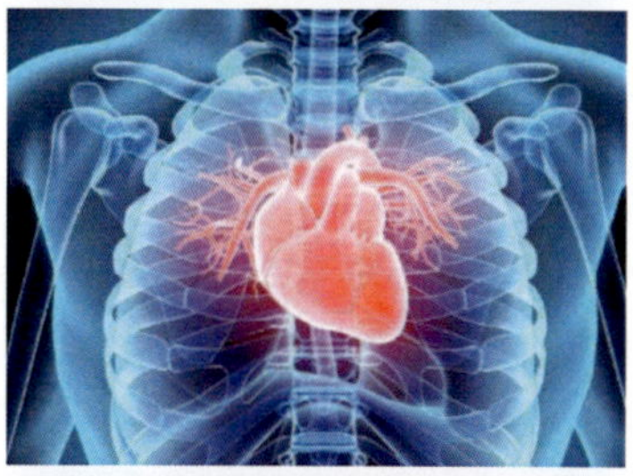
Cardiovascular disease	Cardiovascular disease is the broad term for problems with the heart and blood vessels. These problems are often due to atherosclerosis.	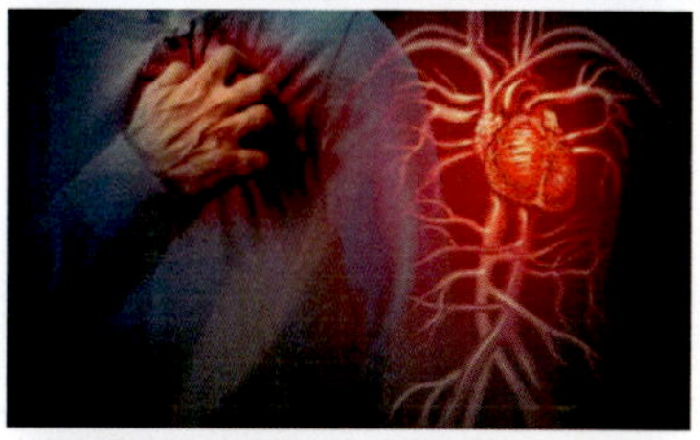
Obstructive sleep apnea	Obstructive sleep apnea occurs when the muscles that support the soft tissues in your throat, such as your tongue and soft palate, temporarily relax. When these muscles relax, your airway is narrowed or closed, and breathing is momentarily cut off.	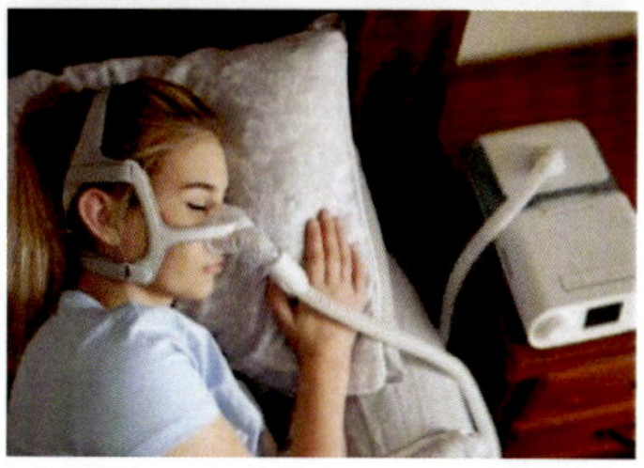

3.1. SLEEP APNEA

A sleep-related breathing disorder called sleep apnea is characterized by frequent pauses in breathing, shallow breathing spells, or upper airway collapses that impair breathing and disturb sleep. Breathing pauses occur frequently throughout the night and can range in duration from a few seconds to several minutes. As breathing starts again, there might be a snort or choking sound. Even with enough sleep, common symptoms include snoring, excessive daytime sleepiness, and non-restorative sleep. People with the disorder may feel sleepy or exhausted during the day because it interferes with their regular sleep patterns. It frequently has a chronic nature. Sleep apnea can be divided into two types: central sleep apnea (CSA), where regular unconscious breathing simply stops, and obstructive sleep apnea (OSA), where breathing is disrupted by a blockage of air flow.

The most prevalent type is OSA. A narrow, congested, or collapsible upper airway, ineffective pharyngeal dilator muscle function during sleep, airway narrowing during sleep, and unstable breathing control (high loop gain) are the four main causes of OSA. When someone has CSA, their basic neurological controls for breathing rate malfunction and don't send the signal to inhale, which results in them missing one or more breathing cycles. Breathing stops for an extended period of time that can cause hypoxaemia, or low blood oxygen percentage, and hypercapnia, or elevated blood carbon dioxide concentration. Consequently, the body will experience further effects like Cheyne-Stokes respiration as a result of these hypoxic and hypercapnic conditions.

It is possible for some sufferers of sleep apnea to be ignorant of their illness. A family member usually notices it for the first time. The recommended procedure for diagnosing sleep apnea is an overnight in-lab sleep study. The apnea-hypopnea index (AHI) is the result of OSA that influences the treatment plan and establishes the severity of the disease. By adding up all breathing pauses and shallow breathing episodes longer than ten seconds and dividing the result by the total number of hours of sleep that have been recorded, this measurement is computed. On the other hand, esophageal pressure or displacement of the thoracic or abdominal cavity serves as an important indicator of the respiratory effort required for CSA, which sets it apart from OSA. Sleep apnea is a systemic disorder that has long been linked to a variety of health problems, such as elevated blood pressure, heart disease, stroke, myocardial infarction, atrial fibrillation, insulin resistance, cancer incidence, and neurodegeneration. More investigation is being done into the possibility of utilizing biomarkers to identify the specific chronic conditions that are linked to sleep apnea (Mehrtash et al., 2019).

Treatment options include surgery, breathing apparatuses, mouthpieces, and lifestyle modifications. A few effective lifestyle adjustments include giving up alcohol, cutting back on calories, quitting smoking, and switching to a side sleep position.

Using a CPAP machine is one type of breathing device. When used correctly, CPAP enhances results. Research indicates that CPAP may enhance blood pressure, insulin sensitivity, and sleepiness. However, long-term compliance is a problem because over half of users do not use the device appropriately. In developed countries, only 15% of prospective patients used CPAP machines in 2017, whereas less than 1% of potential patients in developing countries used CPAP. In the absence of treatment, sleep apnea raises the risk of heart attacks, strokes, diabetes, heart failure, arrhythmias, obesity, and car accidents. One common sleep ailment is OSA. According to a comprehensive analysis of the estimated prevalence of OSA in 2019, up to 30% of the elderly and 936 million—1 billion people worldwide between the ages of 30-69—are affected by the condition. This represents approximately one in ten people worldwide. Men are slightly more likely than women to have sleep apnea (about a 2:1 ratio), and obesity and advanced age are generally associated with a higher prevalence of the condition. Allergies, enlarged tonsils, being overweight, and a family history of the illness are additional risk factors.

3.1.1. Signs and Symptoms

Patients are often questioned about common symptoms like snoring, breathing pauses during sleep, and excessive daytime sleepiness as part of the screening process for sleep apnea. Patients with sleep apnea can present with a wide range of symptoms, from being asymptomatic to nodding off while operating a motor vehicle. Owing to the wide variation in how sleep apnea presents clinically, some people are unaware that they have the condition and are either misdiagnosed or choose to ignore their symptoms completely. Finding distinct sleep apnea subtypes based on patients who frequently present with various clusters or groupings of specific symptoms is a current area that needs more research. Due to frequent arousals during sleep, OSA may increase the risk of work-related and driving accidents by fragmenting sleep. People with untreated OSA are more likely to experience oxidative stress due to frequent decreases in oxygen saturation and excessive daytime sleepiness. They also run the risk of developing diabetes, hypertension, and cardiovascular disease. Treatment-resistant hypertension and cardiac arrhythmias are examples of subtle sleep apnea manifestations. As the condition worsens over time, more overt symptoms may also surface. There may be behavioral effects as a result of the disruption of the daytime cognitive state. These may manifest as aggression, irritability, and a decline in energy and attentiveness. Depression may result from these impacts getting out of control (Yeghiazarians et al., 2021).

3.1.2. Risk factors

Obstructive sleep apnea can affect people regardless of sex, race, or age. However, risk factors include:

- Male gender;
- Obesity;
- Age over 40;
- Large neck circumference;
- Enlarged tonsils or tongue;
- Narrow upper jaw;
- Small lower jaw;
- Tongue fat/tongue scalloping;
- A family history of sleep apnea;
- Endocrine disorders such as hypothyroidism;
- Lifestyle habits such as smoking or drinking alcohol.

Central sleep apnea is more often associated with any of the following risk factors:

- Transition period from wakefulness to non-REM sleep;
- Male gender;
- Older age;
- Heart failure;
- Atrial fibrillation;
- Stroke;
- Spinal cord injury.

3.1.3. Mechanism

3.1.3.1. Obstructive Sleep Apnea

Narrow pharyngeal anatomy and craniofacial structure are common risk factors for obstructive sleep apnea, though the exact causes are varied and complex. The severity of OSA rapidly increases as more factors are present when anatomical risk factors are combined with non-anatomical contributors like weak pharyngeal dilator muscle function during sleep, unstable breathing control (high loop gain), and premature awakening to mild airway narrowing. Carbon dioxide accumulates in the bloodstream when breathing is stopped because of upper airway obstruction. The elevated carbon dioxide levels are detected by chemoreceptors in the blood. The brain sends a signal to wake the person up, opening the airway and enabling breathing to return. The person will return to sleep when their oxygen levels are restored through regular breathing. This build-up of carbon dioxide could be brought on by a decrease in the brainstem's output controlling the muscles of the chest wall or pharynx. Sleep apnea sufferers spend less time in REM sleep and have less or no slow-wave sleep (Dominguez et al., 2022).

3.1.3.2. Central Sleep Apnea

The disease process of CSA is primarily driven by two mechanisms: post-hyperventilation hypocapnia and sleep-related hypoventilation. Heart failure-related post-hyperventilation hypocapnia is the most frequent cause of CSA. This happens when the ventilatory control system briefly malfunctions but the alveolar ventilation remains normal. On the other hand, hypoventilation linked to sleep happens when the brain's urge to breathe is disrupted. A wide range of illnesses, from severe kyphoscoliosis to strokes, are the root cause of the loss of the wakefulness drive to breathe.

3.1.4. Complications

Patients with untreated OSA have a higher mortality risk from cardiovascular disease than those receiving the proper treatment. OSA is a serious medical condition with systemic effects. Hypertension, atrial fibrillation, congestive heart failure, coronary artery disease, stroke, and type 2 diabetes are additional complications. The prevalence of daytime tiredness and drowsiness as a symptom of sleep apnea raises serious public health concerns about drowsiness-related transportation crashes. Another possible risk factor for COVID-19 is OSA. A higher chance of experiencing serious COVID-19 complications exists in individuals with OSA. White matter damage and elevated beta-amyloid protein levels are associated with Alzheimer's disease and severe obstructive sleep apnea. These are the primary symptoms of Alzheimer's disease, which in this instance is caused by neurodegeneration brought on by insufficient sleep or ineffective sleep. In addition to increasing the risk of Alzheimer's later in life, sleep apnea increases the likelihood of Alzheimer's in those who have it in their middle years. Examples of sleep apnea even being misdiagnosed as dementia serve as evidence for this. There is a reversible risk factor in terms of the amyloid proteins with treatment using CPAP. This typically lessens cognitive impairment and restores brain structure.

When sleep apnea is treated effectively, major complications can usually be avoided or resolved. However, if the condition is not treated, it can have a significant negative impact on overall health and wellbeing. Sleep apnea lowers the quality of sleep, and because it alters oxygen levels in the body, the consequences of inadequate sleep are exacerbated. As a result, there is a correlation between obstructive sleep apnea and an increased risk of various health issues, such as:

- Car accidents from drowsy driving
- Cardiovascular diseases like high blood pressure, stroke, heart failure, heart disease, and an abnormal heartbeat
- Metabolic disorders including type 2 diabetes
- Pulmonary hypertension, which is high blood pressure in the arteries

of the lungs that places excess strain on the heart

- Thinking problems such as impaired memory and concentration
- Mood disturbances including irritability and a higher risk of depression
- Nonalcoholic fatty liver disease, which is an increase in fat deposits in the liver that can contribute to serious liver damage
- Anesthesia-related complications during surgery

In central sleep apnea, the complications that can occur depend largely on the underlying medical issue causing breathing to be disordered.

3.1.5. Diagnosis and Tests

To diagnose sleep apnea, a medical professional will typically inquire about your medical history and symptoms. Based on your responses and symptoms, if they think you may have sleep apnea, they will probably want you to get tested.

The most common tests for sleep apnea include:

- **Overnight Sleep Study (Polysomnogram)**: This is an overnight test where you sleep in a medical facility that is specifically designed to monitor your sleep while keeping you as comfortable as possible. The facility is commonly referred to as a "sleep lab." Sensors that track your blood oxygen levels, respiration, heart rate, brain waves, and other parameters are used in this test. This test is regarded by experts as the gold standard for identifying sleep apnea.
- **Home Sleep Apnea Testing**: A sleep study can be finished at home with this type of testing. Though brain wave monitoring is not used, it is comparable to an overnight sleep study. This test cannot identify central sleep apnea, and it is typically not recommended if you have other sleep disorders or medical conditions, or if your doctor suspects more severe cases of sleep apnea. In many cases, experts advise doing an overnight sleep study to confirm the results of a home study if sleep apnea is not detected (Sankri-Tarbichi et al., 2009).

3.1.6. Who Does Sleep Apnea Affect?

Sleep apnea can happen to anyone, ranging from infants and children to older adults. Obstructive sleep apnea is more common in certain circumstances and groups of people:

- Male-assigned birth individuals and men are more likely to experience it before the age of 50 (AMAB). Following the age of fifty, the rate of impact is the same for both women and individuals assigned female at birth (AFAB).
- People are more likely to develop it as they get older.
- Having excess weight or obesity strongly increases the risk of developing it.
- It is more common in people who are Black, Hispanic or of Asian descent.

Central sleep apnea is most common in certain groups of people:

- People who take opioid pain medications.
- Adults over 60 years old.

- People with heart conditions such as atrial fibrillation or congestive heart failure.
- Treatment-emergent central sleep apnea is a condition that can develop in certain individuals with obstructive sleep apnea or CPAP users as a result of this.
- When people live at high altitudes, this can cause central apneas to occur.

3.1.7. How Does Sleep Apnea Affect My Body?

To understand how sleep apnea works, it helps to know a little bit about the human sleep cycle. Sleep happens in multiple stages:

- **Stage 1**: Light sleep. This is a short stage that begins right after you fall asleep. It accounts for about 5% of your total sleep time.
- **Stage 2**: Deeper sleep. This stage is deeper and makes up about 45% to 50% of all the time you spend sleeping (this number goes up as you get older).
- **Stage 3**: Sleeping in waves. You spend roughly 25% of your sleep time in this, the deepest sleep stage (though this percentage decreases with age). A person in stage 3 sleep is extremely difficult to wake up from, and waking up straight out of it typically results in "sleep inertia," a condition characterized by "mental fog" and slowed thought. Sleepwalking and sleeptalking are examples of parasomnias that occur during this phase.
- **REM Sleep**: REM stands for "rapid eye movement." This stage is when you dream. When a person is in REM sleep, you can see their eyes moving beneath their eyelids.

Usually, when you go to sleep, you start in Stage 1 and then cycle through Stages 2 and 3. Following a cycle through those phases, you will eventually enter REM sleep and begin to dream. You enter Stage 1 or 2 again and begin a new cycle after the first REM cycle. Typically, a cycle lasts between 90 and 110 minutes before starting again. If they get eight hours of sleep, most people go through four or five cycles every night.

3.1.8. How Sleep Apnea Disrupts the Sleep Cycle

Your brain constantly monitors your body's status and adjusts your heart rate, blood pressure, breathing, etc. Your blood oxygen levels can drop when you stop breathing because of either apnea or hypopnea.

- **Apnea**: This is when you stop breathing while asleep or have almost no airflow. It combines the Greek roots "a," which means "not" and "pnea," which refers to breathing. Combined, it means "breathless."
- **Hypopnea**: This combines the Greek word roots "hypo" and "pnea." The root "hypo" means "low" or "under." Combining these root words means "under-breathing" or "low breathing," which means you aren't breathing enough to maintain oxygen levels in your blood.

When blood oxygen levels fall due to apnea or hypopnea, your brain responds by initiating a reflex similar to a failsafe, which helps you wake up long enough to resume breathing. Your brain attempts to automatically resume your sleep cycle as soon as you start breathing again. The frequency of these disruptions increases with the severity of your sleep apnea. The average hourly number of apnea or hypopnea events—times when a person stops breathing—is known as the apnea/hypopnea index, or AHI.

The primary determinant of sleep apnea severity is the AHI. The severity is as follows:

- **Mild Sleep Apnea**: At this level, an individual's AHI falls between 5 and 15. This indicates that they experience 5 to 15 episodes of apnea or hypopnea every hour. At this level, though, medical professionals also take symptoms into account. They could decide it is not serious enough to treat if you don't have any more symptoms.
- **Moderate Sleep Apnea**: People with moderate sleep apnea have between 15 and 29 events per hour. That means a person who sleeps eight hours stops breathing and/or wakes up between 120 and 239 times.
- **Severe Sleep Apnea**: People with severe sleep apnea wake up 30 or more times in an hour. That means they stop breathing and/or wake up 240 times or more during a full eight hours of sleep.

Obstructive events can occur at any stage of sleep and are very brief. They are more prevalent during REM, Stage 1, and Stage 2 sleep. Because of this, it is typical for people to forget apnea episodes, which implies they might not be aware of a problem until symptoms become apparent. Although they can happen at any stage of sleep, central events are more frequent in Stages 1 and 2 (Russell et al., 2014).

3.1.9. Treatments for Sleep Apnea

The goal of treatment for sleep apnea is to reduce breathing disruptions and improve sleep. The approach to treatment varies between obstructive sleep apnea and central sleep apnea.

3.1.9.1. Treatments for Obstructive Sleep Apnea

Most patients with obstructive sleep apnea receive treatment with positive airway pressure or PAP. Using pressurized air pumped from a machine via a hose and a face mask, PAP therapy maintains the airway open. A common form of PAP therapy involves the use of a continuous positive airway pressure (CPAP) device, which delivers a constant stream of air at a predetermined pressure. Variability in air pressure is provided by other PAP device types, such as auto-titrating positive airway pressure (APAP) and bi-level positive airway pressure (BiPAP). People with specific anatomical features and less severe OSA may benefit from treatment with certain types of mouthpieces that hold the jaw or tongue in a particular position. While these mouthpieces can lessen snoring and may be preferred by those who find using PAP devices uncomfortable, they frequently do not improve breathing as much as PAP therapy. Patients who have tissue obstructing their airway may benefit from surgery to remove the tissue in their throat and widen their airway. Implanting a device to stimulate a nerve that aids in breathing control is necessary for another kind of surgical treatment.

An additional component of treatment for obstructive sleep apnea involves lifestyle changes to help manage symptoms. These suggestions may include:

- Reducing BMI by losing weight;
- Getting regular exercise, which may decrease OSA symptoms even without weight loss;
- Altering sleeping position to avoid back sleeping;
- Reducing alcohol consumption.

1. Treatments for Central Sleep Apnea

The medical condition causing the irregular breathing is often the main focus of treatment for central sleep apnea. Treatment for the underlying cause may be sufficient if sleep disturbances are mild. To improve breathing while simultaneously attempting to address the underlying issue, further treatment may be suggested if the symptoms of central sleep apnea are severe or persistent. This can entail using PAP machines to encourage more consistent breathing while you sleep. Supplemental oxygen therapy and the use of drugs that quicken breathing are two more potential treatments.

3.2. SLEEP APNEA AND DIABETES

Sleep apnea has far more effects than just making you feel exhausted in the morning. Sleep apnea can affect a person's blood sugar levels throughout the day, alter how the body reacts to insulin, and increase the risk of developing complications from diabetes in later life. An estimated 6% to 17% of adults in the general population suffer from sleep apnea. However, that number is significantly higher among those who have diabetes, as over half of those who have type 2 diabetes also have obstructive sleep apnea. Studies reveal that people with type 1 diabetes also have relatively high levels of it (Morgenstern M, 2014). Sleep apnea can complicate diabetes management for those who have it. This is because there's a rise in blood carbon dioxide levels during sleep when you're breathing pauses.

This leads to:

- Insulin resistance so that the body doesn't use insulin effectively. This causes more sugar in the blood stream leading to high blood sugars.
- Chronic elevated blood pressure.
- A higher incidence of heart problems or cardiovascular disease.
- Early morning headaches.

Lack of desire to work out or prepare meals can also result from getting too little sleep or rest. This frequently results in irritability, which can harm friendships, family ties, and professional relationships. Those who are sleep deprived may also neglect to take their prescriptions, which can worsen their diabetes. Sleep apnea is most frequently found in people over 40, who smoke, and who have a BMI of over 25 (overweight) or over 30 (obesity). It may also be genetically linked.

3.2.1. Diabetes and Sleep Apnea: Awareness and Prevention

The relationship between sleep apnea and diabetes is complex and interconnected. While there is no guarantee that having one condition will lead to the other, there is a significant overlap between the two. It is important to be aware of the increased likelihood of developing diabetes if you have sleep apnea, and vice versa. Health professionals are advised to consider the possibility of both conditions when diagnosing a patient, as they often coexist and can worsen each other's symptoms and complications. Understanding the shared risk factors, such as obesity, and the impact they have on each other is crucial for effective management (Young et al., 2004). By focusing on prevention and raising awareness, individuals can take proactive steps to improve their quality of life and outcomes. Managing both conditions involves ensuring healthy sleep habits for those with diabetes, and closely monitoring risk factors for diabetes in those with sleep apnea. By addressing the interconnected nature of diabetes and sleep apnea, individuals can significantly improve their overall health and well-being.

Campaigns to raise awareness should stress how crucial it is to identify the signs of both conditions. Diabetes manifests as thirstiness, weariness, unexplained weight loss, and frequent urination. The symptoms of sleep apnea include loud snoring, episodes of stopping breathing while you sleep, sudden awakenings that cause gasping or choking, and daytime tiredness. Knowing about these symptoms can encourage people to get checked out by a doctor as soon as possible, which can result in prompt diagnosis and treatment. The main goal of preventive strategies should be to modify lifestyle choices to reduce common risk factors. It is critical to maintain a healthy weight because obesity plays a significant role in the development of both diabetes and sleep apnea. Blood sugar levels and weight can be controlled by promoting a balanced diet low in processed carbohydrates and fats and high in whole grains, lean proteins, and vegetables. In addition to helping with weight management, regular physical activity also improves insulin sensitivity and cardiovascular health. It should be common practice to screen people with diabetes for sleep apnea and vice versa. When diagnosing patients with diabetes for sleep apnea symptoms, medical professionals should be alert and should suggest sleep studies when appropriate. In a similar vein, people with sleep apnea diagnoses ought to have their diabetes symptoms closely watched. Regular screening can help detect problems early, which can improve management and prevent complications (Morgenstern et al., 2014).

Public health campaigns that encourage healthy lifestyle choices and offer resources for diabetes education and weight management can make a big difference in prevention. Particularly helpful are community initiatives that provide assistance with dieting, exercising, and giving up smoking. One way that employers can help is by developing workplace wellness initiatives that promote regular physical activity and offer guidance on managing diabetes and sleep. And last, it is critical to create a supportive environment for people with these conditions. Patients can receive practical guidance and emotional support from support groups and counseling services as they navigate the difficulties of managing chronic conditions. Teaching caregivers and family members about the relationship between diabetes and sleep apnea can also improve support at home.

3.2.2. Could You Have an Obstruction?

Obstructive sleep apnea, or OSA, is one of the various forms of sleep apnea in which there is a physical obstruction to airflow that causes breathing to be disrupted. Snoring is typical in those with OSA. According to the NIH, 12 million Americans suffer from OSA, and type 2 diabetics are more likely to have the disorder. Research indicates a correlation between poorer glucose control and an increase in OSA severity. You should discuss having a sleep study done to determine whether you have sleep apnea with your doctor if you have diabetes and any of the following symptoms:

- Daytime sleepiness.
- Depression.
- Irritability.
- Sexual dysfunction.
- Snoring.
- Feeling tired or fatigued most of the time.

A polysomnogram, a type of sleep test that records bodily functions while you sleep, can be used to diagnose sleep apnea. The test tracks blood oxygen levels, heart rate, breathing patterns, muscle activity, eye movements, and electrical brain activity. A treatment option for sleep apnea is continuous positive airway pressure, or CPAP. When you sleep, you cover your mouth and nose with this mask. The machine's air pressure pushes air through the nose. This prevents the throat from constricting while you sleep. The Food and Drug Administration recently approved the use of an implantable nerve stimulator as a treatment for sleep apnea, providing you with yet another option for managing your condition. In summary, if you have diabetes, you should find out if you have sleep apnea because managing your diabetes requires managing your sleep apnea.

3.2.3. Manage Sleep Apnea with Diabetes

Since diabetes and sleep apnea frequently worsen each other, managing both disorders at the same time calls for a diversified strategy. Precise diagnosis and customized treatment regimens are the foundation of effective management. To treat sleep apnea, Continuous Positive Airway Pressure (CPAP) therapy is usually used. This opens the airways while you sleep, enhancing your quality of sleep and lowering the frequency of apnea episodes. Regular CPAP use can dramatically raise blood oxygen levels and enhance general sleep, both of which are vital for diabetics who require restful sleep to effectively control blood sugar levels. Diabetes management needs to be strict in parallel. It is crucial to keep blood sugar levels within the desired range by following a healthy diet, exercising, and taking medication. Blood sugar levels can be stabilized with a balanced diet low in refined sugars and carbohydrates and high in fiber, lean proteins, and healthy fats. Frequent exercise helps improve glucose metabolism and sleep patterns, both of which can lessen the symptoms of sleep apnea. It is important to take medications exactly as directed, and to promptly discuss any changes in symptoms or side effects with a healthcare provider to modify the treatment plan as necessary (Senaratna et al., 2017).

Another essential element is weight control, since obesity is a common risk factor for type 2 diabetes and sleep apnea. Losing weight can improve airflow during sleep by reducing fat deposits around the upper airway, which can lessen the severity of sleep apnea. Furthermore, losing weight can improve insulin sensitivity, which facilitates easier blood sugar regulation. It can be helpful to follow a comprehensive weight loss plan that incorporates dietary adjustments, increased physical activity, and behavioral changes. It is also crucial to keep an eye on and take care of other related health issues. Both conditions share hypertension, which must be managed with medication and lifestyle modifications to lower the risk of cardiovascular disease. Frequent check-ups and monitoring of blood pressure and cholesterol levels can help reduce these risks. Making changes to one's lifestyle is essential to managing both conditions. Improving sleep quality can be achieved by establishing a regular sleep schedule and making a sleep-friendly environment. It is advisable to stay away from sedatives and alcohol as they can exacerbate sleep apnea. Stress reduction methods like yoga, meditation, and mindfulness can lower stress levels, which is good for blood sugar regulation and sleep quality.

Education and assistance for patients are crucial. Patients can more successfully follow treatment regimens if they are aware of how diabetes and sleep apnea interact. To help deal with the day-to-day difficulties of managing these chronic conditions, support groups and counseling can offer extra encouragement. It is critical to work closely with medical providers. Maintaining good management of both sleep apnea and diabetes requires routine follow-ups with both an endocrinologist and a sleep specialist. On the basis of continuing evaluations and patient input, treatment plans should be modified. To effectively manage sleep apnea, it is a good idea to start with the same strategies used to effectively manage diabetes: maintaining blood sugar levels within range, eating healthily, exercising frequently, and taking prescription drugs as directed. Still, more can be done in this regard.

- Begin with addressing any sinus or allergy issues that interfere with breathing clearly. This might include taking medication to keep the sinuses open and uncongested.
- In addition to treating sleep apnea, treating obesity or being overweight is another issue. Losing weight relieves pressure on the chest and lowers the risk of fat accumulating in the airway. The chance of having clear breathing while you sleep is reduced when you take care of these two.
- One can prescribe a continuous positive airway pressure (CPAP) machine either before or following the conclusion of an overnight sleep study. The individual sleeps with a mask on. A hose and a pressurized air delivery device are fastened to that mask. The pressurized air prevents breathing disturbances by maintaining the airway open.
- An additional option is surgery. In these surgeries, the tissue at the back of the mouth or top of the neck is either removed or reduced in size. There is a decreased chance of an obstruction of the airway during sleep after this soft tissue is removed.

3.2.4. Using Fitness Trackers for Monitoring Sleep Quality

A formal sleep study, in which the patient sleeps with sensors attached to their body and is observed throughout the night, is necessary for a medical diagnosis of sleep apnea. The prevalence of fitness trackers and smartphone apps, however, has made it easier for people to monitor and document their sleep quality. In cases where sleep apnea is suspected, this can be especially beneficial. It is vital to remember that a fitness or sleep tracker cannot replace a doctor's diagnosis of sleep apnea. However, it can be useful in identifying sleeping habits to discuss with a physician. Fitness trackers track the quality of sleep by using a combination of sensors to measure heart rate, breathing rate, and body movement (restlessness). After that, their app analyzes and reports these readings.

What the app reports varies by device, but can include things like:

- How long it took to fall asleep;
- How long the person remained asleep;
- How many times the person woke up through the night;
- How long they stayed awake before going back to sleep;
- How long the person stayed in various stages of sleep (light, deep, and REM).

A composite score that represents the overall quality of sleep (poor, fair, and good, excellent) is frequently created by combining these individual readings. Frequently, the applications also offer guidance on enhancing overall sleep quality. This can include notifications to support a regular bedtime and daily schedule for winding down, as well as tips on how to improve sleep hygiene. The most well-known fitness trackers, Fitbit, Apple Watch, Amazon Halo, and Oura Ring, can all measure sleep to some extent. They all provide information on how long a person sleeps and how well that sleep is done overall.

3.3. OBSTRUCTIVE SLEEP APNEA

The hallmarks of obstructive sleep apnea (OSA) are episodes of total or partial airway collapse, which are accompanied by a drop in oxygen saturation or an increase in arousal from sleep. Additional symptoms include excessive daytime sleepiness, heard apneas during sleep, and loud, disruptive snoring. Sleep that is fragmented and unrestorative is the result of this disruption. OSA significantly affects mental health, driving safety, quality of life, and cardiovascular health. Participants in the activity investigate the pathophysiology, evaluation, treatment options, and cause of obstructive sleep apnea. Students acquire knowledge about the most recent developments in evidence-based treatment modalities, such as oral appliances, continuous positive airway pressure therapy, and surgical interventions, as well as diagnostic techniques, such as polysomnography and home sleep apnea testing. By working together across interdisciplinary fields, medical professionals become more proficient in treating OSA patients, promoting efficient communication and teamwork between pulmonologists, otolaryngologists, sleep specialists, dentists, and other pertinent professionals. With regard to managing obstructive sleep apnea, this collaborative approach guarantees comprehensive care delivery and enhances patient outcomes (Rosen et al., 2003).

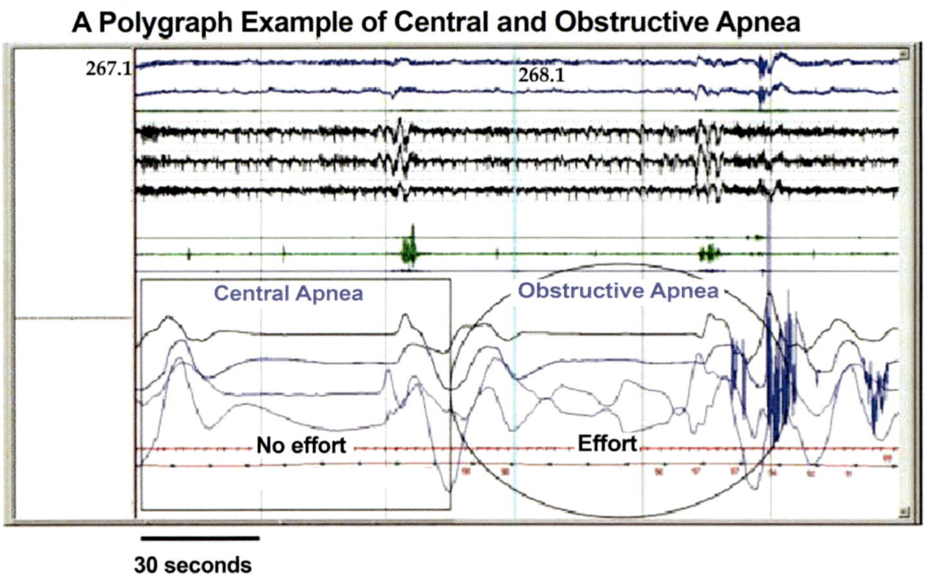

Figure 3.1. *Central and obstructive apnea, polygraph. The image depicts an example of central and obstructive apnea.*

Source: https://www.ncbi.nlm.nih.gov/books/NBK459252/bin/Polygraph_Apnea.jpg.

According to Sankri-Tarbichi AG (2012), obstructive sleep apnea (OSA) is defined as episodes of complete (apnea) or partial (hypopnea) collapse of the upper airway, accompanied by a drop in oxygen saturation or an increase in arousal from sleep. A fragmented, nonrestorative sleep is the outcome of this disturbance. Observed apneas during sleep, loud, disruptive snoring, and excessive daytime sleepiness are additional symptoms. OSA significantly affects quality of life, mental health, cardiovascular health, and driving safety (See Figure 3.1).

3.3.1. Etiology

The pathophysiology of pharyngeal narrowing and closing during sleep is a complex phenomenon with several contributing factors. Upper airway obstruction during sleep is probably largely caused by a combination of anatomic risk factors, sleep-related reduced ventilatory drive, and neuromuscular factors. Anatomical elements such as soft tissue, bone, vessels, and large neck circumference can all contribute to pharyngeal narrowing. A lot of these structures can cause the upper airway's surrounding pressure to rise, which can cause pharyngeal collapsibility and leave the upper airway's portion too small for airflow to pass through while you sleep. A recurring total or partial airway collapse occurs when the tone of the muscles that surround the upper airways diminishes (Young et al., 2003). Male sex, aging, and obesity are the three main causes of OSA in adults. When controlling for body mass index, the severity of OSA decreases with age.

- Anatomic Factors:
  - Micrognathia, retrognathia;
  - Facial elongation;
  - Mandibular hypoplasia;
  - Adenoid and tonsillar hypertrophy;
  - Inferior displacement of the hyoid.
- Nonanatomic Risk Factors:
  - Central fat distribution;
  - Obesity;
  - Advanced age;
  - Male gender;
  - Supine sleeping position;
  - Pregnancy.
- Additional Factors:
  - Alcohol use;
  - Smoking;
  - Use of sedatives and hypnotics.
- Associated Medical Disorders:
  - Endocrine disorders (e.g., diabetes mellitus, metabolic syndrome, acromegaly, and hypothyroidism);
  - Neurological disorders (e.g., stroke, spinal cord injury, and myasthenia gravis);
  - Prader Willi syndrome;
  - Down Syndrome;
  - Congestive heart failure;
  - Atrial fibrillation;
  - Obesity hypoventilation syndrome.

These relationships between OSA and various medical disorders are based mainly on observational studies and not necessarily randomized clinical trials.

3.3.2. Epidemiology

Obstructive sleep apnea is a prevalent ailment that can lead to serious negative outcomes. About 1 billion people worldwide suffer from OSA, with 425 million adults between the ages of 30 and 69 having moderate to severe OSA (15 or more events per hour), according to the definition of 5 or more events per hour. According to reports, between 25% and 30% of men and 9% to 17% of women in the US fit the criteria for obstructive sleep apnea. Asian, Black, and Hispanic populations have a higher prevalence. In addition, the disorder is more common in people 50 years of age and older, and it affects equally as many women as men. The rising rates of obesity, which range from 14% to 55%, are linked to the increasing prevalence of OSA. Obesity and the soft tissue structure of the upper airways are two risk factors that are inherited genetically (Young et al., 2003).

3.3.3. Pathophysiology

Positive collapsing pressure during inspiration is frequently the cause of upper airway obstruction during sleep; however, progressive expiratory narrowing in the retropalatal area also plays a significant part. Anatomical and neuromuscular factors may be involved in airway obstruction, as evidenced by the correlation between the degree of upper airway narrowing during sleep and body mass index. Understanding the pressure-flow relationship through collapsible tubes is useful in comprehending how OSA works.

3.3.4. History and Physical

Patients who may have OSA typically exhibit excessive daytime sleepiness, noisy snoring, and breathing cessation, gasping, or choking during sleep that is observed by a bed partner. Oversleeping during the day is among the most prevalent signs. Still, the majority of patients have no symptoms. Many patients only mention feeling tired during the day, either with or without other related symptoms. As such, it is important to evaluate the distinction between fatigue and sleepiness objectively. The degree of sleepiness can be quantitatively assessed using the Epworth Sleepiness Scale (ESS). The ESS score runs from 0 to 24, with more than 9 points denoting excessive daytime sleepiness and the need for further evaluation. The degree of fatigue symptoms can also be evaluated using the fatigue severity scale (FSS). When symptoms of fatigue and drowsiness coexist, ESS and FSS are typically beneficial. Additional symptoms can include nocturia, self-reported insomnia, and morning headaches. Women reported experiencing symptoms of both sleep-onset and sleep-maintenance insomnia more frequently.

The STOP-BANG questionnaire is one of OSA's most widely accepted screening tools.

- **Snoring:** Do you snore loudly (louder than talking or loud enough to be heard through closed doors)?
- **Tired:** Do you often feel tired, fatigued, or sleepy during the daytime?
- **Observed:** Has anyone observed you stop breathing during your sleep?
- **Pressure:** Are you having or being treated for high blood pressure?
- **BMI:** BMI greater than 35 kg/m^2
- **Age:** age greater than 50
- **Neck circumference:** Neck circumference greater than 40 cm
- **Gender:** Males

To determine whether there is a high likelihood of a moderate-to-severe disease, use STOP-BANG. If "YES" was selected for three or more items, there was a high risk; if "YES" was selected for fewer than three items, there was a low risk. The most prevalent condition in people with OSA is obesity. Large neck circumference (17 inches or 43 cm in men and 16 inches or 40.5 cm in women), crowded oropharynx (Mallampati 3 to 4), tonsilar hypertrophy, retrognathia, micrognathia, low-lying palate, overjet, and a large tongue are additional physical findings. However, after accounting for neck size and body weight, only lateral narrowing remains an independent predictor of OSA.

3.3.5. Evaluation

A sleep apnea evaluation is recommended for any adult patient exhibiting unexplained symptoms during the day or related to sleep, such as excessive sleepiness, fatigue, or unrefreshing sleep. However, aside from those who are at risk of occupational hazards like driving or piloting, universal screening for OSA is not advised in asymptomatic patients. Furthermore, patients with particular comorbidities like resistant hypertension, refractory atrial fibrillation, and a history of stroke can be screened for sleep apnea regardless of symptoms because of the high prevalence of OSA and disease burden. The gold standard test for obstructive sleep apnea diagnosis is nighttime in-laboratory level 1 polysomnography (PSG) (Dominguez and Habib, 2022). Patients are monitored using respiratory impedance plethysmography belts around the chest and abdomen to detect motion, an electrocardiogram lead, electromyogram sensors to detect muscle contraction in the chin, chest, and legs, and electroencephalogram (EEG) leads, temperature, pressure, and pulse oximetry sensors to detect nasal and oral airflow (See Figure 3.2).

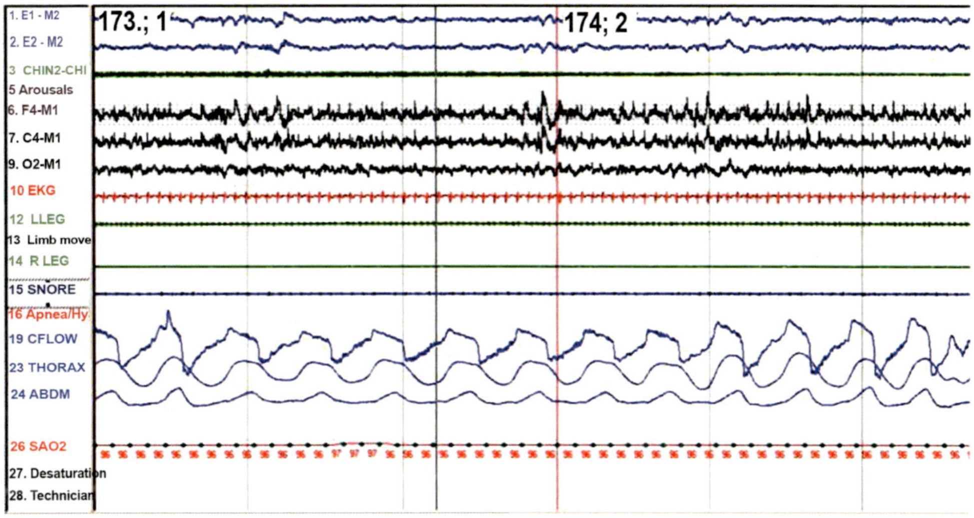

Figure 3.2. *Sleep polygraph, 30-second window. A polygraph recording during sleep; the panel shows electroencephalogram, electrooculogram, electrocardiogram, in addition to chin electromyogram signals from the lower limbs and respiratory signals, chest and abdomen respiratory plethysmography, and oxygen saturation during a 30-second window.*

Source: https://www.ncbi.nlm.nih.gov/books/NBK459252/bin/Picture1.jpg.

Scoring respiratory events in adults relies on 4 channels:

- Oronasal thermal sensor ;
- Nasal air pressure transducer ;
- Inductance plethysmography (esophageal manometry or pressure catheter may be used instead) ;
- Pulse oximetry.

*A snoring monitor is a required channel but is not used to score any respiratory events.

The American Academy of Sleep Medicine (AASM) defines hypopnea as meeting one of two criteria: either a minimum 30-percent decrease in airflow for a duration of more than 10 seconds, or a minimum 4-percent desaturation of oxygen (e.g., G. Medicare criteria) or a decrease in airflow of at least 30% for longer than ten seconds linked to a minimum of 3% oxygen desaturation, or an awakening from sleep as detected by an EEG (recommended AASM criteria) (Morgenstern et al., 2014).

Scoring apnea requires both of the following criteria to be met:

- Drop in the peak signal excursion by ≥90% of pre-event baseline flow.
- Duration of the drop in flow is ≥10 seconds.
  - Apneas are usually further classified based on effort (respiratory inductance plethysmography signals).
  - Obstructive apnea, if there is increased effort throughout the entire apnea.
  - Central apnea, if there is no effort throughout the entire apnea.

Mixed apnea occurs if there is *no effort* in the first part and there *is an effort* in the second part of the apnea. See Figure 3.3. Polygraph depicting an example of central and obstructive apnea.

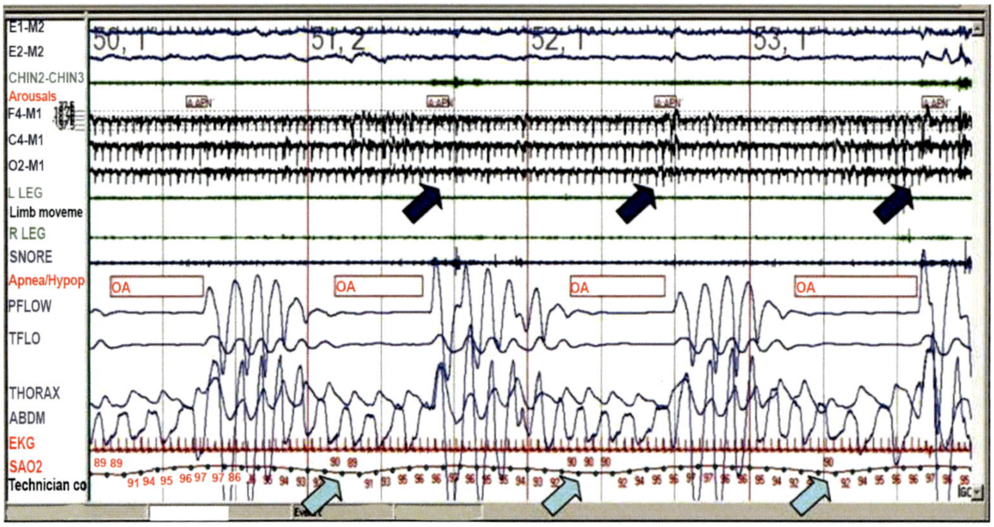

Figure 3.3. *Sleep polygraph, 120-second window. The polygraph, recorded during sleep, shows electroencephalogram, electrooculogram, electrocardiogram, in addition to chin electromyogram during a 120-second window. Note the repetitive obstructive apnea with persistent effort during cessation of both flow channels (nasal pressure flow and thermester followed by desaturation [light blue arrows] and arousals [dark blue arrows]).*

Source: https://www.ncbi.nlm.nih.gov/books/NBK459252/bin/Repetitive_OSA_polygraph.jpg.

Home sleep tests or portable monitoring (PM) have gained popularity due to their relative accessibility and lower cost. PM, however, should be used with specific rules and procedures based on the AASM unattended PM task force guidelines (Rosen et al., 2003). These guidelines outlined the following criteria:

At a minimum, the PM must record airflow, respiratory effort, and blood oxygenation.

- The airflow, effort, and oximetric biosensors conventionally used for in-laboratory PSG should be used in PM.
- PM testing must be performed under the auspices of an AASM-accredited comprehensive sleep medicine program with written policies and procedures.
- An experienced sleep technologist/technician must apply the sensors or directly educate patients on sensor application.

- The PM device must allow for the display of raw data with the capability of manual scoring or editing of automated scoring by a qualified sleep technician/technologist.
- A board-certified sleep specialist or someone who fulfills the eligibility criteria for the sleep medicine certification examination must review the raw data from PM using scoring criteria consistent with current published AASM standards. Under the specified conditions, PM may be used for unattended studies in the patient's home.
- A follow-up visit should be performed to review test results for all patients undergoing PM.
- Negative or technically inadequate PM tests should prompt in-laboratory polysomnography in patients with a high pretest probability of moderate to severe OSA (Figure 3.4).

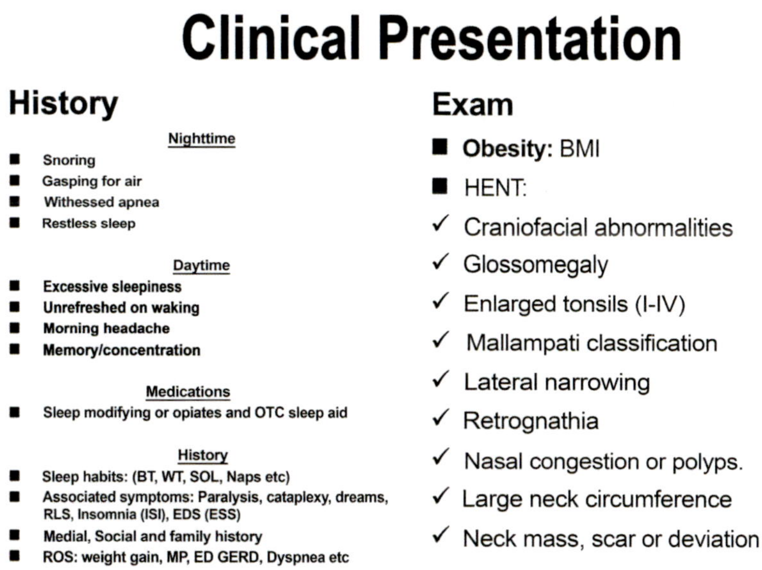

Figure 3.4. *Sleep apnea clinical assessment. The image demonstrates the clinical assessment of patients with suspected sleep apnea.*

Source: https://www.ncbi.nlm.nih.gov/books/NBK459252/bin/Screen__Shot__2022-06 18__at__11.29.17__PM.jpg.

In adults with a high pretest probability of sleep apnea and no major medical comorbidities (advanced congestive heart failure, chronic obstructive pulmonary disease, and neurologic disorders), unattended PM and home sleep tests are appropriate. These are level 3 sleep tests that include temperature, pressure, pulse oximetry, heart rate monitoring, resistance belts around the chest and abdomen to detect motion, and a sensor to determine body position in addition to sensors to detect nasal and oral airflow. Sleep apnea, both moderate and severe (Russell et al., 2014) is found on these tests; however, mild sleep apnea may remain undiagnosed and a repeat in-lab study may be required because of the possibility of underestimating the apnea-hypopnea index relative to the total recording time (which may be longer than the total sleep time measured in an in-lab study). Figure 3.5 presents a suggested algorithm for the proper application of in-lab PSG and portable monitoring. Sleep Apnea, Sleep Testing Methods.

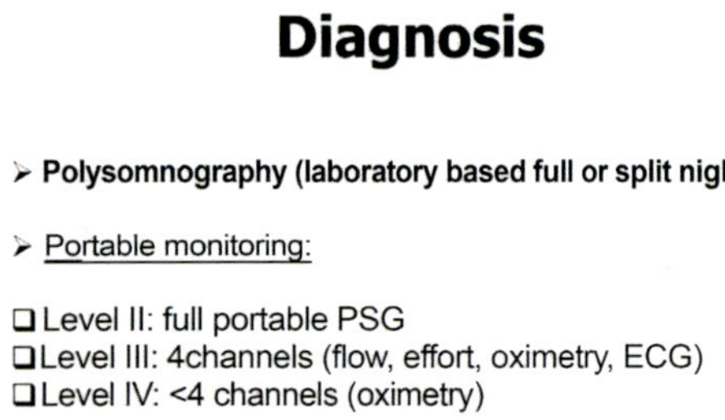

Figure 3.5. *Sleep testing modalities, sleep apnea. The available types of sleep apnea testing from level I (in-lab PSG) to portable monitoring devices (level II, III and IV). Note that only level II and III are acceptable for obstructive sleep apnea testing by the American academy of sleep medicine guidelines.*

Source: https://www.ncbi.nlm.nih.gov/books/NBK459252/bin/Screen__Shot__2022-06-19__at__7.23.21__AM.jpg.

Adults without major medical comorbidities (advanced congestive heart failure, chronic obstructive pulmonary disease, and neurologic disorders) who have a high pretest probability of sleep apnea should do unattended PM and home sleep tests. Level 3 sleep tests with temperature, pressure, pulse oximetry, heart rate monitoring, resistance belts around the chest and abdomen to sense motion, and a body position sensor in addition to sensors for oral and nasal airflow and motion detection. A sleep apnea that is moderate to severe (Russell MB, et al., 2014) is shown on these tests, but mild sleep apnea may go undiagnosed and a repeat in-lab study may be required because of the possibility of underestimating the apnea-hypopnea index in relation to the total recording time (which may be longer than the total sleep time measured in an in-lab study). In Figure 3.5, an algorithm is proposed for the proper application of in-lab PSG and portable monitoring. Modes of Sleep Testing and Sleep Apnea.

The severity of OSA in adults is based on AHI, REI, or pAHI as follows:

- Mild: 5 to 15 events per hour
- Moderate: greater than 15 to 30 events per hour
- Severe: greater than 30 events per hour

The disease burden in mild OSA is controversial and based on associated clinical sequelae (such as excessive daytime sleepiness, sleep maintenance insomnia, and cognitive dysfunction). Recent studies challenged the traditional definition and scoring criteria of OSA in adults due to its limitations in capturing the pathophysiological impact in individual patients. Different metrics have been proposed to increase precision in diagnosing individuals with OSA. These metrics include hypoxic burden, nocturnal heart rate changes, total sleep time with SpO_2 <90% (TST90), duration of obstructive events, sleep arousal burden, and even genetics.

3.3.6. Treatment / Management

The multifaceted approach to treating OSA should be tailored to the specific needs of each patient. The effects of therapy for mild OSA on neurocognition, mood, car accidents, cardiovascular events, stroke, and arrhythmias are poorly or inconsistently supported, although treatment for moderate to severe OSA has been demonstrated to improve clinical outcomes.

3.3.6.1. Lifestyle Changes and Treating Underlying Medical Conditions

Patients with OSA who are overweight or obese should be reminded of the significance of losing weight. While it is generally not curative, losing weight is advised and can frequently lessen the severity of obstructive sleep apnea. Patients should prioritize getting at least 7 to 8 hours of sleep every night and be informed about the effects that sleep duration has on their health. Alcohol, benzodiazepines, opiates, and some antidepressants should be avoided by patients as they may exacerbate their condition. Use nasal steroids for allergic rhinitis or surgery for nasal valve collapse to treat any concurrent nasal obstruction. Optimizing the management of lung or heart disease (including heart failure or asthma) is crucial for patients.

3.3.6.2. Positional Therapy

OSA that is more prominent in the supine position can be treated with a positioning device to keep a patient on their side, which can be an option.

3.3.6.3. Positive Airway Pressure Therapy

For adults, the most successful treatment is continuous positive airway pressure, or CPAP. For patients who need higher pressure settings (>15 cm H2O), bilevel PAP is also more tolerated. But even though CPAP is very effective at preventing respiratory events, its efficacy is hampered by patients not using it enough at night and by poor adherence. About half of patients with OSA do not sufficiently adhere to treatment after the first month, making CPAP adherence among these patients a significant challenge (Mehrtash et al., 2019). A recent statement regarding the best monitoring techniques and outcome measures for adults, as well as CPAP adherence tracking systems, was released by the American Thoracic Society. It is important to standardize the CPAP adherence report to include residual apnea and hypopnea index, mask leakage, and the number of hours used above 4 hours per night (>70% of nights). What is the ideal CPAP adherence rate, though, given that CPAP adherence rates have been demonstrated to rise with the use of telemedicine adherence interventions, remote CPAP monitoring, and more interactive features with individual patients and their families?

Conflicting results have been reported from many studies evaluating the impact of CPAP therapy on cardiovascular outcomes in OSA patients. Acute myocardial infarction, non-fatal stroke, hospital admission for heart failure, and new hospitalizations for unstable angina or transient ischemic attack are defined as cardiovascular events. A recent randomized control trial found that using CPAP for at least a year in patients with acute coronary syndrome (ACS) and OSA without excessive daytime sleepiness did not reduce the incidence of cardiovascular events. This study had two major limitations: the adherence to CPAP therapy was low (2.78 hours/night), and the follow-up period was insufficient. In a different long-term follow-up observational cohort study, patients with severe OSA who used CPAP around years 6 or 7 of follow-up had a lower all-cause mortality rate. In a more recent study, CPAP therapy was more beneficial for patients with coronary artery disease and OSA who did not experience excessive sleepiness and who showed larger changes in heart rate.

3.3.6.4. Oral Appliance

For patients who cannot or do not wish to use CPAP, or who have unreliable access to electricity, custom-fitted oral appliances or mandibular advancement devices (MAD) can be used to bring the lower jaw forward and alleviate airway obstruction. This approach is most effective for individuals with suitable dentition and mild to moderate sleep apnea. In a study involving 126 patients with moderate to severe OSA, it was found that after one month of therapy, the 24-hour mean arterial pressure was similar between CPAP and MAD. However,

MAD was shown to be more effective than CPAP in improving quality of life measures. A more recent study also demonstrated long-term improvement in self-reported neurobehavioral outcomes with both CPAP and MAD over a 10-year follow-up period. The American Academy of Sleep Medicine (AASM) and the American Academy of Dental Sleep Medicine (AADSM) have developed guidelines for the use of MAD in patients with OSA.

The AASM/AADSM guidelines recommend the following:

- Oral appliances can be considered rather than no treatment for adult patients with snoring (without OSA) or those with OSA who do not tolerate CPAP therapy or prefer alternate treatment.
- When a sleep physician prescribes oral appliance therapy for an adult patient with obstructive sleep apnea.
- A qualified dentist should use a custom, titratable appliance.
- A follow-up with a qualified dentist after oral appliance therapy is initiated in adult patients with OSA to assess for dental-related side effects.
- A follow-up with sleep testing to confirm treatment efficacy is necessary.

3.3.6.5. Surgical Treatments

To increase the amount of space in the oropharynx, uvulopalatopharyngoplasty (UPPP) involves surgically removing the uvula and tissue from the soft palate. This can occasionally be combined with an adenoidectomy and tonsillectomy. However, less than 50% of patients experience a meaningful improvement in the apnea-hypopnea index after the first year, indicating that the long-term effectiveness of UPPP is quite limited. To create more room in the oropharynx, maxillomandibular advancement (MMA) necessitates the surgical advancement of the lower and upper jaws anteriorly. Patients with retrognathia respond to this the best; older patients or those with larger neck circumferences find it less effective. Drug-induced sleep endoscopy has been used more recently for preoperative planning to determine whether these patients are candidates for surgical treatment such as hypoglossal nerve stimulators and MMA and to identify multiple levels of obstruction in these patients. This enables surgeons to treat obstructions of the nose, soft palate, and hypopharynx in a single surgical procedure. The implantable hypoglossal nerve stimulator (HNS) is a more recent option. It is typically implanted unilaterally, though reports of bilateral implantation have been made recently. During apneas, this device stimulates the genioglossus, or upper airway dilator muscle, which causes the tongue to protrude and relieves the obstruction (Young et al., 2008). In patients with moderate to severe OSA who are not responding to CPAP treatment, HNS effectively lowers the AHI (median AHI score at 12 months decreased by 68%, from 29.3 events per hour to 9.0 events per hour) and improves symptoms related to sleepiness. Short- and long-term adverse events following HNS are not frequently reported. Over the course of five years, 132 patient reports yielded 134 adverse events, according to one study. Following HNS, tongue abrasion (11%), pain (6.2%), and device malfunction (3% to 6%) are the most frequently reported adverse events.

The eligibility criteria for HNS adopted from the original randomized trial include the following characteristics:

- Adults older than 18 years;
- Moderate to severe OSA (AHI between 20 to 50 with <25% central or mixed apneas);

- Inability to tolerate CPAP;
- No complete concentric collapse at the palate on drug-induced sleep endoscopy.

Exclusion criteria for HNS include the following:

- Body mass index greater than 32.0 kg/m2;
- Neuromuscular disease;
- Hypoglossal-nerve palsy;
- Severe restrictive or obstructive pulmonary disease;
- Moderate-to-severe pulmonary arterial hypertension;
- Severe valvular heart disease;
- Heart failure, New York Heart Association class III or IV;
- Recent myocardial infarction or severe cardiac arrhythmias (within the past 6 months);
- Persistent uncontrolled hypertension despite medication use;
- Active psychiatric disease and coexisting nonrespiratory sleep disorders.

A tracheostomy can be used to treat OSA in severe cases to get around the oropharyngeal blockage. The best places to address this management option are academic or specialty sleep centers that have a history of treating tracheostomy patients. These patients face many difficulties with home health care, durable medical equipment, and educating partners and family about managing a tracheostomy. Furthermore, comorbidities are common in patients with severe OSA who need tracheostomy (Senaratn et al., 2017).

3.3.7. Differential Diagnosis

Differential diagnoses for OSA include the following:

- Asthma;
- Central sleep apnea;
- Chronic obstructive pulmonary disease;
- Depression;
- Gastroesophageal reflux;
- Hypothyroidism;
- Narcolepsy;
- Periodic limb movement disorder.

3.3.8. Prognosis

With treatment, the prognosis for OSA is favorable in the short term but uncertain in the long run. The largest issue is non-adherence to CPAP; despite education, almost 50% of patients discontinue using CPAP within the first month. Comorbidities and the risk of adverse cardiac events and stroke are common among patients. As a result, people who do not use CPAP run the risk of experiencing adverse cardiac and brain events, as well as higher annual healthcare costs. In addition, pulmonary hypertension, hypercapnia, hypoxemia, and daytime drowsiness are linked to OSA, and those who have these conditions are more likely to be involved in auto accidents. Patients with OSA have a shorter life expectancy overall than people without the condition. It is well known that OSA impairs cardiac function, especially in obese people. It has recently been discovered that CPAP therapy improves the mechanics of the left and right ventricles in OSA patients.

3.3.9. Complications

Complications from OSA can include the following:

- Hypertension;

- Myocardial infarction;
- Cerebrovascular accident;
- Depression;
- Sleeplessness-related accidents.

3.3.10. Deterrence and Patient Education

Patients with OSA should be encouraged to lose weight. Alcohol, benzodiazepines, opiates, and some antidepressants should be advised against as these substances may exacerbate their condition. They should also be educated about the dangers of driving while intoxicated, the significance of maintaining good sleep hygiene, and the necessity of getting enough sleep each night. Encouragement of CPAP adherence and emphasis on the significance of routinely cleaning and maintaining the machine are important.

3.3.11. Enhancing Healthcare Team Outcomes

An interdisciplinary team comprising a sleep specialist, primary care physician, cardiologist, otolaryngologist, dietitian, pulmonologist, neurologist, and nursing staff is optimal for managing obstructive sleep apnea. There are numerous ways to treat OSA, with CPAP being the main one. Nurses and sleep assessment specialists play a crucial role in helping clinicians oversee overall therapy. Nurses should encourage the clinician to address the issue and make sure the right diagnostic algorithms are followed because they are often able to identify therapeutic failure or non-compliance (such as with CPAP machines). Patients with OSA will benefit most from the interprofessional care model, especially considering how challenging it is to manage the condition. Regrettably, there is still little CPAP compliance. An oral or nasal device might help some patients, but patient compliance is still a problem. The final option, surgery, should only be discussed following a comprehensive assessment of the patient. Surgery is costly, doesn't treat the illness, and may have serious side effects. For the majority of OSA patients, the prognosis is uncertain. Most therapies are ineffective until the patient begins to lose weight.

3.4. HYPERTENSION IN PEOPLE WITH SLEEP APNEA

In the US, obstructive sleep apnea (OSA) is very common; 1 in 4 people are thought to be at risk. A substantial amount of research has been conducted in the last few years to evaluate OSA's potential as a stand-alone risk factor for hypertension. Age and the type of elevated blood pressure are two patient characteristics that may increase the likelihood that the hypertension is secondary to underlying sleep apnea. In addition, patients with hypertension, especially those whose hypertension is poorly controlled, may benefit from early detection and treatment of OSA. This succinct review centers on current advancements in the nature and management of hypertension linked to sleep apnea. Owing to spatial constraints, a restricted number of references are offered (Perfect et al., 2012).

3.4.1. Interdependence between OSA and Hypertension

The Joint National Committee's seventh report named OSA as a significant, verifiable cause of hypertension. Up to 50% of patients with underlying hypertension may also have sleep apnea, and many patients with hypertension—especially resistant hypertension—may also have OSA. Indeed, there appears to be a relationship between the severity of OSA and the inability to respond to antihypertensive drugs. Even in patients with normotension, elevated nocturnal blood pressure and decreased blood pressure "dipping" during sleep also point to a greater chance of underlying sleep apnea. It is unclear if hypertension plays a role in OSA.

3.4.2. Systolic and Diastolic Hypertension

Individuals with OSA may not always have high systolic pressures, but they may also frequently experience isolated diastolic hypertension. According to one study, there was no significant correlation found between isolated systolic hypertension and sleep apnea in either age group, and there was a significant correlation between the incidence of combined systolic and diastolic hypertension and the presence of sleep apnea in younger patients (<60 years of age) but not in older patients. These studies imply that when examining epidemiologic interactions, pathophysiologic trends, and treatment options in sleep apnea-associated hypertension, the type of hypertension may need to be taken into account.

3.4.3. Effects of Gender

It is yet unclear how different sexes' blood pressure reactions to OSA are explained. Studies based on a population have not shown that gender has a different impact on the prevalence of hypertension linked to sleep apnea in middle-aged individuals. There is some evidence in rat models for a sex-dependent difference in response to intermittent hypoxic insults, but most studies have focused primarily on men with OSA. Compared to male or ovariectomized female rats, female rats exposed to intermittent hypoxic insults had a lower chance of experiencing hypertension. However, it has been suggested that factors such as advancing age, body mass index, a family history of hypertension, and female gender—regardless of menopause and obesity—may put patients with OSA at risk for developing hypertension. Additionally, it has been proposed that women's apnea-hypopnea index is more strongly linked to compromised conduit and resistance vessel function than it is to men's. Thus, human research on any correlation between female gender and sleep apnea-induced hypertension is still inconclusive, despite animal models suggesting a reduced hypertensive response to intermittent hypoxia in females.

3.4.4. Age

Additionally, age may influence how OSA and hypertension interact. Patients with sleep apnea under 60 years of age were more likely to show a significant correlation between minimum oxygen saturation and the onset of hypertension, according to a subgroup analysis of the Sleep Heart Health Study. This specific study also showed that there was only a significant correlation between blood pressure elevations and abnormal breathing patterns in younger patients. Compared to controls with a similar body mass, children with sleep apnea have higher diastolic blood pressure during the day and fewer nocturnal blood pressure dips. Therefore, younger OSA patients may be more vulnerable than older patients to the ensuing hypertension (Koren et al., 2015).

3.4.5. Nocturnal Nondipping Blood Pressure Patterns

A non-dipping nocturnal blood pressure profile is one feature of OSA. This is probably the consequence of increased sympathetic drive during sleep, which is brought on by four primary stimuli: hypoxemia, hypercapnia, lack of lung inflation, and microarousals at the conclusion of apneic episodes. The daytime hypertension observed in these patients may be the consequence of a combination of excessive sympathetic activation and other vasoactive factors released in response to hypoxia, such as endothelin. However, because of apnea-induced sympathetic activation, patients with sleep apnea may not experience the typical nocturnal dip in blood pressure during sleep, even in the absence of daytime hypertension. Independent of hypertension during the day, higher blood pressure at night may be a major factor in the development of cardiovascular problems. Therefore, a nocturnal non-dipping blood pressure profile may indicate elevated cardiovascular risk even in patients with normotension. To determine the prognostic significance of elevated nocturnal blood pressure in sleep apnea, more research is required.

3.4.6. Subclinical OSA and Prehypertension

Understanding the interaction between OSA and hypertension has been aided by criteria for identifying early or subclinical manifestations of each condition. Guidelines for the designation of patients as "prehypertensive" were established in the seventh Joint National Committee report. Although these patients do not currently meet the clinical criteria for hypertension, they are more likely to develop other cardiovascular diseases and established hypertension in the future. Similarly, subclinical syndromes such as upper airway resistance syndrome and snoring that are suggestive of OSA but do not meet criteria have been identified. Studies based on population data have indicated a possible interaction between hypertension and snoring, but more research is required to fully understand the relationship. Therefore, the connection between OSA and hypertension might be more complex than just OSA and could represent a wider interaction between blood pressure and disrupted sleep. Studies that have thoroughly investigated any possible causal relationship between these conditions have only recently been conducted. Independent of other variables, one of these studies showed a direct relationship, lasting four years, between the severity of sleep-disordered breathing and the occurrence of incident hypertension. It is unknown if early detection and treatment of sleep disordered breathing or OSA contributes to the long-term prevention of hypertension and other cardiovascular problems, even though treating OSA may lower blood pressure.

3.4.7. Sleep Duration and Hypertension

Frequent nocturnal arousals are the cause of decreased sleep quality in patients with sleep apnea. A sizable patient cohort from the First National Health and Nutrition Examination Survey was used to describe the effects of sleep duration on hypertension. Even after adjusting for diabetes and obesity, patients under 60 years old who slept for less than five hours a night had a significantly higher risk of developing hypertension (Lavie and Hoffstein 2001). The Sleep Heart Health Study results, which indicate that sleep duration above or below a median of 7 to 8 hours per night is associated with a higher prevalence of hypertension, lend support to these findings. Therefore, increasing the quantity and quality of sleep in individuals with sleep apnea may theoretically help lower the chance of hypertension.

3.4.8. Mechanisms Mediating OSA-Associated Hypertension

Other recent reviews have gone into great detail about the mechanisms through which patients with OSA may develop cardiovascular complications. The etiology of hypertension resulting from open-ended boats (OSA) could be complex, involving factors such as oxidative stress, endogenous vasoactive factors, endothelial dysfunction, elevated sympathetic activation, and metabolic dysregulation. Increased adrenergic tone, vascular injury, improper vasoconstriction, and increased atherosclerosis are possible examples of the underlying maladaptive physiology causing hypertension.

3.4.9. Hypertension, OSA, and Changes in Cardiac Structure and Function

An increasing amount of research indicates that sleep apnea and obesity may have long-term effects on adult and pediatric cardiac structure and function, partly through effects on blood pressure and partly through direct effects on the heart. OSA may be a separate risk factor for the emergence of left ventricular hypertrophy and atrial enlargement even after blood pressure has been taken into account. Independent of hypertension, impaired right ventricular systolic and diastolic function has also been linked to sleep apnea. Even in children with OSA, there are obvious structural alterations to the heart. Continuous positive airway pressure (CPAP) therapy has also been demonstrated to improve the effects of OSA on left ventricular systolic function and right ventricular myocardial performance index, systolic function, and free wall diameter. These findings imply that OSA may have a major effect on the structure and function of the heart, which may be somewhat reversed with CPAP therapy.

3.4.10. Management

Treating OSA and taking antihypertensive drugs as prescribed is the first line of treatment for hypertension caused by OSA. The best ways to treat OSA are with postural corrections, weight control, and continuous positive airway pressure (CPAP). When treating medically complex, difficult-to-treat OSA, tracheostomy is thought to be the last option. It is unclear which antihypertensive medication class in OSA has better blood pressure control. Treatments for sleep apnea, such as oral appliances, positional therapy, and bariatric surgery, have been proposed to improve hypertension in patients with OSA. The primary antihypertensive effect is presumably attained by relieving concurrent OSA.

3.4.11. Continuous Positive Airway Pressure

CPAP is the cornerstone of treatment for patients with sleep apnea; it is delivered through a face mask or nasal mask while the patient is asleep. When CPAP is used to treat OSA, it may lessen inflammation, endothelial dysfunction, and metabolic dysfunction—some of the mechanisms thought to be behind the development of hypertension in these patients. Research on the effects of short-term CPAP therapy on blood pressure control during the day has been inconsistent, but long-term, consistent CPAP treatment is generally thought to be beneficial in lowering blood pressure.

In hypertensive patients, CPAP can significantly lower systemic blood pressure at night. In normotensive patients, it appears to have less of an effect. However, the kind of CPAP therapy used and the extent of OSA improvement may have an impact on the antihypertensive effect. In fact, to lower blood pressure, the apnea-hypopnea index may need to be lowered by more than 50%. Moreover, a study comparing CPAP and nocturnal supplemental oxygen therapy suggests that CPAP may lower blood pressure through mechanisms other than increasing oxyhemoglobin saturation (Figure 3.6). However, there is some inconsistent data regarding the antihypertensive effect of CPAP therapy, with some studies failing to find any such effect. Many recent meta-analyses revealed that although some subgroups may respond more robustly, CPAP only has very minor effects, lowering blood pressure by about 2 mm Hg. Patients with more severe OSA and better nightly CPAP use had greater reductions in blood pressure (Figure 3.7). Therefore, more research is required to understand the function of CPAP therapy, the efficacy of various devices in treating OSA-associated hypertension, and the clinical significance of this degree of blood pressure reduction in the context of OSA (Polotsky et al., 2003).

3.4.12. Clinical Perspectives

While OSA has been linked to various cardiovascular diseases, it is most strongly associated with hypertension. Research suggests that treating sleep apnea can lower blood pressure in both the short and long term, particularly in those with more severe hypertension.

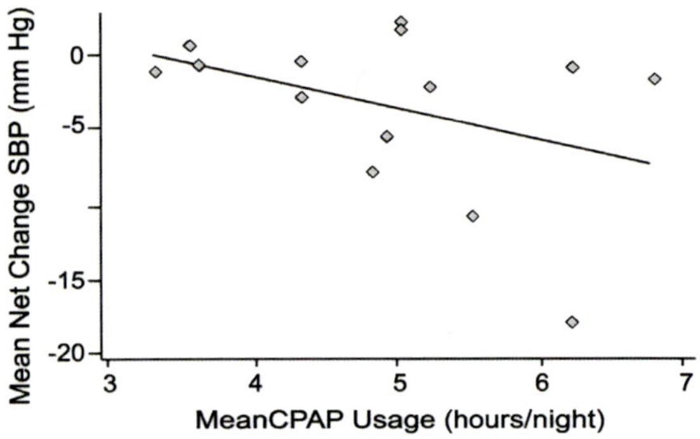

Figure 3.6. *Effect of CPAP vs supplemental oxygen on 24-hour ambulatory blood pressure. Use of CPAP was associated with a significant decrease in blood pressure compared with patients treated with placebo or supplemental oxygen. The change was measured from the mean pretreatment minus posttreatment values.*

Source: https://www.ahajournals.org/cms/asset/a640af96-fcf4-46e5-8335-91d1c6e1f299/11ff2.jpg.

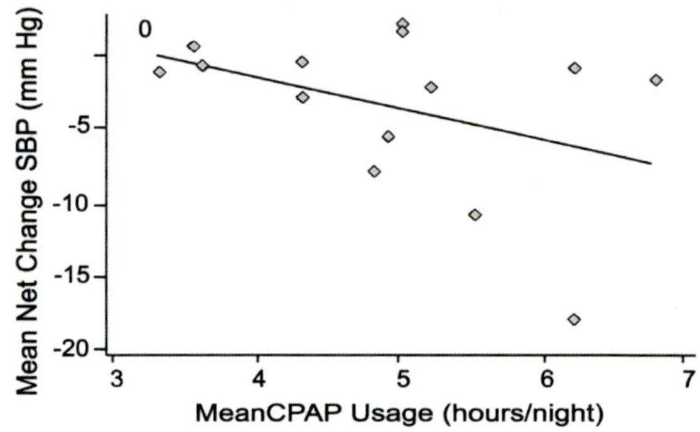

Figure 3.7. *Effect of CPAP usage on change in blood pressure. Shown is the relationship between the mean net change in systolic blood pressure (SBP) and the corresponding mean nocturnal CPAP usage based on a meta-analysis of CPAP. This suggests that longer nightly CPAP use may offer greater benefit in reducing SBP ($r2=0.40$; $P=0.13$).*

Source: https://www.ahajournals.org/cms/asset/a640af96-fcf4-46e5-8335-91d1c6e1f299/11ff2.jpg.

Patients with resistant hypertension often have undiagnosed OSA, indicating the importance of treating both conditions simultaneously. While it is logical to assume that treating sleep apnea can reduce the risk of cardiac and vascular events by improving oxygen levels and lowering blood pressure, conclusive evidence from long-term randomized controlled studies is still needed to confirm this hypothesis. The impact of treating obstructive apnea on reducing cardiovascular events through blood pressure reduction is also not yet fully understood.

A Closer Look

Continuous Positive Airway Pressure (CPAP) Therapy

Continuous Positive Airway Pressure (CPAP) therapy is a primary treatment for obstructive sleep apnea (OSA), a condition characterized by repeated interruptions in breathing during sleep due to airway obstruction. CPAP therapy involves using a machine that delivers a constant stream of air through a mask worn over the nose, or sometimes the nose and mouth. This steady airflow keeps the airway open, preventing the apneas and hypopneas (partial blockages) that disrupt sleep.

The CPAP machine consists of several components: the main unit which generates the air pressure, a flexible tube that conveys the air, and a mask that the user wears. There are different types of masks available, including nasal masks, full-face masks, and nasal pillows, allowing users to choose the most comfortable option.

The benefits of CPAP therapy are significant. By keeping the airway open, CPAP eliminates the apneas and hypopneas that characterize sleep apnea. This leads to improved oxygenation of the blood, better sleep quality, and a reduction in the daytime sleepiness and fatigue that often accompany sleep apnea. For individuals with diabetes, the benefits extend further. Improved sleep quality can enhance insulin sensitivity and blood sugar control, which are often adversely affected by the fragmented sleep patterns seen in untreated sleep apnea.

Adherence to CPAP therapy is crucial for its effectiveness. Initial discomfort is a common barrier, but most users find that with proper mask fitting, humidification to reduce dryness, and gradual acclimatization to the air pressure, they can adapt successfully. Regular follow-ups with a sleep specialist can help address any issues with CPAP use, ensuring that users receive the maximum benefit from the therapy.

CPAP therapy can also have positive effects on other health aspects. It can lower blood pressure, reduce the risk of cardiovascular events, and improve overall quality of life. For individuals with both sleep apnea and diabetes, these benefits are particularly important as they help mitigate the compounded health risks associated with both conditions.

Summary

- A sleep-related breathing disorder called sleep apnea is characterized by frequent pauses in breathing, shallow breathing spells, or upper airway collapses that impair breathing and disturb sleep. Breathing pauses occur frequently throughout the night and can range in duration from a few seconds to several minutes. As breathing starts again, there might be a snort or choking sound.
- Narrow pharyngeal anatomy and craniofacial structure are common risk factors for obstructive sleep apnea, though the exact causes are varied and complex. The severity of OSA rapidly increases as more factors are present when anatomical risk factors are combined with non-anatomical contributors like weak pharyngeal dilator muscle function during sleep, unstable breathing control (high loop gain), and premature awakening to mild airway narrowing.
- Sleep apnea has far more effects than just making you feel exhausted in the morning. Sleep apnea can affect a person's blood sugar levels throughout the day, alter how the body reacts to insulin, and increase the risk of developing complications from diabetes in later life.
- The hallmarks of obstructive sleep apnea (OSA) are episodes of total or partial airway collapse, which are accompanied by a drop in oxygen saturation or an increase in arousal from sleep. Additional symptoms include excessive daytime sleepiness, heard apneas during sleep, and loud, disruptive snoring.
- The pathophysiology of pharyngeal narrowing and closing during sleep is a complex phenomenon with several contributing factors. Upper airway obstruction during sleep is probably largely caused by a combination of anatomic risk factors, sleep-related reduced ventilatory drive, and neuromuscular factors.
- A sleep apnea evaluation is recommended for any adult patient exhibiting unexplained symptoms during the day or related to sleep, such as excessive sleepiness, fatigue, or unrefreshing sleep.
- To increase the amount of space in the oropharynx, uvulopalatopharyngoplasty (UPPP) involves surgically removing the uvula and tissue from the soft palate. This can occasionally be combined with an adenoidectomy and tonsillectomy.
- Patients with OSA should be encouraged to lose weight. Alcohol, benzodiazepines, opiates, and some antidepressants should be advised against as these substances may exacerbate their condition. They should also be educated about the dangers of driving while intoxicated, the significance of maintaining good sleep hygiene, and the necessity of getting enough sleep each night.

References

1. Dominguez, J. E., & Habib, A. S. (2022). Obstructive sleep apnea in pregnant women. *International Anesthesiology Clinics, 60*(2), 59–65.
2. Koren, D., O'Sullivan, K. L., & Mokhlesi, B. (2015). Metabolic and glycemic sequelae of sleep disturbances in children and adults. *Current Diabetes Reports, 15*(2), 562.
3. Lavie, P., & Hoffstein, V. (2001). Sleep apnea syndrome: A possibly contributing factor to resistant hypertension. *Sleep, 24*(6), 721–725.
4. Mehrtash, M., Bakker, J. P., & Ayas, N. (2019). Predictors of continuous positive airway pressure adherence in patients with obstructive sleep apnea. *Lung, 197*(2), 115–121.
5. Morgenstern, M., Wang, J., Beatty, N., Batemarco, T., Sica, A. A. L., & Greenberg, H. (2014). Obstructive sleep apnea: An unexpected cause of insulin resistance and diabetes. *Endocrinology and Metabolism Clinics of North America, 43*(2), 187–204.
6. Perfect, M. M., Patel, P. G., Scott, R. E., et al. (2012). Sleep, glucose, and daytime functioning in youth with type 1 diabetes. *Sleep, 35*(1), 81–88.
7. Polotsky, V. Y., Li, J., Punjabi, N. M., et al. (2003). Intermittent hypoxia increases insulin resistance in genetically obese mice. *Journal of Physiology, 552*(1), 253–264.
8. Rosen, C. L., Larkin, E. K., Kirchner, H. L., et al. (2003). Prevalence and risk factors for sleep-disordered breathing in 8- to 11-year-old children: Association with race and prematurity. *Journal of Pediatrics, 142*(4), 383–389.
9. Russell, M. B., Kristiansen, H. A., & Kværner, K. J. (2014). Headache in sleep apnea syndrome: Epidemiology and pathophysiology. *Cephalalgia, 34*(10), 752–755.
10. Sankri-Tarbichi, A. G. (2012). Obstructive sleep apnea-hypopnea syndrome: Etiology and diagnosis. *Avicenna Journal of Medicine, 2*(1), 3–8.
11. Sankri-Tarbichi, A. G., Rowley, J. A., & Badr, M. S. (2009). Expiratory pharyngeal narrowing during central hypocapnic hypopnea. *American Journal of Respiratory and Critical Care Medicine, 179*(4), 313–319.
12. Senaratna, C., et al. (2017). Prevalence of obstructive sleep apnea in the general population: A systematic review. *Sleep Med, Rev., 34*, 70–81. https://pubmed.ncbi.nlm.nih.gov/27568340/ (accessed on 5 September 2024).
13. Yeghiazarians, Y., Jneid, H., Tietjens, J. R., Redline, S., Brown, D. L., El-Sherif, N., Mehra, R., Bozkurt, B., Ndumele, C. E., & Somers, V. K. (2021). Obstructive sleep apnea and cardiovascular disease: A scientific statement from the American Heart Association. *Circulation, 144*(3), e56–e67.
14. Young, T., Finn, L., Peppard, P. E., et al (2008). Sleep-disordered breathing and mortality: Eighteen-year follow-up of the Wisconsin sleep cohort. *Sleep, 31*(8), 1071–1078.
15. Young, T., Palta, M., Dempsey, J., Skatrud, J., Weber, S., & Badr, S. (1993). The occurrence of sleep-disordered breathing among middle-aged adults. *New England Journal of Medicine, 328*(17), 1230–1235.
16. Young, T., Skatrud, J., & Peppard, P. E. (2004). Risk factors for obstructive sleep apnea in adults. *JAMA, 291*(16), 2013–2016.

Chapter

RESISTANT HYPERTENSION: ETIOLOGY, EVALUATION AND MANAGEMENT

4

Contents

INTRODUCTION

Because resistant hypertension, a subtype of high blood pressure, stubbornly resists standard treatment approaches, it poses a significant challenge in clinical management. It affects a large percentage of the hypertensive population and is defined as blood pressure that stays above target levels even when three antihypertensive medications, including a diuretic, are taken concurrently. This increases the risk of cardiovascular morbidity and mortality. To find the best course of treatment and uncover its underlying causes, this condition requires careful assessment. Correctly identifying and treating the factors that contribute to resistant hypertension is one of the main challenges in managing the condition. Comorbid conditions like obesity, diabetes, chronic kidney disease, and obstructive sleep apnea are common in patients, which can worsen hypertension and reduce the efficacy of standard treatments. Treatment resistance may also be influenced by lifestyle choices like drinking alcohol, consuming too much salt, and not getting enough exercise. Thus, to make informed therapeutic decisions, a thorough evaluation of the patient's medical history, medication compliance, and lifestyle choices is crucial (Calhoun et al., 2008).

A multimodal approach is usually used to treat resistant hypertension, with the goal of addressing both modifiable and non-modifiable risk factors. In clinical practice, two common strategies used are optimizing medication adherence and intensifying pharmacological therapy by adding or adjusting antihypertensive agents. To improve blood pressure control, combination therapies that target various pathways of blood pressure regulation, such as diuretics, calcium channel blockers, beta-blockers, and renin-angiotensin-aldosterone system inhibitors, may be prescribed. Nonetheless, possible drug interactions, side effects, and unique patient characteristics should all be taken into account when choosing medications.

Lifestyle changes are essential for managing resistant hypertension in addition to medication. Blood pressure can be lowered with dietary interventions that emphasize limiting sodium intake, eating more fruits and vegetables, and consuming alcohol in moderation. In addition to being essential elements of managing hypertension, regular physical activity and weight control also enhance cardiovascular health and general well-being. Invasive treatments like renal denervation or baroreceptor activation therapy may be taken into consideration as adjunctive therapies for specific patients with resistant hypertension. These operations seek to interfere with the neural pathways that control blood pressure, which may be therapeutically beneficial for some patients who have not responded to traditional treatments.

The management of resistant hypertension requires a comprehensive and customized approach due to its significant clinical challenge. Healthcare professionals can work to improve blood pressure control and reduce the associated cardiovascular risks in affected individuals by addressing underlying causes, optimizing pharmacotherapy, and encouraging lifestyle modifications. Working together, patients and medical teams can better navigate the complex treatment of resistant hypertension and achieve better long-term results.

Orientation and Directional Terms

Term	Definition	Illustration
Blood Pressure	Blood pressure is the amount of force your blood uses to get through your arteries. When your heart pumps, it uses force to push oxygen-rich blood out to your arteries.	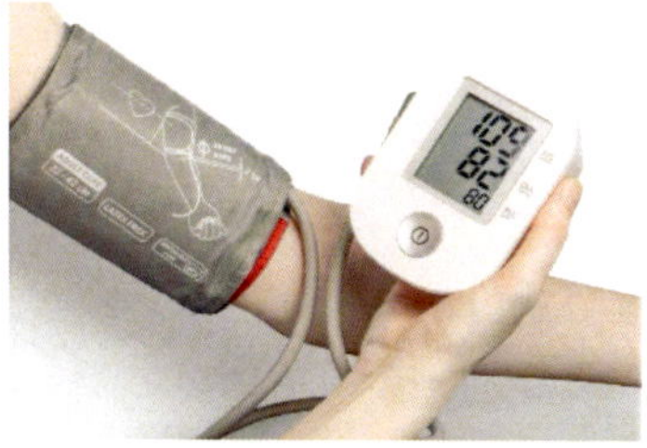
Hyperaldosteronism	Hyperaldosteronism is a disorder in which the adrenal gland releases too much of the hormone aldosterone into the blood.	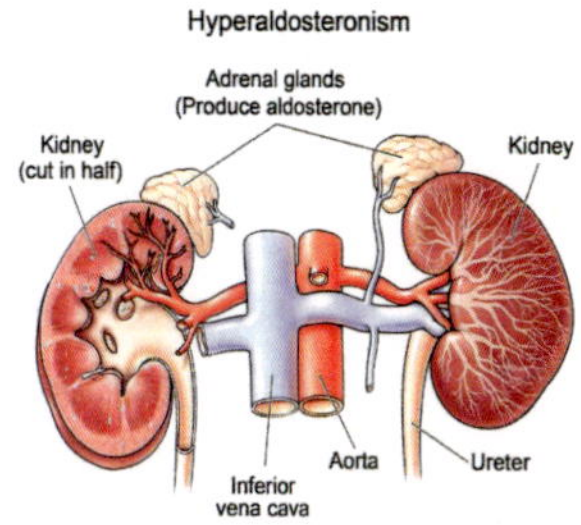
Pheochromocytoma	Pheochromocytoma is a type of neuroendocrine tumor that grows from cells called chromaffin cells.	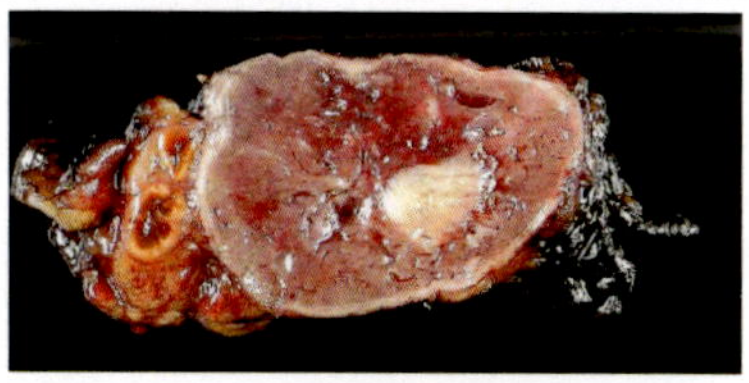
Rheumatoid arthritis	Rheumatoid arthritis (RA) is a chronic (long-lasting) autoimmune disease that mostly affects joints. RA occurs when the immune system, which normally helps protect the body from infection and disease, attacks its own tissues.	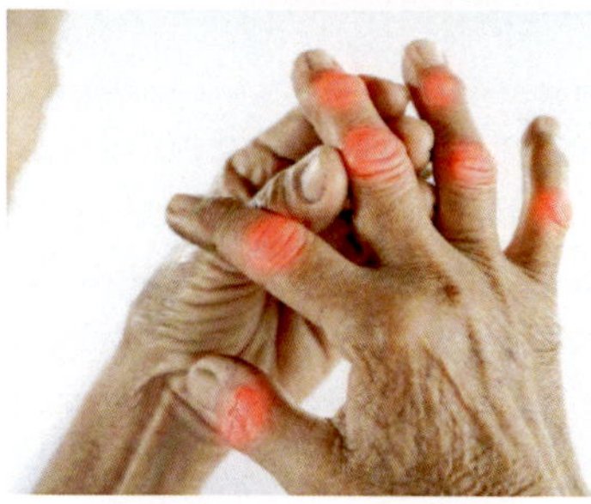
Chronic kidney disease	Chronic kidney disease (CKD) is when the kidneys have become damaged over time (for at least 3 months) and have a hard time doing all their important jobs.	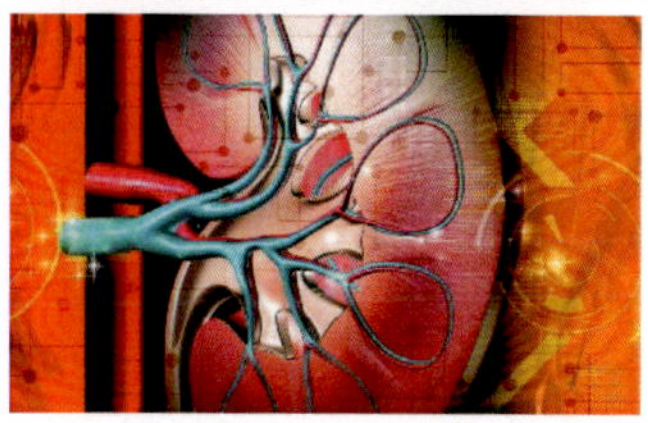

4.1. CONCEPT OF RESISTANT HYPERTENSION: DETECTION, EVALUATION, AND MANAGEMENT

The greatest risk factor in the world for heart disease (CVD), stroke, disability, and death is hypertension. A significant percentage of hypertensive adults, despite diligent clinical management, still fail to meet their recommended blood pressure (BP) treatment targets on three antihypertensive medications or require four or more medications to meet their targets, despite a steady improvement in hypertension awareness, treatment, and control rates over the past thirty years. Despite receiving continuous antihypertensive medication therapy, these people—who are classified as having treatment-resistant hypertension (RH)—remain at elevated risk for harm to target organs, morbidity, and death (Calhoun et al., 2008).

The 2017 American College of Cardiology/American Heart Association (AHA) clinical practice guideline for the prevention, detection, evaluation, and management of high blood pressure in adults contains new recommendations for the identification, assessment, and treatment of hypertension. The 2017 guideline lowers the BP goal of treatment to <130/80 mm Hg for the majority of people and the BP threshold for starting antihypertensive therapy to ≥130/80 mm Hg for adults with pre-existing CVD or a 10-year atherosclerotic CVD risk of ≥10%. These recommendations will raise the prevalence of RH in the hypertensive population by influencing the blood pressure threshold for diagnosis. The American College of Cardiology/American Heart Association 2017 guideline is congruent with the current scientific statement.

4.1.1. Definitions of RH

RH is defined as a patient's blood pressure that stays elevated above goal even after taking three different classes of antihypertensive medications at the same time. These medications typically include long-acting calcium channel blockers (CCBs), angiotensin receptor blockers (ARBs) or ACE inhibitors, which block the renin-angiotensin system, and diuretics. Every agent should be used at the highest dosage or the highest amount that can be tolerated, along with the recommended frequency of dosage.

This definition of RH, though arbitrary in terms of the quantity of drugs needed, identifies patients who are more likely to experience fatalities and morbid CVD events. In addition, compared to hypertensive patients without drug resistance, they are more likely to experience medication side effects, have a secondary cause of hypertension, and may benefit from specialized diagnostic or therapeutic approaches to control their blood pressure. RH also includes patients whose blood pressure reaches target values while taking four or more antihypertensive medications; this condition has been called controlled RH in the literature. Hence, depending on the quantity of antihypertensive medications taken, the term "hypertension" can refer to both uncontrolled and controlled hypertension.

Misdiagnosis of RH may be due to measurement errors in blood pressure. The patient's preparation, the surrounding circumstances, the size of the cuff, and the BP measurement method can all significantly affect the readings. Specifically, because of intrinsic blood pressure variability, diagnostic blood pressure recordings must contain an average of two or more readings taken at least twice. Therefore, it is crucial to make sure that the blood pressure is measured accurately before making the diagnosis of RH. Both self-monitored and out-of-office blood pressure require appropriate techniques. Any site should measure blood pressure in accordance with current recommendations.

The term "white-coat effect" describes a patient taking three or more antihypertensive medications whose office blood pressure is above goal but their home blood pressure, as determined by ambulatory blood pressure monitoring (ABPM) or by home blood pressure monitoring, is below goal. Patients with a white-coat effect have a risk of CVD complications that is comparable to that of hypertensive patients whose blood pressure is under control. True RH diagnosis usually requires out-of-office blood pressure monitoring.

Before RH is diagnosed, nonadherence to the prescribed antihypertensive medication regimen must be ruled out. Nonadherence to medication is very common in patients who appear to have RH. Up to 50–80% of hypertensive patients who are prescribed antihypertensive medications are thought to exhibit suboptimal adherence. The large pill burden, complicated dosing, high cost, frequent adverse reactions with multidrug antihypertensive regimens, poor patient-clinician relationship, and clinician inertia with reduced insistence on adherence when patients are consistently nonadherent are all contributing factors to this relatively high proportion of nonadherence that may mimic RH. A candid and nonjudgmental conversation between a clinician and patient, tracking of medication counts and prescription refills, and, if possible, a biochemical assay of the drugs or their metabolites in urine or plasma should all be included in the process of ruling out nonadherence (Diaz et al., 2014).

The 2008 AHA scientific statement's definition of RH has been modified in four significant ways:

- Patients should take a blood pressure measurement, and the blood pressure threshold for diagnosis and treatment goals should follow current clinical practice guidelines;
- Patients should be taking at least three antihypertensive medications, commonly a diuretic, an ACE inhibitor, or a long-acting CCB, at maximum or maximally tolerated doses;
- Patients with the white-coat effect should not be included in the definition of RH; and
- The diagnosis of RH necessitates the exclusion of antihypertensive medication nonadherence.

4.1.2. Prevalence of RH

As previously mentioned, RH demands that patients take their medications as directed and that the uncontrolled subset has elevated blood pressure when they are not in the office. When ≥1 of the following data elements is missing—medication dose, adherence, or out-of-office blood pressure—the term apparent treatment RH (aTRH) is used; pseudoresistance cannot be ruled out in this scenario. Prevalent aTRH is found in approximately 12–15% of population-based and 15–18% of clinic-based reports of treated adults with hypertension. When an at-risk group is chosen, such as patients with treated hypertension and chronic kidney disease (CKD), prevalent aTRH occurs in a higher percentage of the population- and clinic-based samples. The increased frequency of aTRH (34–39%) among treated hypertensive adults in clinical trials can probably be attributed to the patient population's selection based on demographic and comorbidity traits that put them at high risk for the desired CVD outcomes, both fatal and nonfatal. Furthermore, some RH cases may remain unidentified in population- and clinic-based studies due to patients not receiving prescriptions for ≥3 drugs at maximal doses in spite of uncontrolled blood pressure. Conversely, forced titration schemes that uncover RH by lowering the frequency of suboptimal treatment are typically a part of clinical trials (Table 4.1) (Diaz et al., 2014).

Table 4.1. *Prevalence of aTRH in Adults with Treated Hypertension as Reported from Selected Population-, Clinic-, and Intervention-Based Studies*

Population Based	**Time Period**	**n**	**Uncontrolled with ≥3 BP Medications, %**	**Controlled with ≥4 BP Medications, %**	**aTRH, %**
NHANES	1988–1994	2755	8.3	1.1	9.4
NHANES	1999–2004	3031	8.8	2.9	11.7
NHANES	2003–2008	3710			12.8
NHANES	2005–2008	2586	9.7	4.8	14.5
REGARDS	2003–2007	14 731	9.1	5.0	14.1
REGARDS (CKD)*	2003–2007	3134			28.1
Clinic Based					
EURIKA (diabetes mellitus)	2009–2010	5220	13.0†	3.1	16.1
Spanish ABPM	2004–2009	68 045	12.2	2.6	14.8
CRIC (CKD)	2003–2008	3939	21.2	19.2	40.4
South Carolina	2007–2010	468877	9.5	8.4	17.9
Clinical Trials					
ALLHAT	1994–2002	14 684	11.5	1.2	12.7
ASCOT	1998–2005	19 527	48.5		
ACCOMPLISH	2003–2006¶	10 704	39		
INVEST	1997–2003#	17 190	25.1	12.6	37.8

Source: https://www.ahajournals.org/doi/10.1161/HYP.0000000000000084

Uncontrolled aTRH is defined as BP ≥140 mm Hg systolic and/or ≥90 mm Hg diastolic on ≥3 BP medications. Controlled aTRH is defined as BP <140 mm Hg systolic and <90 mm Hg diastolic on ≥4 BP medications unless otherwise specified.

4.1.3. Prognosis of RH

Patients with RH are more likely to experience negative outcomes than patients without RH, according to observational studies that used the 2008 criteria. Those with RH had a 47% higher chance of experiencing the combined outcomes of death, myocardial infarction, heart failure, stroke, or chronic kidney disease (CKD) during the median 3.8 years of follow-up, according to a retrospective study of over 200,000 patients with incident hypertension. A higher risk of developing CKD was the primary driver of differences in CVD events in this study. In an additional study involving over 400 000 patients, those with RH had a higher risk of end-stage renal disease by 32%, an ischemic heart event by 24%, heart failure by 46%, stroke by 14%, and death by 6% when compared to patients without RH. According to ABPM-based prospective studies, patients with true RH had an almost two-fold higher risk of CVD events than patients with hypertension that responds to treatment. When taken as a whole, these studies point to RH as a significant public health issue and a risk factor for unfavorable outcomes.

In patients with certain comorbid conditions, RH is linked to worse outcomes. Compared to patients without RH, those with CKD are more likely to experience heart failure, peripheral arterial disease, myocardial infarction, stroke, and all-cause mortality if they have RH. Similarly, RH is linked to an increased risk of adverse events such as death, myocardial infarction, and stroke in patients with ischemic heart disease. On the other hand, RH may reduce the risk of rehospitalization due to heart failure and is not linked to an increase in adverse clinical events in patients with heart failure who have a reduced ejection fraction (Calhoun et al., 2008).

Lower blood pressure among patients with resistant hypertension is linked to a decreased risk of certain cardiovascular events. In the REGARDS study, individuals with uncontrolled resistant hypertension had a higher risk of developing coronary heart disease compared to those with controlled resistant hypertension. However, control status did not impact the likelihood of stroke or mortality. Another study involving over 118,000 treated hypertensive adults found that blood pressure control was linked to lower rates of stroke and coronary heart disease, with no significant difference in rates of heart failure. Among patients with resistant hypertension, blood pressure control led to a 13% reduction in risk for stroke, coronary heart disease, or heart failure, whereas individuals without resistant hypertension had a 31% lower risk of these outcomes. While blood pressure control has benefits in preventing certain cardiovascular events, the advantages may be lesser in individuals with resistant hypertension compared to those without it.

4.1.4. Patient Characteristics

Three demographic factors are associated with RH: male sex, older age, and black race. Variable clustering of different demographics, comorbidities, physiological aberrations, and metabolic abnormalities are characteristics of RH. These elements, however, are not exclusive of one another since they may actually be highly interdependent (e.g., hyperactivity of the sympathetic nervous system, non-dipping or reverse-dipping blood pressure, visceral obesity, and elevated aldosterone).

There are several comorbidities linked to RH. Compared to non-RH, RH patients are more likely to have obesity, left ventricular hypertrophy, albuminuria, diabetes mellitus,

CKD, a higher Framingham 10-year risk score, and obstructive sleep apnea (OSA). A significant percentage (60%–84%) of people with RH also suffer from sleep apnea. Compared to people with controlled hypertension or normotensives, RH also exhibits other abnormalities related to sleep, such as shorter sleep duration, decreased efficiency, and less rapid eye movement sleep.

Vascular disease/dysfunction, as demonstrated by high rates of peripheral and carotid artery atherosclerosis, impaired endothelial function, decreased arterial compliance, and elevated systemic vascular resistance, are among the physiological abnormalities in RH. These abnormalities may be more severe in RH than in non-RH individuals. The typical nocturnal drop in blood pressure is also diminished in a significant percentage (43% to 65%) of people with RH. When compared to controlled RH, the attenuated nocturnal decline in blood pressure is even more noticeable in uncontrolled settings. In people with RH, nondipping ambulatory blood pressure has been associated with decreased heart rate variability, a sign of hyperactivity of the sympathetic nervous system. The nocturnal BP paradoxically rising during reverse dipping may be linked to an increase in subclinical organ damage and potentially CVD events. Additionally linked to increased sympathetic nervous system activity at night is reverse dipping. Renal denervation reduced office systolic blood pressure (SBP) at 6 months more effectively than sham controls in adults with severe uncontrolled RH and self-reported sleep apnea in the SYMPLICITY HTN-3 trial (Renal Denervation in Patients With Uncontrolled Hypertension) (−17.0 mm Hg versus −6.3 mm Hg; P<0.01). Patients without sleep apnea did not see a reduction in office SBP with renal denervation.

Additionally, hyperuricemia, excess aldosterone, and suppressed circulating renin levels (approximately 60% of individuals with RH have suppressed renin levels) have all been associated with RH. RH is typically characterized by exceptional BP salt sensitivity. Cutting back on sodium consumption in food to considerably lower levels than what is typically consumed in Western countries (e.g., 50 mmol/d) quickly and significantly decreased blood pressure in a large number of RH patients. Furthermore, dietary sodium intake is positively correlated with the severity of sleep apnea in individuals with RH, at least in those who have hyperaldosteronism. People with RH have nearly twice the plasma osmolality-adjusted copeptin concentrations—a proxy for vasopressin release—than people with nonresistant, controlled blood pressure (Diaz et al., 2014).

People with RH have different prescription and administration patterns for antihypertensive medications. Inadequate antihypertensive medication regimens significantly raise the risk of developing a diagnosis of RH. Because of this, medication regimens for RH rarely include either of the two very effective BP-lowering medications, spironolactone or chlorthalidone, in this high-risk group of hypertensives. Due to the fact that bedtime dosing of once-daily antihypertensive medications results in higher rates of nocturnal normalization of blood pressure and fewer patients with nondipping of blood pressure and >24-hour blood pressure control than morning or twice-daily dosing, it appears to significantly affect diurnal blood pressure patterns.

4.1.5. Genetics/Pharmacogenetics

The heritability of blood pressure in family-based research indicates that blood pressure has a genetic basis. Estimates for long-term average blood pressure suggest that additive genetic factors may account for as much as 50–60% of the variability in blood pressure. The heritability of RH or the BP-lowering response to particular antihypertensive medications, however, has not received much research. Although genetic factors may play a role in the disproportionately higher prevalence of RH among Blacks, other potential explanations include environmental or psychosocial determinants of BP control.

Although common genetic variants affecting blood pressure have been found at over 300 distinct loci, it takes scores from hundreds of thousands of people to detect them. The order of 1.0 mm Hg diastolic blood pressure and 1.0 mm Hg SBP per BP-raising allele is usually affected by these genetic variations. Each of these variations accounts for ≤0:1% of BP variability, while taken as a whole, they only account for 3% of the variance in BP. This is in line with the complicated nature of blood pressure regulation, which involves numerous compensatory systems, including myocardial function, autonomic nervous system function, sodium excretion and plasma volume, vascular tone, and numerous other as-yet-unknown factors.

The bulk of RH genetic research has focused only on candidate genes and hasn't used large enough sample sizes to withstand the burden of multiple testing that comes with conducting so many of these studies. Further extensive investigations involving well-characterized RH patients as well as individuals both before and after treatment with particular antihypertensive medications are required to more precisely identify the contribution of common and uncommon genetic variations to RH and drug response modulation.

4.1.6. Etiology

Resistant hypertension has a complex etiology that involves multiple factors, including genetic, environmental, and lifestyle factors. Comprehending the fundamental reasons behind the issues is crucial in directing treatment choices and enhancing results for impacted persons. Inadequate adherence to medication is a significant factor in resistant hypertension. Antihypertensive patients may not follow their prescribed regimens for a variety of reasons, such as forgetfulness, adverse drug reactions, insufficient funds, or a lack of awareness of the significance of treatment. Treatment resistance can be exacerbated and blood pressure control compromised by nonadherence.

Resistant hypertension is frequently linked to comorbid conditions like obesity, diabetes mellitus, chronic kidney disease, and obstructive sleep apnea (Calhoun et al., 2008). Through processes like insulin resistance, sodium retention, sympathetic nervous system activation, and endothelial dysfunction, these disorders frequently make hypertension worse. Improving blood pressure control and lowering the risk of cardiovascular problems require treating underlying comorbidities. Consuming too much salt is another important factor in resistant hypertension. Increased vascular resistance, blood pressure, and fluid retention can all result from a high-sodium diet. Dietary changes intended to lower sodium intake, such as switching to a low-salt diet or avoiding processed foods high in sodium, may be beneficial for patients with resistant hypertension.

Genetic predisposition contributes to the development of resistant hypertension in addition to lifestyle factors. Gene variations encoding sodium transporters, sympathetic nervous system, and renin-angiotensin-aldosterone system components may affect how each person reacts to antihypertensive drugs and lead to treatment resistance. Personalized medicine techniques and genetic testing could be useful in identifying patients who are more likely to develop resistant hypertension and in tailoring treatment plans to their unique genetic profiles. In the differential diagnosis of resistant hypertension, other conditions such as renal artery stenosis, atherosclerosis, and secondary hypertension brought on by diseases like Cushing's syndrome, pheochromocytoma, or primary aldosteronism should be taken into account. To find and treat the underlying etiologies causing treatment resistance, these conditions might need specialized diagnostic evaluations like hormone testing or renal artery imaging.

All things considered, there are many different factors contributing to the heterogeneous etiology of resistant hypertension. As such, a thorough evaluation and customized management strategies are necessary. Healthcare professionals can work to lower blood pressure by treating underlying causes, maximizing drug regimens, and encouraging lifestyle changes, managing and enhancing the course of treatment for individuals with resistant hypertension. (Mancia et.al., 2013)

4.2. DIAGNOSING RH

RH is defined as a patient's blood pressure that stays elevated above goal even after taking three different classes of antihypertensive medications at the same time. These medications typically include long-acting calcium channel blockers (CCBs), angiotensin receptor blockers (ARBs) or ACE inhibitors, which block the renin-angiotensin system, and diuretics. Every agent should be used at the highest dosage or the highest amount that can be tolerated, along with the recommended frequency of dosage.

The 2008 AHA scientific statement's definition of RH has been modified in four significant ways:

- Patients should take a blood pressure measurement, and the blood pressure threshold for diagnosis and treatment goals should follow current clinical practice guidelines;
- Patients should be taking at least three antihypertensive medications, commonly a diuretic, an ACE inhibitor, or a long-acting CCB, at maximum or maximally tolerated doses;
- Patients with the white-coat effect should not be included in the definition of RH; and
- The diagnosis of RH necessitates the exclusion of antihypertensive medication nonadherence.

4.2.1. Identifying and Correcting Medication Nonadherence

Adherence, as opposed to compliance, which is defined as yielding to a request, desire, or demand, is the state of continuing to adhere to a medication regimen. One significant factor influencing the management of hypertension is medication adherence. Unfortunately, 25% of patients who start antihypertensive therapy for the first time don't finish their prescribed medication. Only 50% of patients on average have antihypertensive medications during the first year of treatment, and only 1 in 5 patients adheres to their treatment plan well enough to see the benefits seen in clinical trials. However, the trend toward better blood pressure control (<140/90 mm Hg) rates among those on antihypertensive treatment to > 70% of respondents believe that recent initiatives to enhance antihypertensive drug adherence and care have been effective.

In the assessment and treatment of patients with RH, measuring and guaranteeing optimal medication adherence are crucial steps. Since these patients are by definition taking three or more antihypertensive medications, knowledge of the degree of adherence to the recommended regimen is essential for directing clinical judgment and decision-making. The patient's ability to adhere to daily instructions (adherence) and continue therapy (persistency) is a key component of success; the latter is especially important in clinical settings. Actually, the patient's compliance with the recommended regimen is the basis for the diagnosis of RH, and the overestimation of the prevalence of "true" RH results from the inability to recognize insufficient adherence. Although the exact scientific basis for this cutoff is unknown, adequate adherence is generally defined as taking at least 80% of prescribed medication for patients to benefit from full exposure to pharmaceutical therapy. A review of studies on medication adherence in aTRH revealed rates of nonadherence in this population that ranged from 7% using pharmacy refill records in a managed care population to >60% using serum drug levels in a referral clinic, despite the paucity of available data.

4.2.1.1. Assessment of Adherence

Finding patients with poor adherence among those with aTRH will prevent needless and possibly hazardous treatment intensification and enable the application of adherence-improving techniques and more economically efficient health resource allocation. Furthermore, in trials evaluating novel RH treatment modalities, evaluation of changes in adherence as a significant potential confounder is crucial. Therefore, a methodical approach that combines practical and trustworthy methods for measuring medication adherence would help providers optimize their antihypertensive regimens (Hameed et al., 2016).

Despite being paradoxical, one analysis discovered that there was no variation in the SBP response to therapeutic intensification for uncontrolled hypertension among adherence quintiles. With each increase in therapy, SBP decreased by an average of 2.1 mm Hg in the quintile with the highest adherence (≥98% adherence) and 2.4 mm Hg in the quintile with the lowest adherence (<80% adherence; mean, 62%). When a clinician determines that a patient is not adhering to their medication regimen, they are less inclined to increase the dosage. Nevertheless, adherence is not well assessed by clinicians. Therefore, clinicians should exercise caution when deciding against therapeutic intensification in a patient with uncontrolled hypertension whom they perceive to be nonadherent, even though work is still being done to optimize methods for assessing medication adherence. It is imperative that healthcare providers employ efficacious tactics to enhance adherence, like the ones outlined below.

Adherence is complex and dynamic, making it challenging to measure, especially with a single assessment. Methods like pill counting and the impression of the clinician are frequently unreliable. Nonetheless, there are more accurate and advanced direct and indirect techniques available for measuring medication adherence. Many hypertensive populations have shown that indirect methods, such as patient self-report medication adherence assessment tools like the Morisky Medication Adherence Scale and the Hill-Bone Compliance Scale, have predictive validity. These tools also identify adherence risk factors that can be used to customize messages aimed at improving adherence. Patients should be interviewed about adherence using a nonthreatening, nonaccusatory approach, which calls for excellent communication skills. Here's an example: "Missing doses during the week is common when taking multiple medications." In a week, how many times do you forget to take your blood pressure medication?

A reliable indicator of adherence is the possession and refill of prescription drug databases. Pharmacodynamic parameter measurement (e.g., limited specificity, such as heart rate in the case of β-blockers, lack of rise in plasma renin activity [PRA] in the case of renin-angiotensin inhibitors, and N-acetyl-serylaspartyl-lysyl-proline measurements in the case of ACE inhibitors. Drug monitoring in bodily fluids, the Medication Event Monitoring System, and observed drug intake are examples of direct methods. Although this method has not been extensively applied in general practice, observed medication taking followed by monitoring of the effect on blood pressure has proven useful in detecting possible nonadherence in trials of innovative treatment modalities. Although ingestion of the medication is not confirmed, Medication Event Monitoring System monitoring of the date and time that a medication bottle is opened and closed has superior sensitivity compared with other methods. Mass spectroscopy measurements of drugs or their metabolites in urine or blood can accurately identify the presence or absence of a drug, but they cannot reveal if a drug was taken consistently or at a therapeutic level. Urine fluorometry is a novel approach that has recently been reported as a simple, safe, and accurate way to measure adherence. Furthermore, a novel technology that is headed for clinical implementation consists of a sensor embedded in the tablet, which when it comes into contact with stomach acid, sends out a signal that is picked up by a skin sensor (Hameed et al., 2016).

There is no gold standard for measuring adherence. Indirect methods such as pill count, self-report, and prescription refill data are simple, inexpensive, and widely used. However, they can easily be manipulated to overestimate adherence. A direct method such as urine or blood measurement of drug or metabolites is considered more robust but is relatively expensive, is of limited availability, and does not perfectly reflect level of adherence. All methods have limitations, and ideally, accurate assessment of adherence should involve a combination of approaches.

4.2.1.2. Multisystem Intervention to Improve Adherence

Lackluster adherence is caused by a wide range of multilevel factors. Adherence obstacles can be found at the patient (e. g. many coexisting illnesses, a lack of resources, inadequate health literacy, and a lack of participation in the treatment decision-making process), a clinician (e.g., the administration of complicated medication regimens, communication obstacles, inadequate disclosure of side effect information, the use of multiple providers for treatment, clinician inertia), and the healthcare system (e.g., restrictions on the length of office visits, restricted access to care, absence of team-based methods, and health information technology). Multifactorial solutions are necessary to improve medication adherence at the population level due to the complexity and variety of barriers to adherence.

The effects of interventions, such as changing antihypertensive therapy, on adherence to antihypertensive medication have been evaluated by many systematic reviews and meta-analyses. There is little data specifically pertaining to enhancing adherence in the RH population. Nonetheless, evidence-based strategies that work for the majority of people with hypertension can be used. There is no one intervention that works for everyone. Instead, the best results usually come from a consistent strategy that employs a variety of tactics, such as addressing the health system's issues and addressing the adherence barriers specific to each patient. This list of interventions, which are arranged according to the health system, clinician, and patient levels, has been shown to be beneficial in enhancing adherence.

Multidisciplinary team-based care is used in health system-level interventions to enhance the standard of care for hypertension, medication adherence, and blood pressure control. It has been shown that a range of patient-centered, team-based hypertension care models raise the percentage of people with controlled blood pressure. A successful, comprehensive strategy frequently incorporates clinical decision-making systems support (i.e., Treatment algorithms), patient-physician cooperation, medication compliance, blood pressure monitoring, and patient self-management. Further systems-level support such as use of electronic health records, registries, clinical decision support (i.e., Team-based care initiatives are enhanced and strengthened by the use of technology-based remote monitoring, self-management support tools, treatment algorithms, and performance monitoring (Diaz et al., 2014).

Effective strategies for improving adherence to antihypertensive medications include: opting for agents that are taken once daily instead of multiple times a day and using fixed-dose combination agents when possible. It is also important to choose low-cost and generic antihypertensives, especially when cost is a barrier for patients with multiple chronic conditions. Consolidating refills can help minimize trips to the pharmacy for all prescribed medications.

Involving patients in decisions about their antihypertensive treatment can also improve adherence, as well as considering the overall adverse effects of the medications and preferring those that are well tolerated. Medication adherence scales may be helpful, and clinicians may benefit from training to improve communication skills and cultural competence in their interactions with patients.

Educating patients, their families, and caregivers about hypertension, its consequences, and potential medication side effects is crucial at the individual patient level. A well-informed patient can work with a clinician to develop a care plan and common therapeutic objectives. Telehealth or mobile communication strategies may be useful in keeping in touch with patients for continued follow-up and monitoring. It is necessary for patients to incorporate the taking of their medications into their regular daily activities by using adherence support tools like packaging, pillboxes, reminders, and other tools. In a busy practice, individual obstacles to adherence, like low health literacy, can be challenging to pinpoint. Furthermore, only 12% of adult Americans possess the health literacy abilities required to meet the demands of our intricate healthcare system. The Health Literacy Universal Precautions Toolkit suggests establishing a supportive system and assuming that all patients may have trouble understanding to provide written and oral communication in plain language that encourages self-management and empowerment for all patients. Two important suggestions are to give a medication list or pictorial medication schedule and to use interactive, visual education. A different strategy called the teach-back method gives medical professionals a non-coercive means of finding out if patients have understood what has been explained to them. A patient can accurately "teach back" the information if they comprehend it. Supporting efforts to modify one's lifestyle and adhere to medication regimens can also be facilitated by motivational interventions. To identify and address nonadherence, it is imperative to create a supportive, blame-free environment where patients are empowered to ask questions, acknowledged for making progress toward treatment goals and given "permission" to honestly respond to questions about their treatment.

4.2.1.3. Poor BP Measurement Technique

Treatment resistance may emerge as a result of inaccurate blood pressure measurement. Triage SBPs were a median of 17 mm Hg higher in a study comparing standard triage blood pressure measurements by clinic staff with an automated device that obtained up to six BP measurements one minute apart while the patient was alone and seated in a quiet room. The difference was greatest in the group of patients with initial SBPs >160 mm Hg. 33% of the patients in this study who were referred for RH had erroneous blood pressure measurements. As oscillometric devices have become widely used to measure blood pressure in hospitals, workplaces, and homes, some aspects of the technique have become standard. For instance, using non-auscultatory techniques eliminates the possibility of measurement confounders like observer bias, end-digit preference, and the existence of an auscultatory gap. However, common characteristics of oscillometric and auscultatory methods that impact the accuracy of blood pressure measurement include cuff size, body and arm positions, and measurement environment. The steps involved in a proper blood pressure measurement procedure are as follows: (1) getting the subject ready by having them empty their bladder completely; (2) selecting a blood pressure cuff with a bladder length of at least 80% and a width of at least 40% of the arm circumference; (3) placing the cuff directly on the skin of the upper arm at the level of the heart on the supported arm; and (4) taking at least two readings, one minute apart, in a quiet room. Ideally, this process is completed five minutes before the first reading is taken.

IABP and cuff-measured blood pressure may not be the same. When blood pressure is measured using the auscultatory method, severe arterial stiffness or medial calcification of the brachial artery may cause an inaccurate detection of Korotkoff sounds. Pseudoxertension is the term used to describe the abnormally high cuff pressure in patients with severe arterial disease. Although the exact impact of brachial artery calcification or arterial stiffness on oscillometric device-based blood pressure measurement is unknown, it is thought to be less significant. Furthermore, it is probable that the auscultatory method's overestimation of diastolic blood pressure in hypertensive individuals is unrelated to calcified arteries.

4.2.2. White-Coat Effect

The white-coat effect occurs when a hypertensive patient taking medication has recurrent episodes of elevated blood pressure in the office and controlled or noticeably lower blood pressure outside the office. The sympathetic nervous system's alerting reflex, which is set off by the healthcare provider or the clinic environment, has been linked to the white-coat effect. Most people experience a slight increase in blood pressure during in-office measurements; however, those who have been diagnosed with hypertension, women, and older people are more susceptible to the white-coat effect. According to office blood pressure measurements, 28 to 39% of people with a TRH may have a clinically significant white-coat effect.

The absence of CKD or diabetes mellitus and short-term hypertension are also linked to pseudoresistance from a white-coat effect. The CVD risk associated with overdiagnosing RH in populations with RH due to the white-coat effect is similar to that of patients with treated controlled hypertension. While office blood pressure had no predictive value, ambulatory blood pressure was an independent predictor of both all-cause death and a composite outcome of CVD events in a Brazilian cohort of patients with RH. These results are in line with general population outcome studies. The International Database on Ambulatory Blood Pressure in Relation to Cardiovascular Outcomes, which comprised over 12,000 participants worldwide, was analyzed, and the results showed that the white-coat effect had no effect on the risk of CVD after age was taken into consideration. Patients whose blood pressure is managed by measurement using either ABPM or home blood pressure monitoring have not been included in randomized clinical trials in RH due to the risk discrepancy between white-coat-related elevated blood pressure and RH. (Diaz et.al., 2014)

The 24-hour ABPM makes it simple to identify the white-coat effect. But not all countries have easy access to ABPM, and it is not even widely used in the US due to insurance reimbursement restrictions. Clinical use of oscillometric digital devices—known as automated office BP—has made it possible to automatically record three to six blood pressure readings without a clinician present in the examination room. The white-coat effect is mitigated by automated office blood pressure monitoring. The white-coat effect can be detected using self-measured home blood pressure (BPs) that have received the proper training in BP measurement technique. These BPs correlate with average daytime BPs determined by 24-hour ABPM. It is crucial to keep in mind, though, that people could falsify their blood pressure records or underreport elevated or lowered readings. Wrist BP monitors are not as good as upper arm cuff-based home blood pressure monitors. Wrist monitors can cause measurement error in people with arrhythmias, during arm movement, or when the wrist is not at heart level, despite their potential convenience, especially for obese patients who need very large cuff sizes. It is not advised to use finger blood pressure monitors due to inaccurate and fictitious readings. Although BP control is <130/80 mm Hg in the office, control by 24-hour ABPM is defined as <125/75 mm Hg.

4.2.2.1. Treatment Inertia

A significant portion of patients do not reach their blood pressure targets due to suboptimal antihypertensive therapy (Figure 4.1). In the United States, only 49.6% of patients with uncontrolled aTRH who were found in a community-based practice network between 2007 and 2010 received the recommended antihypertensive medication.

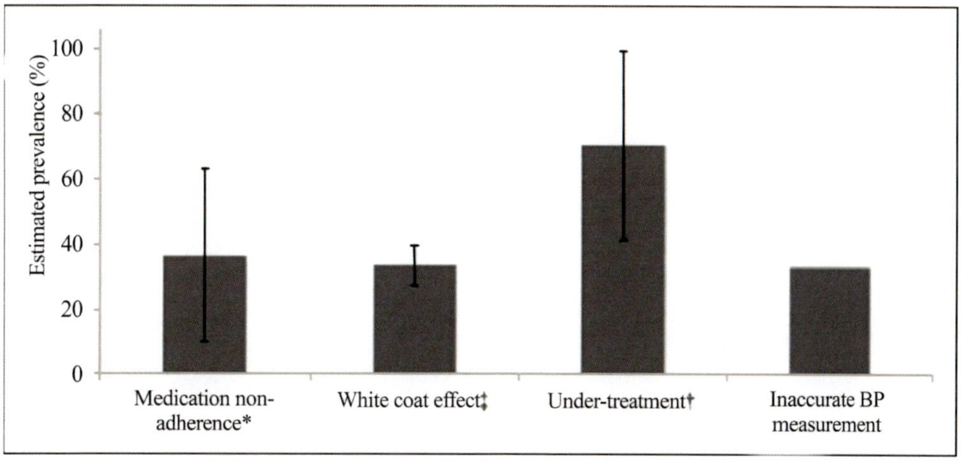

Figure 4.1. *Estimated prevalence of each of the causes of pseudoresistant hypertension. BP indicates blood pressure.*

Source: https://www.ncbi.nlm.nih.gov/corecgi/tileshop/tileshop.fcgi?p=PMC3&id=371651&s=88&r=2&c=3.

Of the 84 193 patients with aTRH, more than 90% received the proper prescription for a diuretic; however, 42.1% of patients with uncontrolled aTRH received antihypertensive drugs at less than half of the recommended dosage. Patients who were diagnosed with coronary heart disease, diabetes mellitus, or chronic kidney disease (CKD) had a higher likelihood of receiving an optimal regimen if they were Black.

By using an integrated health system model of care, clinician treatment inertia can be overcome. The Veterans Affairs and Kaiser Permanente health systems, where BP control is approached in a systematic and multidisciplinary manner, have rates of hypertension control that are higher than the national average. By identifying patients with hypertension, standardizing blood pressure measurements, and applying a stepwise treatment algorithm, the Kaiser Permanente Southern California health system's blood pressure control rates increased from 54% in 2004 to 84% in 2010 (Hameed et al., 2016).

4.2.2.2. Lifestyle Factors

The 2017 American College of Cardiology/AHA clinical practice guideline for the prevention, detection, evaluation, and management of high BP in adults provides a detailed discussion of the relationships between several lifestyle factors and high BP.

4.2.2.3. Obesity

One of the key contributing factors to the rising incidence of hypertension is excess body fat. Particularly visceral obesity is a major contributor to high blood pressure through many pathways that end in increased sensitivity to salt, vascular dysfunction, and stimulation of the sympathetic nervous system and renin-angiotensin system. Growing data emphasizes the significance of increased mineralocorticoid activity in RH. Recent findings from the NHANES (National Health and Nutrition Examination Survey) of 13 375 hypertensive adults demonstrate that body mass index (BMI) ≥30 kg/m^2 approximately doubles the risk for aTRH. In 14 461 patients with RH in the Spanish Ambulatory Blood Pressure Monitoring Registry, a BMI ≥30 kg/m^2 was also an independent risk factor for RH (odds ratio, 1.62; 95% CI, 1.32–1.99). Even among 3367 hypertensives with CKD, increasing levels of obesity were independently associated with higher risks of aTRH, ranging from an odds ratio of 1.52 (BMI ≥30 kg/m^2) to 2.26 (BMI ≥40 kg/m^2). Finally, in a large data set (>470 000) from the Kaiser Permanente Southern California health system, obesity (BMI ≥30 kg/m^2) was also found to be an independent risk factor for RH (odds ratio, 1.62; 95% CI, 1.42–1.51). Although obesity has the potential to promote spurious elevations in BP (e.g., use of a smaller-than-optimal BP cuff), these findings nonetheless strongly support a direct role for excess adiposity in promoting RH.

4.2.3. Dietary Sodium

There is no doubt that higher dietary sodium intake causes arterial blood pressure to rise. Nonetheless, there are sizable interindividual differences in the "salt sensitivity" of blood pressure. The processes are intricate and probably involve a wide range of reactions in addition to excessive volume retention, such as immune cell modulation, renin-angiotensin axis suppression impairment, arterial stiffness, sympathetic activation, vascular dysfunction, and mineralocorticoid receptor activation.

It is more challenging to determine with precision how much excess dietary sodium contributes to RH for many reasons, including the challenges associated with precisely characterizing routine intake in the relevant populations. Still, many recently released studies point to a possible involvement. While 24-

hour urine sodium levels were not elevated, brain natriuretic peptide was higher and PRA was lower in 279 RH patients compared to control patients, suggesting a relative volume excess component. One-third of 204 patients with genuine RH determined by ambulatory monitoring showed signs of excessive sodium consumption (i.e., >200 mEq in 24-hour urine levels). Large population studies that have consistently connected aTRH to chronic renal insufficiency—a known cause of elevated salt sensitivity of blood pressure—provide additional indirect evidence. Possibly the strongest evidence comes from the few clinical trials showing significant drops in blood pressure in RH patients after a low-sodium diet (Diaz et al., 2014).

4.2.3.1. Alcohol

Drinking alcohol has been associated with elevated blood pressure and an increased risk of hypertension. Men and women may exhibit different dose-response associations (linear and J-shaped, respectively), and metabolic genes may influence this relationship. However, excessive alcohol consumption (>30–50 g/d) is a known risk factor for hypertension.

4.2.4. Physical Inactivity

Lower physical fitness and less physical activity are two separate risk factors for hypertension. Research on young adults, men, and women has demonstrated graded inverse associations between activity and fitness level and the risk of developing high blood pressure. Additional evidence suggests that leading a sedentary lifestyle (e.g., increased television viewing) separately encourages the development of hypertension. On the other hand, few studies have documented links between physical inactivity and RH. Among patients in the REGARDS cohort, self-reported inactivity was not associated with RH in addition to other poor lifestyle factors. However, a randomized study showing that a thrice-weekly treadmill walking exercise program for 8 to 12 weeks significantly lowered daytime ambulatory BP (6±12/3±7 mm Hg; P=0.03) among 50 treated patients with RH provides indirect support for the important role of activity.

4.2.5. Dietary Pattern and Other Risk Factors

According to a recent meta-analysis, the Dietary Approaches to Stop Hypertension (DASH) eating pattern is well-established to lower blood pressure by 6/7 mm Hg. However, a low DASH diet questionnaire score was not independently linked to aTRH, similar to other lifestyle factors in the REGARDS cohort. To precisely determine how a poor diet contributes to the pathophysiology of RH, more research is required. stresses related to psychology (e.g., negative personality traits (anxiety, anger, depression), low social support, occupational stress, and decreased sleep duration/quality have also been linked to high blood pressure; however, there is a dearth of data specifically connecting these factors to recurrent headaches. Lastly, exposure to a range of environmental factors, such as loud noises (e.g., traffic), and chilly weather (e.g., high altitudes, air pollution, and winter) all encourage elevated blood pressure. Further research is necessary to clarify the possible influence of these often-encountered environmental factors on relative humidity (RH) (Coulhon et al., 2008).

4.2.6. Drug-Related RH

Drug-induced RH can be exacerbated by many pharmacologic agent classes that raise blood pressure (Table 4.2). However, it is discovered that these agents' effects are highly individualistic, with some people experiencing significant elevations in blood pressure and the majority exhibiting little to no effect at all.

Table 4.2. *Drugs and Other Substances with Potential to Induce or Exacerbate Elevated BP and Hypertension*

NSAIDs
Oral contraceptives
Sympathomimetic
Cyclosporine, tacrolimus
Erythropoietin
VEGF inhibitors
Alcohol
Cocaine
Amphetamines
Antidepressants
Glucocorticoids, mineralocorticoids

Source: https://www.ahajournals.org/doi/10.1161/HYP.0000000000000084

4.2.6.1. Nonsteroidal Anti-Inflammatory Agents

Because they decrease the synthesis of prostaglandins E_2 and I_2, nonsteroidal anti-inflammatory drugs (NSAIDs) raise blood pressure by reducing vasodilation and sodium excretion. NSAIDs are regarded as one of the most frequent offending agents affecting BP control due to their extensive use. Generally speaking, both normotensive and hypertensive people's blood pressure can be impacted by nontopical NSAIDs when taken in doses high enough to minimize inflammation and pain. Meta-analyses have shown that there is considerable variability in the average rise in mean arterial pressure, with reports varying from 2 to 5 mm Hg. Moreover, NSAIDs have an impact on how well various antihypertensive drug classes, such as β-blockers, ACE inhibitors, diuretics, and ARBs, work. It is crucial to remember that interactions between antihypertensive medications and CCBs have generally not been demonstrated, and using NSAIDs may have little to no impact on the effectiveness of α- and β-blockers.

There are notable differences in the extent of blood pressure changes in hypertensive patients on antihypertensive medications, despite reports of the impact of NSAIDs on the incidence of hypertension as previously discussed. NSAIDs had no effect on blood pressure in patients taking diuretics, according to multiple studies. For ACE inhibitor users, the SBP increase with NSAIDs varied from 5 to 10 mm Hg. The mechanism by which NSAIDs inhibit prostaglandins is thought to account for the ACE inhibitors' diminished ability to lower blood pressure (Mancia et al., 2013).

Different NSAID types have different blood pressure effects; for example, selective COX-2 (cyclooxygenase-2) inhibitors, like celecoxib, have a lower blood pressure effect than conventional NSAIDs. The kidneys' inhibition of COX-2 is thought to be the dose-dependent BP effect, which also results in an increase in intravascular volume and a decrease in sodium excretion. In contrast, the HOT study's (Hypertension Optimal Treatment) findings show that low-dose aspirin has no effects on blood pressure or COX-2 inhibition. These findings, however, cannot be applied to higher aspirin dosages.

4.2.6.2. Oral Contraceptives and Hormone Replacement

By increasing the biosynthesis of angiotensin, oral contraceptives cause hypertension and elevated blood pressure. In comparison to women who did not use oral contraceptives, women who used oral contraceptives had an 80% higher risk of developing hypertension, according to the Nurses' Health Study, which followed up on over 60,000 normotensive women for four years. Nevertheless, the use of oral contraceptives was only responsible for 41.05 cases of hypertension per 10,000 person-years, and this number quickly decreased when treatment was stopped. Comparably, a different study on hypertensive women found that those who used oral contraceptives experienced more severe hypertension and had worse rates of blood pressure control than those who used other forms of contraception. The kind of oral contraceptive is crucial; higher rates of blood pressure elevation have been linked to combined oral contraceptives (progestin and estradiol) than to lower-dose oral contraceptives that contain only progestin or estradiol. The use of high-dose estrogen was linked to mean elevations in SBP of 3 to 6 mm Hg and ≈5% of women developing new hypertension, according to epidemiological studies. When estrogen use is stopped, blood pressure usually returns to normal in two to twelve months, although proteinuria may linger. Because estrogen increases the production of angiotensinogen, the renin-angiotensin system may be the mechanism underlying the hypertensive effect of oral contraceptives.

4.2.6.3. Other Agents

1. Recombinant Human Erythropoietin

In a dose-dependent manner, recombinant human erythropoietin can raise blood pressure through intricate mechanisms, leading to hypertension in 20–33% of patients. Long-term erythropoietin use maintains elevated blood pressure while promoting the growth of vascular smooth muscle cells, vascular remodeling, and medial hypertrophy. Antihypertensive drugs can be used to treat erythropoietin-induced hypertension, frequently with just one medication.

2. Tyrosine Kinase Inhibitors

Antineoplastic medications that block the VEGF (vascular endothelial growth factor) pathway have been shown to cause hypertension in cancer patients undergoing treatment. For instance, patients on VEGF inhibitor therapy frequently developed hypertension. Many explanations are put forth, such as decreased bioavailability of prostacyclin and nitric oxide, increased systemic vascular resistance, and vascular stiffness, which has been seen in animals given VEGF tyrosine kinase inhibitors.

3. Cocaine

Tachycardia and BP elevation are common clinical manifestations of cocaine use. BP elevation is caused by increased central sympathetic outflow and blockade of neuronal norepinephrine reuptake, resulting in neurotransmitter accumulation in the synaptic cleft with intense sympathetic activation.

4. Amphetamines

Amphetamines enhance the sympathetic nervous system's activation by producing more norepinephrine. Similar to the side effects of cocaine, amphetamines can cause tachycardia and hypertension. Children receiving treatment for attention deficit disorder have been linked to the development of hypertension when given methylphenidate. Mescaline can raise blood pressure and has effects that are strikingly similar to amphetamines (Mancia et al., 2013).

5. Antidepressants

When people who take monoamine oxidase inhibitors eat foods high in tyramine, their blood pressure can become dangerously elevated. By lengthening norepinephrine's half-life at sympathetic nerve terminals, the medications themselves can worsen hypertension; however, this effect is frequently amplified when amine precursors are also ingested. When comparing triadlcypromine to moclobemide and brofaromine, it is the agent that is most likely to increase blood pressure. It has been observed that tricyclic antidepressants raise blood pressure in people with panic disorders. Similarly, in patients receiving therapeutic doses of venlafaxine, reports of dose-dependent increases in blood pressure have been made. Furthermore, individuals receiving antidepressant medications like fluoxetine have been found to have severe hypertension.

4.2.7. Sleep Disorders and Pseudopheochromocytoma

4.2.7.1. Sleep Deprivation and Pseudopheochromocytoma

Sleep disturbances and a related condition called pseudopheochromocytoma are contributing factors to RH. This term was first used in 1999 to describe a syndrome similar to pheochromocytoma. Pseudochemocytoma is a syndrome that presents with three distinct features of paroxysmal hypertension: abrupt elevation of blood pressure, equally abrupt onset of physically distressing symptoms, and absence of reported fear or panic at the onset of attacks. It should be considered after true pheochromocytoma has been ruled out. Patients who had previously denied an emotionally traumatizing event were included in the original description; many of them recovered with antidepressant therapy, β-blockers, and counseling. Numerous case reports of pseudopheochromocytoma have been published since then, and a recent update summarizes the syndrome.

Poor sleep quality is a related issue that many people with pseudopheochromocytoma experience. Long-term poor sleep quality, particularly in the afternoon and evening, results in the same symptoms of elevated blood pressure and paroxysmal hypertension. Not only can OSA lead to poor sleep quality, but many other sleep disorders as well, such as insomnia and restless legs syndrome. These various sleep disorders frequently coexist and keep the patient from getting the rest they need.

The activation of both the sympathetic nervous system and the renin-angiotensin-aldosterone system is the mechanism by which low-quality sleep leads to elevated blood pressure and paroxysmal episodes of extremely high blood pressure. Restless legs syndrome, OSA, and sleep deprivation all result in increased sympathetic activity. Data from a post hoc analysis of the SYMPLICITY HTN-3 trial assessed the impact of renal denervation versus sham control on office and ambulatory (including nocturnal) SBP in patients with OSA, which lends additional support to this in RH. Renal denervation decreased the 6-month office SBP in OSA subjects when compared to sham control.

Individuals without OSA who experience sleep deprivation—which is defined as getting fewer than six hours of uninterrupted sleep—also exhibit elevated sympathetic activity. In this instance, the nocturnal drop in blood pressure is also influenced by a result of less time spent in slow-wave or non-rapid eye movement sleep. This lends support to the theory that sleep deprivation or restless legs syndrome cause an increase in sympathetic tone through disrupted non-rapid eye movement sleep quantity or quality.

The day following a sleepless night is associated with elevated heart rate, diastolic blood pressure, and SBP in comparison to the day following a typical sleep; norepinephrine excretion in the urine is also elevated. Peripheral vascular resistance, heart rate, and blood pressure also gradually drop during non-rapid eye movement sleep. As a result, any decline in the quantity or quality of sleep may be linked to an increase in nocturnal blood pressure, which may have a role in the development of inadequate hypertension control.

The increase in sympathetic activity linked to OSA is a result of intermittent hypoxia, as opposed to decreased sleep duration and quality; the degree of oxygen desaturation at night is reflected in the short-term rise in blood pressure. Indeed, both animal models that are exclusively exposed to intermittent hypoxia and healthy human volunteers who are exposed to intermittent hypoxia in a "tent" exhibit increased sympathetic activity. A meta-analysis provides additional evidence that the renin-angiotensin system contributes to respiratory event-related intermittent hypoxia in addition to the adrenergic system's hyperactivity. It is also noteworthy that treatment with continuous positive airway pressure (CPAP) only marginally lowers hypertension associated with OSA. Nonetheless, when taking into account the risk of either developing or controlling preexisting hypertension, treating sleep disorders or habits is important.

There is a strong correlation between OSA and poor blood pressure control, particularly in patients whose apnea/hypopnea index is at least 30 events per hour. When sleep apnea is treated with CPAP, adherents experience a reduction in blood pressure. However, since the reduction in SBP ranges only from 2 to 5 mm Hg, adjunctive medications are nearly always required. BP control is improved by using ARBs, some β-blockers, and central α-agonists like guanfacine, a longer-acting medication with comparable activity, or clonidine before bed. The risk of developing hypertension rises when one does not spend enough time in the deep stages of sleep.

Self-reported sleep duration and the prevalence of hypertension are correlated in a U-shaped way, with 7 to 8 hours of uninterrupted sleep per night representing the nadir of the U. Hypertension is more common when sleep duration is either lowered or raised beyond this range. Additionally, the length of sleep of. <5 hours is associated with incident hypertension in subjects <60 years of age, whereas sleep duration of > In subjects over 60, 9 hours per night is linked to incident hypertension. Larger, more recent studies and meta-analyses have further confirmed these initial findings (Mancia et al., 2013).

The length and quality of sleep play a crucial role in regulating blood pressure in RH. Because sleep quality and duration activate the sympathetic and renin-angiotensin systems, which further exacerbate the effects of hypertension, clinicians should regularly inquire about these factors. A clinical indicator that may be connected to poor sleep quality is the elevated heart rate that many of these patients will have in relation to their blood pressure. Restoring normal sleep patterns and using agents that block the systems causing the issue are crucial in this situation. It should be noted that the patient will experience nocturnal micturition and disrupted sleep if they are taking diuretics and do not follow a low-sodium diet. Additionally, diuretics raise sympathetic tone; ARBs do not blunt this activation, but spironolactone does.

4.2.8. Secondary Hypertension: Diagnosis and Management

4.2.8.1. Primary Aldosteronism

Primary aldosteronism is a group of disorders characterized by excessive production of aldosterone, which is independent of the renin-angiotensin system and unaffected by sodium levels. This condition can lead to hypertension, hypokalemia, metabolic alkalosis, and complications such as cardiovascular and renal disease. The harmful effects of aldosterone on the heart and blood vessels contribute to a higher risk of cardiovascular events, including stroke, myocardial infarction, and atrial fibrillation, compared to primary hypertension. Primary aldosteronism is also associated with various cardiovascular issues, such as left ventricular hypertrophy, diastolic dysfunction, heart failure, arterial stiffness, oxidative stress, inflammation, fibrosis, and vessel remodeling.

Most research suggests that a particularly common cause of RH is primary aldosteronism. Numerous observational studies conducted in various countries have revealed that patients with confirmed RH have a prevalence rate of approximately 20% for primary aldosteronism. In primary hypertension, the overall prevalence of primary aldosteronism is approximately 8%, which is in contrast to this comparatively high prevalence. Nonetheless, only 7.1% of the 1656 hypertensive Chinese patients with RH had confirmed primary aldosteronism, demonstrating a notable variation in prevalence across populations. In light of the prevalence of primary aldosteronism, it is critical to confirm the findings of this screening test with one of the four suggested confirmatory tests rather than merely accepting positive plasma aldosterone:renin ratio as the disease's diagnosis. To confirm the diagnosis, saline infusion was administered to every patient in the Chinese study (Hameed et al., 2016).

All patients with RH should be screened because primary aldosteronism is comparatively common in these individuals. The ratio of plasma aldosterone concentration to PRA (aldosterone/renin ratio [ARR]) from a blood sample drawn in the morning, with the patient seated for at least 30 minutes before sampling, should be used to screen for primary aldosteronism. An ARR of >30 is needed for a positive screening test, or >20 if the plasma aldosterone level is less than 16 ng/dL. Adequate patient preparation before the test is crucial for maintaining the validity of the screening test. Before testing, hypokalemia (which lowers aldosterone secretion) should be treated with oral K+ supplements. At least one month before testing, pharmacological agents such as eplerenone, high-dose amiloride, and spirolactone that significantly alter plasma ARR should be stopped. It is also critical to understand that antihypertensive drugs other than amiloride, eplerenone, and spironolactone can affect the outcomes of screening tests. For instance, ACE inhibitors, ARBs, dihydropyridine CCBs, non-potassium-sparing diuretics, and β-adrenergic receptor blockers and renin inhibitors suppress PRA, while dihydropyridine CCBs, ACE inhibitors, and ARBs increase PRA and change plasma ARR values. In the event that the results of the initial screening test are unconvincing, these drugs may be selectively stopped for a minimum of two weeks while other agents that do not affect the renin-angiotensin-aldosterone system—such as hydralazine, slow-release verapamil, or an α1-adrenergic receptor antagonist—are used to control blood pressure (prazosin, doxazosin, or terazosin).

The patient is typically referred to an endocrinologist or hypertension specialist for additional evaluation if the screening test for primary aldosteronism comes back positive. A confirmatory test (such as captopril, fludrocortisone, oral salt-loading, or saline suppression tests) may be administered as a next step. Adrenal venous sampling is typically used for subtype classification if one of these tests confirms the presence of primary aldosteronism. Individuals who have unilateral disease (50%; either aldosterone-producing adenoma or, less commonly, unilateral hyperplasia) react well to unilateral laparoscopic adrenalectomy, with 50% or more achieving complete cure or 50% improving in terms of blood pressure control. When taking spironolactone or eplerenone, patients with bilateral idiopathic hyperaldosteronism typically experience a significant improvement in the control of their hypertension.

4.2.9. Other Causes of Secondary Hypertension

In addition to the above, other unusual/rare endocrine causes of secondary hypertension are included in Table 4.3.

Table 4.3. *Other Endocrine Causes of Secondary Hypertension*

Disorder	Major Clinical Findings	Physical Examination	**Screening Tests**	**Additional/ Confirmatory Tests**
Hypothyroidism	Dry skin; cold intolerance; constipation; hoarseness; weight gain	Delayed ankle reflex; periorbital puffiness; coarse skin; cold skin; slow movement; goiter	High TSH; low or normal fT4	
Hyperthyroidism	Warm, moist skin; heat intolerance; nervousness; tremulousness; insomnia; weight loss; diarrhea; proximal muscle weakness	Lid lag; fine tremor of the outstretched hands; warm, moist skin	Low TSH; high or normal fT4 and T3	Radioactive iodine uptake and scan
Hypercalcemia and primary hyperparathyroidism	Hypercalcemia	Usually none	Serum calcium	Serum parathyroid hormone
Congenital adrenal hyperplasia (excess DOC)	Hypertension and hypokalemia; virilization (11-β-OH deficiency); incomplete masculinization in males and primary amenorrhea in females (17-α-OH deficiency)	Signs of virilization (11β) or incomplete masculinization (17α)	Hypertension and hypokalemia with low or normal aldosterone and renin	11-β-OH: elevated DOC, 11-deoxycortisol and androgens; 17-α-OH: decreased androgens and estrogen; elevated DOC and corticosterone
Other mineralocorticoid excess syndromes caused by DOC	Early-onset hypertension, hypokalemia	Arrhythmias (with hypokalemia)	Low aldosterone and renin	DOC; urinary cortisol metabolites; genetic testing
Acromegaly	Acral features; enlarging shoe, glove, or hat size; headache; visual disturbances; diabetes mellitus	Acral features; large hands and feet; frontal bossing	Serum growth hormone ≥1 ng/mL during oral glucose load	Elevated age- and sex-matched IGF-1 level; MRI scan of the pituitary

DOC indicates deoxycorticosterone; fT4, free thyroxine; IGF-1, insulin-like growth factor-1; MRI, magnetic resonance imaging; OH, hydroxylase; T3, triiodothyronine; and TSH, thyroid-stimulating hormone.

Source: https://www.ahajournals.org/doi/10.1161/HYP.0000000000000084

4.3. EVALUATION OF RH

When evaluating patients with RH, the goals should be to confirm that they are truly resistant to treatment, find the reasons behind their resistance (such as secondary causes of hypertension), and record any complications that arise from the course of their hypertensive disease (refer to Figure 4.2 for the evaluation algorithm).

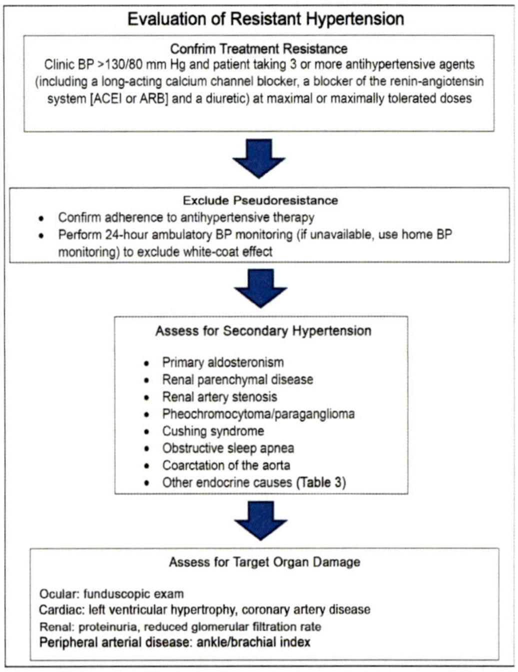

Figure 4.2. *Algorithm depicting the evaluation of resistant hypertension. ACEI indicates angiotensin-converting enzyme inhibitor; ARB, angiotensin receptor blocker; and BP, blood pressure.*

Source: https://www.ncbi.nlm.nih.gov/pmc/articles/PMC6530990/bin/nihms-1016897-f0002.jpg.

To verify RH, assessments of treatment adherence and ABPM use (or home blood pressure monitoring if ABPM is not available) are required. True RH typically has several underlying causes, such as obesity, CKD, OSA, and excessive salt consumption in the diet. The evaluation of comorbidities and hypertensive complications is important because it affects the choice of pharmacological agent class and blood pressure targets for antihypertensive treatment.

4.3.1. Medical History

Along with adherence to doctor's appointments and antihypertensive treatment, clinical and adverse event responses to previous antihypertensive medication, and current prescription and over-the-counter medications that may raise blood pressure or interfere with the effects of antihypertensive drugs, documentation of the duration, severity, and behavior of the hypertension is crucial. Accurate self-reported medication adherence is uncommon in the clinical setting. Therefore, physicians need to politely ask patients about how frequently they might forget to take their medications every week, whether side effects could be contributing to their nonadherence, or whether they are facing financial difficulties that make it difficult for them to pay for their antihypertensive medications out of pocket (Diaz et al., 2014).

4.3.1.1. Physical Examination

The goal of an RH patient's examination should be to determine any target organ damage and any potential secondary causes. As previously mentioned, blood pressure should be measured. When investigating the possibility of vascular disease, including in the retina, fundoscopic evaluation, meticulous assessment of the carotid and peripheral pulse quality, and bruit auscultation should all be done. Abdominal bruits are not specific, but they raise the risk of obstructive renal artery disease. BP should be measured in both arms and in the thigh (in patients <30 years of age) if aortic occlusive disease or aortic coarctation is suspected. If the thigh SBP is >10 mm Hg lower than the arm SBP while the patient is supine, imaging studies for coarctation should be performed. Hypercortisolism may be suspected in patients with obesity, diabetes mellitus, hypertension, depression, and bone loss accompanied by abdominal striae, "moon" facies, and intrascapular fat deposition.

4.3.1.2. Out-of-Office BP Monitoring

The differences in BP between in-office and out-of-office readings ought to be resolved. Self-measurements (at home or at work), unattended automated office measurements, and ABPM are useful in figuring out whether there could be a white-coat effect that gives the impression of treatment resistance. Since ABPM has been shown to be a more reliable indicator of CVD morbidity and mortality than clinic measurements and has been recommended for use in the diagnosis of hypertension in both the United States and the United Kingdom, it is the most objective and robust way to define the white-coat effect among these methods.

In patients with normal or lower self-measured blood pressure, in those without target organ involvement (e.g., retinopathy, CKD, left ventricular hypertrophy), and in cases where symptoms of excessive antihypertensive therapy are present, a white-coat effect (office blood pressure above goal but ambulatory blood pressure below goal) should be taken into consideration. If a white-coat effect is verified, drug therapy adjustments and the confirmation of BP goal achievement should be made using out-of-office measurements (ambulatory or self-measured values if ABPM is unavailable).

4.3.2. Biochemical Evaluation

A basic metabolic profile (serum sodium, potassium, chloride, bicarbonate, glucose, blood urea nitrogen, and creatinine), as well as a urinalysis and a paired morning plasma aldosterone and PRA to screen for primary aldosteronism, should be part of the laboratory examination for a patient with RH. Certain antihypertensive medications, such as direct renin inhibitors and β-adrenergic blocking drugs (which lower renin levels) or mineralocorticoid receptor antagonists (which raise aldosterone levels), make the interpretation of the ARR more difficult. Due to its high negative predictive value for primary aldosteronism screening, the ratio is a useful screening tool. Due to the prevalence of low-renin states (such as volume expansion, dietary salt excess, or sensitivity), the specificity for a high ARR is low. In patients taking an ACE inhibitor or ARB, which elevates PRA and increases the sensitivity of the ratio if renin is still suppressed, a high ratio (> 20) when serum aldosterone is >16 ng/dL and PRA is <0.6 ng/mL per hour is suggestive of primary aldosteronism. However, additional assessments are necessary to confirm the diagnosis. Assessing plasma metanephrine levels or 24-hour urine metanephrine levels is a useful screening test for individuals who may have paraganglioma or pheochromocytoma (Parati et al., 2010).

4.3.2.1. Noninvasive Imaging

Patients with a high probability of renovascular disease, such as young individuals with possible fibromuscular dysplasia and older patients with a history of smoking or vascular disease who are atherosclerosis-prone, should be the only ones undergoing imaging for the assessment of renal artery stenosis in patients with RH. The typical initial test is duplex ultrasonography of the renal arteries to calculate the velocities of the aortic and renal arteries. This method is preferred as a screening tool over computerized tomography and magnetic resonance angiography, especially in cases where patients have CKD (e.g., eGFR <60 $mL \cdot min^{-1} \cdot 1.73\ m^{-2}$). It is not advised to perform a direct renal arteriography in the absence of suspicious noninvasive imaging. High-resolution CT or magnetic resonance imaging of the abdomen is recommended for the imaging of the adrenal glands only in cases where there is biochemical evidence of hormonally active tumors (e.g., elevated aldosterone, catecholamines, or cortisol).

4.3.3. Management of RH

An algorithm for managing RH is depicted in Figure 4.3.

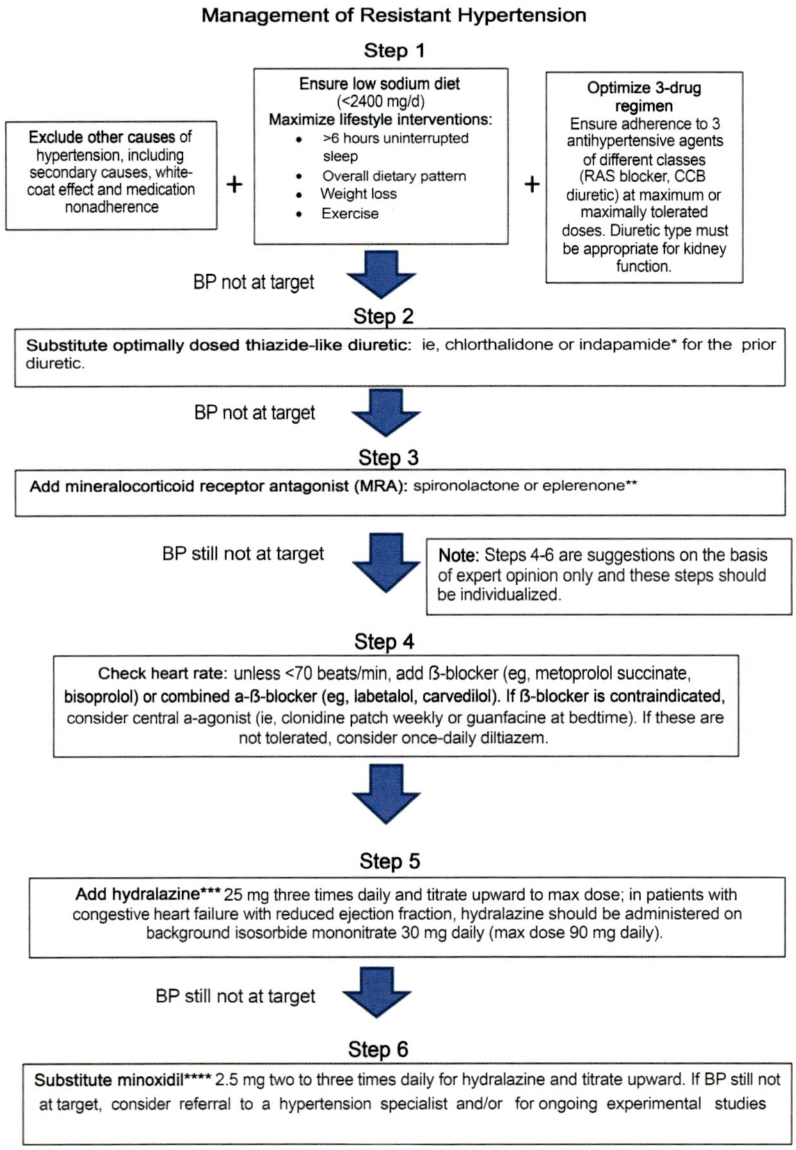

Figure 4.3. *Algorithm depicting the management of resistant hypertension. BP indicates blood pressure; CCB, calcium channel blocker; and RAS, renin-angiotensin system. *These diuretics maintain efficacy down to estimated glomerular filtration rates (eGFRs) of 30 mL·min−1·1.73 m−2. **Use caution if eGFR is <30 mL·min−1·1.73 m−2. ***Requires concomitant use of a β-blocker and diuretic. ****Requires the concomitant use of a β-blocker and loop diuretic.*

Source: *https://www.ncbi.nlm.nih.gov/pmc/articles/PMC6530990/bin/nihms-1016897-f0003.jpg.*

4.3.4. Lifestyle Interventions

4.3.4.1. Weight Loss

According to the most recent meta-analysis, it is well established that weight-reducing diets can lower blood pressure in patients with hypertension by 4.5/3.2 mm Hg. However, the results of pharmaceutically assisted weight loss are inconsistent; while some drugs, like orlistat, have some benefit, others, like sibutramine, may even increase blood pressure. Despite the fact that obesity is a known risk factor for RH, there aren't many studies showing how effective weight loss is for these patients. To help lower blood pressure, guidelines consistently promote a healthy lifestyle, which includes caloric restriction. For overweight and obese adults, the goal should be to lose between >5% and -10% of their body weight. Despite the paucity of published research involving these patients, the same guidelines ought to be followed by those who have RH. This is especially true given that losing weight can successfully result in medication withdrawal, which will ease the control of hypertension. It is crucial to remember that the long-term persistence of weight loss (>1 year) and the corresponding drop in blood pressure are not well understood and call for more research (Parati et al., 2010).

4.3.4.2. Dietary Salt Restriction

A reduced-sodium diet is well-proven to decrease BP. In a recent meta-analysis, an estimated 1-g (43.5-mmol) reduction in daily sodium intake produces a 2.1– and 1.2–mm Hg decrease in SBP among hypertensive and normotensive patients, respectively. In addition to hypertensives, other subgroups of individuals (e.g., those with CKD and obesity, blacks) are often more sensitive and can derive particularly robust benefits from sodium restriction. In patients with RH, 2 recent small studies have demonstrated the efficacy of a reduced dietary sodium intake for BP lowering. In 12 patients with true RH (taking 3.4±0.5 antihypertensive medications), a low-sodium (50 mmol/d) versus a high-sodium (250 mmol/d) diet resulted in a profound reduction in average office BP (−22.7/−9.1 mm Hg) over a 7-day period. The low-sodium diet also led to significant reductions in daytime, nocturnal, and 24-hour BP levels (−20.1/−9.8 mm Hg). In a 6-week-long double-blind placebo-controlled crossover trial of 20 patients with stage 3 to 4 CKD, many of whom had RH (average, 3.2 ± 1.1 antihypertensive medications), a low-sodium (75 mmol/24-hour urine) versus a high-sodium (168 mmol/24-hour urine) diet significantly reduced 24-hour ambulatory BP (−9.7/−3.9 mm Hg).

The ideal sodium intake for preventing CVD morbidity and mortality is still up for debate. Although blood pressure continues to drop linearly with even greater reductions to 173 to 217 mmol/d (4–5 g/d), there is concern that a U-shaped relationship may exist, with the greatest risk reductions being achieved by adhering to only moderate restrictions in sodium intake. <65 mmol/d (1.5 g/d). It has been posited that the sympathetic nervous system and renin-angiotensin system activation may counter the health benefits derived from the additional BP lowering at the lower range of sodium intake <130 mmol/d (3 g/d). AHA recommendations have continued to promulgate that an ideal daily sodium intake is <65 mmol/d (1.5 g/d), particularly among high-risk populations. Moreover, it is possible that the meta-analysis findings do not apply specifically to individuals with RH and that the additional BP lowering achieved through sodium restriction may offset putative risks of achieving low levels of sodium intake. Evidence-based recommendations on the optimal sodium intake among patients with RH must await more definitive clinical trial data. For the time being, the available studies (albeit of short-term duration) support that sodium restriction, even to low levels <65 to 100 mmol/d (1.5–3.0 g/d), yields significant linear reductions in BP among patients with high BP and RH. Therefore, it seems prudent to continue to support the prior AHA recommendations for patients with RH to reduce daily sodium intake to <100 mmol/d (2.3 g/d) and to consider more stringent restrictions to <65 mmol/d (1.5 g/d) on a case-by-case basis. Future trials testing the efficacy of this approach, particularly over longer-term durations (> 3-6 months), are essential.

4.3.4.3. DASH Diet and Other Dietary Factors

A DASH-style eating pattern, alcohol restriction to <10 g/d (women) and <20 g/d (men), and a variety of other dietary modifications can each yield significant reductions in BP among patients with hypertension. There are no studies examining diet interventions specifically for RH patients. Patients with RH should adhere to the established dietary guidelines supported by the American Heart Association and American Society of Hypertension, which are described in detail elsewhere, due to their proven safety and effectiveness in lowering blood pressure in the general hypertensive population. Patients with more advanced (stages 4 and 5) CKD should proceed cautiously when implementing a potassium-rich DASH diet, as they are susceptible to severe hyperkalemia and its aftereffects.

1. Exercise

Exercise has been shown in numerous clinical trials to be an effective way to lower blood pressure, especially in patients who already have hypertension. A range of endurance (aerobic) exercise programs reduced blood pressure in hypertensive patients by 8.3/5.2 mm Hg over several weeks, according to the largest meta-analysis to date. Furthermore, it has been demonstrated that dynamic resistance exercise lowers blood pressure in hypertensive patients by 1.8/3.2 mm Hg. As was previously mentioned, one study found that a treadmill walking exercise program was both safe and effective in lowering blood pressure in patients with RH. A water-based aerobic exercise program may be safe and effective for lowering blood pressure in this population, according to a recent small pilot study (n= 16). Despite the paucity of evidence, it would seem reasonable for patients with RH to adhere to the latest exercise guidelines, which are supported by multiple expert guidelines, such as the 2017 American College of Cardiology/AHA guideline, to lower their blood pressure. Generally speaking, this entails ≥150 minutes per week (division into 3–5 sessions of 30–40 minutes) of moderate–intense aerobic activity, best complemented by 2–3 sessions of mild resistance training. Some people may not be able to engage in moderate-to-intense aerobic activity because RH is more prevalent in older and obese adults. In sedentary people, low-intensity exercise, 6 minutes per hour over an 8-hour period, decreased blood pressure (14/8 mm Hg) and improved metabolic syndrome variables. Low-intensity exercise may also be just as beneficial as moderate-to-intense exercise in preventing type 2 diabetes mellitus, which is a concern for non-diabetic adults with RH, according to available data (Coulhon et al., 2008).

4.3.4.4. Alternative Approaches

The evidence proving alternative methods are effective at lowering blood pressure was examined in a recent scientific statement from the American Heart Association. While many therapies, like acupuncture and yoga, lacked sufficient scientific backing, some were thought to have potential for use in clinical settings. These included transcendental meditation, slow breathing guided by a device, and isometric handgrip exercises. More recent data keeps proving that isometric handgrips in particular are effective. According to the most recent meta-analysis, isometric handgrip reduces blood pressure by 5.2/3.9 mm Hg when done for 12 minutes, three to five times a week. Nevertheless, no trials involving RH patients have been carried out. More research is necessary to determine whether any alternative strategy can effectively control blood pressure in this population as an adjuvant. Additionally, the effectiveness of addressing other lifestyle factors that have been connected to elevated blood pressure or relative humidity, like enhancing sleep quality and reducing environmental triggers (e.g., noise, pollution, and cold) are still unknown. An intensive multifaceted lifestyle intervention program versus routine care is being investigated in at least one ongoing randomized clinical trial (TRIUMPH [Triple Pill vs Usual Care Management for Patients with Mild-to-Moderate Hypertension]) to determine which is more effective for patients with RH.

4.3.5. Pharmacological Treatment of RH

4.3.5.1. General Principles

Therapeutic approaches to improved blood pressure control in RH can start once all identifiable forms of hypertension, especially those with endocrine causes excluded, have been ruled out and contributions from the white-coat effect (office BP at least 20/10 mm Hg higher than home or ABPM measurements) and masked uncontrolled hypertension (office BP measurements suggesting adequate BP control but out-of-office readings elevated above goal) have been taken into consideration. Three mechanistically complementary antihypertensive agents, commonly including a long-acting CCB, a blocker of the renin-angiotensin system (ACE inhibitor or ARB), and a diuretic, should already be prescribed and taken by the patient to ensure a proper diagnosis of RH (Figure 4.3, step 1). Hydrochlorothiazide does not induce a predictable natriuresis below a GFR of 45 $mL \cdot min^{-1} \cdot 1.73\ m^{-2}$, but chlorthalidone induces natriuresis down to an eGFR of 30 $mL \cdot min^{-1} \cdot 1.73\ m^{-2}$. Thiazide or thiazide-like diuretics are appropriate down to an eGFR of 25 to 30 $mL \cdot min^{-1} \cdot 1.73\ m^{-2}$. Below this eGFR level or in hypoalbuminemia states (i.e., serum albumin < 3.0 g/L), a long-acting loop diuretic such as torsemide should be used over shorter-acting agents such as bumetanide or furosemide. These 3 separate pharmacological classes of antihypertensive agents must be given at maximally tolerated doses such as amlodipine 10 mg, chlorthalidone 25 mg, and one of the ACE inhibitors or ARBs at maximal dose. Suboptimal medication regimens are common in patients with hypertension resistant to antihypertensive therapy (Hameed et al., 2016).

4.3.5.2. Specific Therapeutic Regimens

The majority of RH cases are associated with either high sympathetic tone, particularly in CKD, or volume excess, so determining the pathogenesis will best aid in selecting the fourth medication. Furthermore, when a fourth agent is added, it is crucial to make sure the best antihypertensive drug from specific pharmacological classes is chosen (Table 4.4).

Table 4.4. *Specific Clinical Issues Associated With Treatment Resistance**

Issue Associated With Treatment Resistance	Management Consideration(s)
Volume control, edema resolution	Thiazide→chlorthalidone→loop diuretic
Heart rate control inadequate	β-Blocker, α,β-blocker, verapamil, diltiazem
Renin and aldosterone levels low	Low-salt diet, avoid nighttime shift work, amiloride

Renin low, aldosterone normal to high normal	Mineralocorticoid receptor antagonist
Would split dosing of medications improve control?	Evaluate BP pattern according to home and ambulatory BP monitoring
Medication adherence questionable	Initiate indirect or direct methods to detect nonadherence; if nonadherence is documented (partial or complete), discuss frankly, nonjudgmentally with the patient and family
Pattern of BP response to medications outside clinician visit times unknown	Identify meal effects on BP, duration of medication effect, relationship of BP to side effects using out-of-office BP monitoring
Sleep disordered breathing; significant anxiety associated with highly variable hypertension	Initiate nondrug strategies concurrently with or separately from antihypertensive drug therapy

4.3.5.3. BP Indicates Blood Pressure

Selecting the right diuretic is crucial in managing resistant hypertension, as volume excess and poor adherence to low-sodium diets are commonly seen in patients. Thiazide-like diuretics such as chlorthalidone and indapamide have the most evidence supporting their efficacy in reducing cardiovascular events. Studies have shown that switching from hydrochlorothiazide to chlorthalidone can lead to an additional reduction in systolic blood pressure by 7 to 8 mm Hg.

Recent reports document the efficacy of mineralocorticoid receptor blockade (Figure 4.3, step 3, and Table 4.4) to improve BP in patients with RH. In patients who are not overtly volume overloaded but who have evidence of low renin status or salt sensitivity of BP, mineralocorticoid receptor antagonists (spironolactone or eplerenone) are more successful than α- or β-blockers. Spironolactone has the advantage of once-daily administration and can be initiated at doses of as little as 12.5 to 25 mg daily. However, the use of spironolactone as a fourth drug is limited by tolerability issues in some patients, including the development of hyperkalemia in those with CKD with an eGFR <45 $mL \cdot min^{-1} \cdot 1.73\ m^{-2}$ or baseline serum potassium >4.5 mEq/L. Approximately 70% of adults with RH are candidates for mineralocorticoid receptor antagonists based on eGFR and serum K^+, yet only a small fraction receive these effective agents. With prolonged use at higher doses, gynecomastia and erectile dysfunction in men and menstrual irregularities in women may limit the use of spironolactone. In such cases, eplerenone may be used successfully. Because of its shorter half-life compared with spironolactone, eplerenone should be administered twice daily for optimal effect.

The choice of ARB may also be important. Studies comparing various ARBs demonstrate clear advantages of certain agents in BP reduction over others. Specifically, 24-hour ABPM studies demonstrate that azilsartan medoximil provides on average an additional 4 to 8 mm Hg of further SBP reduction over other ARBs (e.g., valsartan and olmesartan) or the ACE inhibitor ramipril.

Dihydropyridine CCBs such as amlodipine and nifedipine extended-release are the most studied in the setting of hypertension. Other drugs in this class such as nicardipine and is radipine are administered 2 or 3 times daily and do not lend themselves to optimal adherence in RH. Some data suggest that long-acting formulations of nifedipine may have slightly greater antihypertensive actions than amlodipine but are associated with more edema. Nondihydropyridine CCBs such as verapamil also may be useful, but the evidence supporting their use in RH is limited (Mancia et al., 2013).

Alteration of the dosing times (e.g., to include a nocturnal dose) or using divided doses of drugs with half-lives of <12 to 15 hours may also improve BP control even when the drug theoretically has a pharmacodynamic effect of up to 24 hours in duration. Dosing at night of certain agents, for example, guanfacine, also helps reduce adverse effects such as drowsiness and may aid in sleeping.

The choice of a fifth drug (to add) depends on the sympathetic drive as assessed in part by heart rate (Figure 4.3, step 4). In 2 post hoc analyses from large outcome trials, patients with heart rates >80 bpm had higher mortality. Thus, agents such as β-blockers or, if medically contraindicated, central α−2 agonists such as transdermal clonidine or guanfacine should be considered (Figure 4.3, step 4). Clonidine tablets should be avoided because of the need for frequent administration and the risk of rebound hypertension during periods of nonadherence and after discontinuation.

If blood pressure remains uncontrolled despite the measures mentioned above, it may be advisable to add hydralazine while also using nitrates for patients with heart failure (refer to Figure 4.3, step 5). Nitrates are the preferred choice because they aid in restoring calcium (Ca^{2+}) cycling, improving cardiac contractile performance, and regulating superoxide production in isolated cardiomyocytes. Additionally, hydralazine can help reduce nitrate tolerance in this situation. It is important to note that hydralazine may increase sympathetic tone and sodium retention, so it should be used alongside appropriate background diuretic and β-blocker therapy (refer to Figure 4.3, step 5). Keep hydralazine daily doses under <150 mg to avoid drug-induced systemic lupus erythematosus.

Finally, if hydralazine is ineffective, minoxidil could be attempted (Figure 4.3, step 6). It is difficult to tolerate minoxidil. It causes hirsutism, which in females may result in stopping the medication. Minoxidil induces severe sodium avidity, fluid retention, and elevated sympathetic tone; it must be administered at least twice daily. Therefore, in almost every situation, a β-blocker and loop diuretic are needed. However, minoxidil usually lowers blood pressure in this situation.

4.3.5.4. Hypertension Specialist

The American Hypertension Specialists Certification Program has established requirements for physicians to become Certified Hypertension Clinicians (accounting for both physicians and allied health professionals) and Certified Hypertension Specialists (limited to physicians). Online is where you can find the prerequisites for both certification programs. Compared to other healthcare professionals, hypertension specialists and clinicians possess a higher level of experience and knowledge in managing patients with renal impairment. Studies conducted in the past have shown that patients with uncontrolled hypertension who were referred to hypertension specialists had better blood pressure control. Referrals are appropriate when the patient's blood pressure control is not improving as the primary care physician believes it should.

4.3.6. Device-Based Treatment of RH

Dysfunction of the human sympathetic nervous system is a key factor in the development and progression of hypertension, heart failure, and chronic kidney disease. In the 1940s, surgical sympathectomy showed promising results in improving blood pressure control, reducing cardiac size, enhancing renal function, and decreasing cerebrovascular events in the absence of antihypertensive medications. However, this approach was soon overshadowed by the side effects of severe orthostatic hypotension, erectile dysfunction, bowel and bladder incontinence, and the availability of antihypertensive drugs. Consequently, lumbar sympathectomy fell out of favor in clinical practice by the mid-1970s. Despite this, these early studies laid the foundation for the development of modern devices aimed at treating resistant hypertension, many of which target reducing sympathetic nervous system activity.

4.3.6.1. Renal Nerve Ablation

Since renal nerve ablation has been researched and used in clinical settings outside of the US for many years, the majority of data on its effects that have been published until recently have come from Australian and European centers. In patients whose blood pressure could not be controlled with four or five antihypertensive medications, early research in this area demonstrated significant reductions in clinic blood pressure. These studies, however, lacked control, and the majority did not use ambulatory blood pressure as their main outcome. Subsequent studies revealed that the effect sizes using ABPM in uncontrolled studies were much smaller (one-third) than the changes measured in the clinical setting.

Renal denervation therapy had little to no effect in a severely drug-resistant population, according to SYMPLICITY HTN-3, the first sham-controlled prospective randomized study in the field of renal ablation therapy. The most meticulously planned randomized sham-control study's inability to achieve the efficacy end points raised many methodological questions, such as changes in patient behavior regarding adherence to multidrug pharmacological regimens and insufficient denervation due to catheter, interventional proceduralist, or both technical failures. Many new catheters and trial designs have been developed to assess the effectiveness of more extensive renal denervation as a result of the methodological issues raised by SYMPLICITY HTN-3 (Parati et al., 2010).

Numerous investigations are still in progress, but as of right now, no findings exist. Data from animal studies demonstrate unequivocally that using radiofrequency and ultrasonic catheters to induce renal artery denervation reduces the rate of norepinephrine spillover and lowers blood pressure. According to SYMPLICITY HTN-3 post hoc analyses, patients with higher degrees of renal nerve ablation had lower blood pressure than those with less complete ablation. Furthermore, patients on three antihypertensive medications who were randomized to renal denervation as opposed to those on four antihypertensive medications showed a statistically significant decrease in daytime ambulatory SBP (−5.9 mm Hg; P=0.03) in the DENERHTN trial (Renal Denervation for Hypertension). Currently, most nations have stopped using renal denervation treatments to treat RH unless the patients are part of research projects.

4.3.6.2. Carotid Baroreceptor Activation Therapy

An implanted pulse generator, an external programming system, and baroreflex activation leads positioned next to the carotid sinus make up the carotid baroreceptor activation therapy system. This modality electronically stimulates baroreceptors, which in turn triggers the brain to coordinate a multisystemic response for conditions like arrhythmias, heart failure, and hypertension that are linked to sympathetic overactivity. Enhanced vagal activity and decreased sympathetic nervous system activity are two effects of carotid sinus stimulation. As a result, the heart rate lowers, extending the time that the left ventricle can fill and lowering the energy and workload required by the heart.

Furthermore, natriuresis is enhanced by arterial dilatation, which lowers cardiac afterload and improves renal blood flow. In intervals of approximately four minutes, the level of stimulation can be adjusted to suit the hemodynamic needs of each patient. A large randomized trial with 322 participants with RH produced preliminary results, but the trial's primary end point—a composite of five individual efficacy and safety end points—was not met. In RH, the gadget was thought to be long-term safe and effective. This has prompted improvements to the apparatus and additional studies using new Rheos systems and single-sided catheters (Mancia et al., 2010).

A tiny endovascular implantable device called the MobiusHD carotid bulb expansion device lowers blood pressure by activating baroreceptors and stretching the carotid artery at the bulb. Results from the completed CALM-FIM_EUR (Controlling and Lowering Blood Pressure with the MOBIUSHD) study in Europe and the ongoing CALM-FIM_US study in the US should be available in a year or two. Recently, CALM-FIM_EUR showed that endovascular baroreflex amplification using the MobiusHD device significantly reduced blood pressure with a tolerable safety profile in patients with RH.

4.3.7. Devices on the Horizon for RH

Other innovative experimental devices are being investigated for the treatment of RH with varying degrees of success and experience in patients, in addition to renal nerve ablation therapy and baroreceptor activation therapy. The majority of studies using these devices up to this point have small sample sizes and lack control. These include the ReCor endovascular ultrasonic renal denervation device, the central arteriovenous anastomosis ROX coupler device, and median nerve stimulation, which lowers sympathetic outflow by means of electroacupuncture.

4.3.8. Research Challenges and Needs

It is critically necessary to understand the prevalence of true RH, which can explain medication nonadherence, white-coat effect, and inaccurate blood pressure measurement. There is little doubt that raising the BP target in the general hypertensive population will lead to a rise in RH prevalence. In addition to the prevalence being documented, the prognosis for RH needs to be verified again. It is likely that when the definition is refined to use lower blood pressure thresholds, the characteristics of patients with RH will shift. More research is required to determine the ideal blood pressure target for RH. Clarification of the pathophysiology of RH is desperately needed, as it is not always evident in individual patients. This covers the effects of the environment, particularly the part played by dietary salt intake and blood pressure's sensitivity to salt.

Even with today's advanced genetics technologies, the underlying genetics of both hypertension and RH remain unclear. The pathophysiology of primary hypertension seems to be controlled by a variety of genes, each of which has a small impact, except the uncommon monogenetic causes. Potential phenotypes to be investigated through genetic analysis include hypertension associated with dysregulation of specific hormonal systems, such as the sympathetic nervous system and the renin-angiotensin-aldosterone system, obesity-induced hypertension, and hypertension sensitive to salt. Finding particular RH phenotypes that could be further investigated for genetic contributions would probably improve our comprehension of the underlying causes of this intricate illness process.

Once the true prevalence of RH is established, preventative measures ought to be taken into account. These could involve starting pharmaceutical treatment earlier in life for people who are at high-risk for RH and preventing comorbidities like renal function loss, arteriolar hypertrophy, and vascular stiffening that could make treating hypertension more challenging. Behavioral and sleep treatments are examples of nonpharmacological tactics (Pickering et al., 2005).

The current strategy for BP control in RH has centered on adding or changing medications or drug classes according to sound pharmacological principles, which is only partially effective in actual RH. Improved individualized antihypertensive medication selection for RH patients should be the focus of future research. For instance, pharmacogenomics and pharmacogenetics are anticipated to offer a more logical and focused therapeutic approach. Establishing the significance of genetic/genomic variation in BP responses to various pharmacological classes in specific populations is necessary, though. Large-scale, carefully monitored studies with participants who are as well phenotypically characterized as possible will be necessary to achieve this. To enhance the currently constrained range of medication alternatives in RH, it will be crucial to develop new classes of pharmacological agents in the interim. It will also be critical to expand the treatment plan to include more effective strategies for enacting long-term, healthful lifestyle changes, identifying and correcting nonadherence, and lowering blood pressure with team-based care and telehealth. Other strategies, like enhancing the quality of sleep, might also aid in lowering the incidence of RH.

A Closer Look

Cardiovascular Disease

Cardiovascular disease (CVD) remains a formidable global health challenge, encompassing a range of conditions affecting the heart and blood vessels. This multifaceted disorder includes coronary artery disease, heart failure, stroke, and hypertension, among others. At its core, CVD often arises from a complex interplay of genetic predisposition, lifestyle factors, and environmental influences.

One of the primary culprits behind CVD is atherosclerosis, the buildup of plaque within arteries, which restricts blood flow and can lead to heart attacks and strokes. Risk factors such as high blood pressure, high cholesterol levels, smoking, obesity, and diabetes significantly contribute to the development and progression of CVD. Moreover, socioeconomic disparities and access to healthcare also play pivotal roles in shaping the prevalence and impact of CVD across populations. Efforts to combat CVD involve a multifaceted approach, encompassing both preventive measures and therapeutic interventions. Lifestyle modifications such as a healthy diet, regular exercise, smoking cessation, and stress management are crucial in reducing CVD risk. Additionally, pharmacological treatments, surgical procedures, and innovative technologies like stents and pacemakers are deployed to manage existing CVD and prevent its complications (Schulz et al., 2016).

However, despite advancements in medical science and public health initiatives, CVD remains the leading cause of death worldwide. Continued research, education, and advocacy are imperative in the ongoing battle against this pervasive and deadly disease.

Summary

- Resistant hypertension, a subset of high blood pressure, presents a formidable challenge in clinical management due to its stubborn resistance to conventional treatment strategies.
- Hypertension is the world's leading risk factor for cardiovascular disease (CVD), stroke, disability, and death.
- Demographic correlates of RH include black race, older age, and male sex. RH is characterized by the variable clustering of distinct demographics, comorbidities, physiological aberrations, and metabolic abnormalities.
- The etiology of resistant hypertension is multifactorial, involving a complex interplay of genetic, environmental, and lifestyle factors. Understanding the underlying causes is essential for guiding therapeutic decisions and improving outcomes in affected individuals.
- Health system-level interventions to improve the quality of hypertension care, medication adherence, and BP control use multidisciplinary team-based care.
- The white-coat effect is the observation of repeated BP elevations in the office with controlled or significantly lower BP outside the office in a hypertensive patient on medication.
- Higher dietary sodium intake is incontrovertibly linked to increases in arterial BP. However, relatively large interindividual variations exist in "salt sensitivity" of BP.
- It is more difficult to precisely quantify the importance of excess dietary sodium specifically in regard to causing RH for several reasons, including the complexities in accurately characterizing routine intake in the relevant populations.
- Primary aldosteronism is defined as a group of disorders in which aldosterone production is inappropriately high, relatively autonomous, and independent of the renin-angiotensin system and in which aldosterone secretion is not suppressed by sodium loading.
- Human sympathetic nervous system dysfunction plays an important role in the development and progression of hypertension, heart failure, and CKD.

References

1. Calhoun, D. A., Jones, D., Textor, S., Goff, D. C., Murphy, T. P., Toto, R. D., White, A., Cushman, W. C., White, W., Sica, D., Ferdinand, K., Giles, T. D., Falkner, B., & Carey, R. M. (2008). Resistant hypertension: Diagnosis, evaluation, and treatment: A scientific statement from the American Heart Association Professional Education Committee of the Council for High Blood Pressure Research. *Hypertension, 51*(6), 1403–1419.
2. Diaz, K. M., Booth, J. N., III, Calhoun, D. A., Irvin, M. R., Howard, G., Safford, M. M., Muntner, P., & Shimbo, D. (2014). Healthy lifestyle factors and risk of cardiovascular events and mortality in treatment-resistant hypertension: The Reasons for Geographic and Racial Differences in Stroke study. *Hypertension, 64*(3), 465–471.
3. Hameed, M. A., Tebbit, L., Jacques, N., Thomas, M., & Dasgupta, I. (2016). Non-adherence to antihypertensive medication is very common among resistant hypertensives: Results of a directly observed therapy clinic. *Journal of Human Hypertension, 30*(2), 83–89.

4. Mancia, G., Bombelli, M., Brambilla, G., Facchetti, R., Sega, R., Toso, E., & Grassi, G. (2013). Long-term prognostic value of white coat hypertension: An insight from diagnostic use of both ambulatory and home blood pressure measurements. *Hypertension, 62*(1), 168–174.

5. Parati, G., Stergiou, G. S., Asmar, R., Bilo, G., de Leeuw, P., Imai, Y., Kario, K., Lurbe, E., Manolis, A., Mengden, T., O'Brien, E., Ohkubo, T., Padfield, P., Palatini, P., Pickering, T. G., Redon, J., Revera, M., Ruilope, L. M., Shennan, A., Staessen, J. A., Tisler, A., Waeber, B., Zanchetti, A., & Mancia, G. (2010). European Society of Hypertension practice guidelines for home blood pressure monitoring. *Journal of Human Hypertension, 24*(12), 779–785.

6. Pickering, T. G., Hall, J. E., Appel, L. J., Falkner, B. E., Graves, J., Hill, M. N., Jones, D. W., Kurtz, T., Sheps, S. G., & Roccella, E. J. (2005). Recommendations for blood pressure measurement in humans and experimental animals, part 1: Blood pressure measurement in humans: A statement for professionals from the Subcommittee of Professional and Public Education of the American Heart Association Council on High Blood Pressure Research. *Circulation, 111*(5), 697–716.

7. Schulz, M., Krueger, K., Schuessel, K., Friedland, K., Laufs, U., Mueller, W. E., & Ude, M. (2016). Medication adherence and persistence according to different antihypertensive drug classes: A retrospective cohort study of 255,500 patients. *International Journal of Cardiology, 220*, 668–676.

Chapter

DIABETES AND CARDIOVASCULAR DISEASE

5

Contents

INTRODUCTION

Diabetes and cardiovascular disease (CVD) are two interrelated chronic conditions that pose significant health challenges globally. Diabetes mellitus, commonly referred to as diabetes, is a metabolic disorder characterized by chronic hyperglycemia, resulting from either the body's inability to produce sufficient insulin (type 1 diabetes) or its inability to effectively use insulin (type 2 diabetes). Over time, persistent high blood sugar levels can lead to various complications, including damage to the blood vessels, nerves, and organs. Cardiovascular disease encompasses a range of conditions that affect the heart and blood vessels, including coronary artery disease, heart failure, stroke, and peripheral arterial disease (Wild et al., 2004).

The link between diabetes and CVD is well-established, with diabetes recognized as a major risk factor for the development of cardiovascular complications. Individuals with diabetes are at a significantly higher risk of experiencing heart attacks, strokes, and other cardiovascular events compared to those without diabetes. This increased risk is attributed to several factors, including the chronic inflammatory state, oxidative stress, and endothelial dysfunction associated with diabetes, which accelerate the process of atherosclerosis—the buildup of plaques in the arteries that impedes blood flow. Furthermore, diabetes often coexists with other cardiovascular risk factors such as hypertension, dyslipidemia, and obesity, compounding the risk of CVD (Aguiree et al., 2013).

Understanding the intricate relationship between diabetes and cardiovascular disease is crucial for effective prevention and management strategies. Comprehensive approaches that address both conditions simultaneously are essential to reduce the burden of these chronic diseases. Lifestyle modifications, such as maintaining a healthy diet, engaging in regular physical activity, and avoiding tobacco use, play a pivotal role in managing diabetes and preventing CVD. Additionally, medical interventions, including blood glucose control, lipid-lowering therapies, antihypertensive medications, and antiplatelet agents, are integral components of reducing cardiovascular risk in individuals with diabetes (Bahia et al., 2011).

Orientation and Directional Terms

Term	Definition	Illustration
Stroke	A stroke can occur when blood flow to the brain is blocked or there is sudden bleeding in the brain.	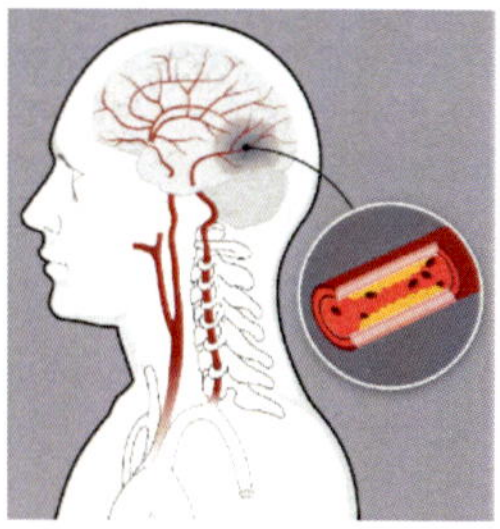
Coronary Artery Disease (CAD)	Coronary artery disease (CAD) limits blood flow in your coronary arteries, which deliver blood to your heart muscle. Cholesterol and other substances make up plaque that narrows your coronary arteries.	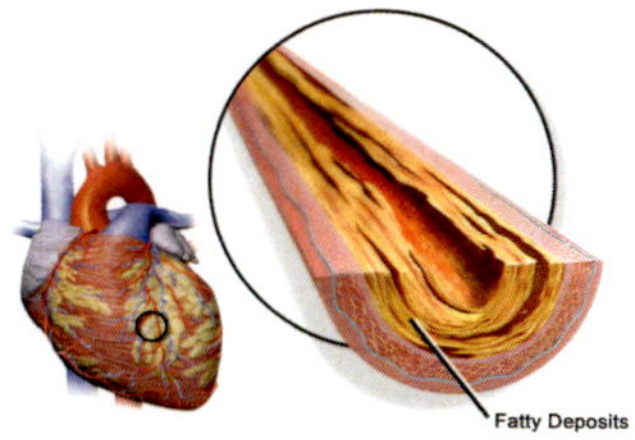
Peripheral Vascular Disease (PVD)	Peripheral vascular disease (PVD) is a slow and progressive circulation disorder caused by narrowing, blockage or spasms in a blood vessel.	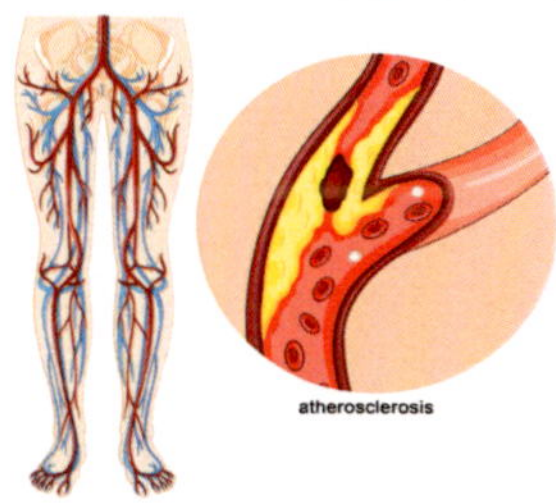
Obesity	Obesity is a chronic complex disease defined by excessive fat deposits that can impair health. Obesity can lead to increased risk of type 2 diabetes and heart disease, it can affect bone health and reproduction, it increases the risk of certain cancers.	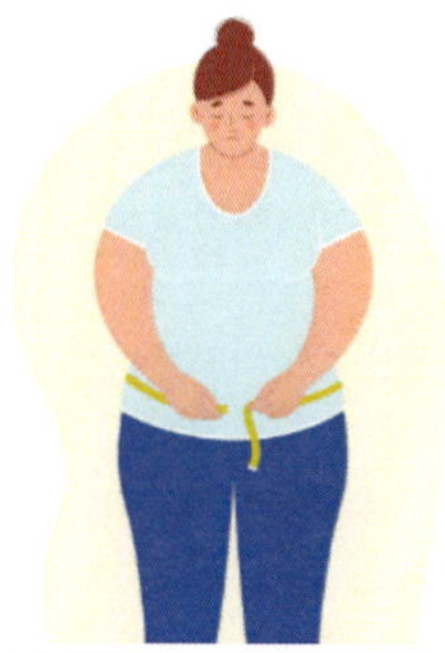
Dyslipidemia	Dyslipidemia is a metabolic disorder characterized by abnormally high or low amounts of any or all lipids (e.g., fats, triglycerides, cholesterol, phospholipids) or lipoproteins in the blood.	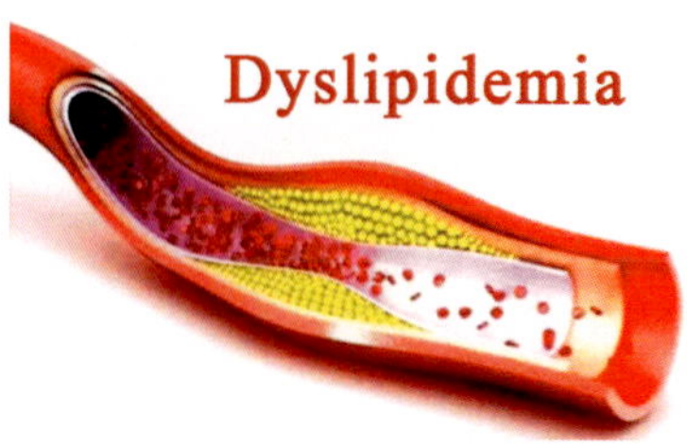

5.1. CARDIOVASCULAR DISEASE

Compared to people without diabetes, those with type 1 and type 2 diabetes are more likely to experience a variety of incapacitating and potentially fatal health issues. High blood glucose levels on a regular basis can cause major illnesses that impact the heart, blood vessels, kidneys, nerves, and eyes. Without efficient methods to encourage improved diabetes management, the prevalence of type 2 diabetes is expected to rise, which could lead to significant increases in the rates of these complications in low- and middle-income nations (Matheus et al., 2013).

It is possible to prevent or delay the complications of diabetes by keeping blood pressure, cholesterol, and glucose levels as close to normal as possible. Screening programs enable the early detection of many complications, allowing for treatment to stop them from getting worse (Rivellese et al., 2010).

One of the leading causes of death and disability among diabetics is cardiovascular disease (CVD), a group of illnesses affecting the heart or blood vessels. Diabetes raises the risk of atherosclerosis, or the narrowing of the arteries, by being linked to elevated blood pressure and cholesterol levels (Li and Aronow, 2011). This may result in symptoms like intermittent claudication or angina pectoris. Blood clot risk can be elevated by high blood glucose because it activates the blood coagulation system more. When combined, these can result in total blockage of an artery, which stops blood flow and causes conditions like myocardial infarction, stroke, and gangrene (Figure 5.1).

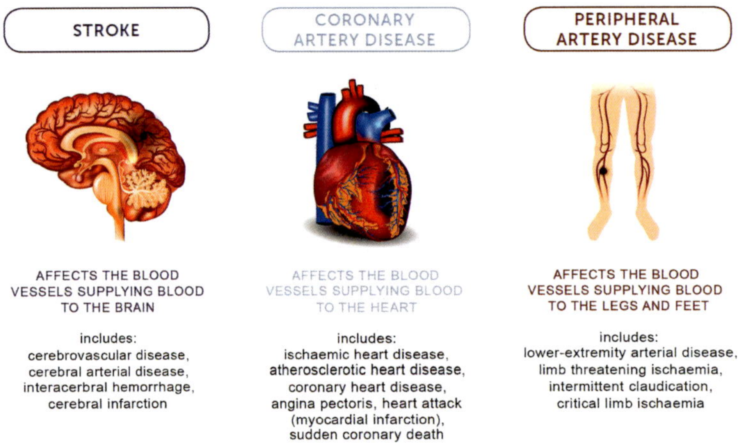

Figure 5.1. *The main types of cardiovascular diseases (CVD) include stroke, coronary artery disease and peripheral artery disease.*

Source: https://idf.org/media/uploads/2023/05/attachments-39.pdf.

5.1.1. Stroke

One type of cerebrovascular disease, also known as cerebral arterial disease, is stroke, which can be brought on by a cerebral hemorrhage or cerebral infarction (Figure 5.2). The two carotid arteries and the two vertebral arteries are the four main arteries that supply blood to the brain.

The specific area of the brain affected by vascular disease will determine the clinical outcomes (Duncan et al., 2003).

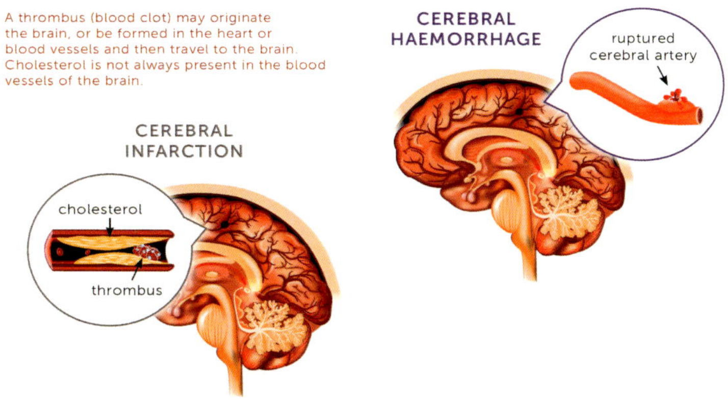

Figure 5.2. *Stroke can arise from cerebral infarction or cerebral haemorrhage.*

Source: https://idf.org/media/uploads/2023/05/attachments-39.pdf.

A stroke happens when a blood vessel bursts or becomes blocked, damaging a portion of the brain. If a large vessel is impacted, the consequences could be extremely serious disability or possibly death very quickly. Smaller blood vessels that are impacted may recover well and the prognosis is less dire (Shoelson et al., 2006). Speech issues and the inability to use one side of the body are the two most prevalent forms of disability. Stroke typically manifests as sudden weakness, numbness, confusion, headache, dizziness, and vision problems (Figure 5.3).

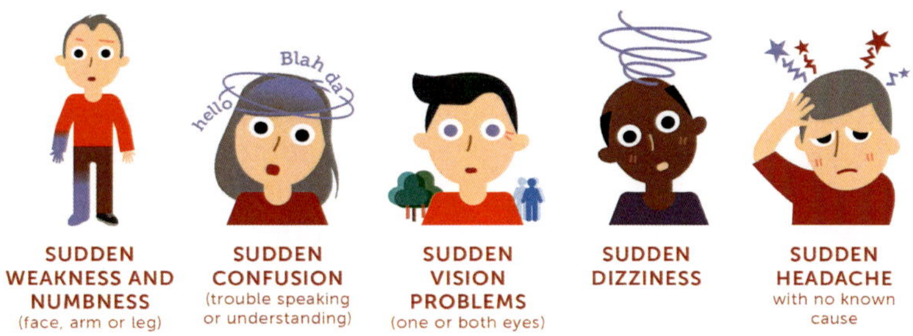
hello
Blah da
SUDDEN WEAKNESS AND NUMBNESS
(face, arm or leg)
SUDDEN CONFUSION
(trouble speaking or understanding)
SUDDEN VISION PROBLEMS
(one or both eyes)
SUDDEN DIZZINESS
SUDDEN HEADACHE
with no known cause

Figure 5.3. *The main symptoms of stroke.*

Source: https://idf.org/media/uploads/2023/05/attachments-39.pdf.

5.1.2. Coronary Artery Disease

The coronary arteries supply the heart's blood supply. Narrowing or blockage of these arteries results in coronary artery disease. Angina pectoris, heart attacks, heart failure, and sudden coronary death are all included in the category of diseases known as coronary artery disease, sometimes referred to as ischemic heart disease, atherosclerotic heart disease, or coronary heart disease (Vicenova et al., 2009).

5.1.2.1. Angina Pectoris

Chest pain brought on by an inadequate blood supply to the heart is known as angina pectoris (ischaemia). Angina pectoris, which can be fatal when unstable, is caused by an inadequate blood supply to the heart's muscle tissue. Angina pectoris typically results in central chest pain that is aggravated by exertion or emotional stress. This pain frequently radiates to the left arm, shoulder, or jaw. Perspiration and dyspnea are also typical. Acute coronary syndromes include both angina pectoris and heart attacks (Barouch et al., 2003).

5.1.2.2. Heart Attack (Myocardial Infarction)

A heart attack, sometimes referred to as a myocardial infarction, is the result of permanently damaging a portion of the heart muscle because of clogged blood vessels. Severe central chest pressure, which can also radiate to the left arm, shoulder, or jaw, is typically the first sign of an impending heart attack (Kim et al., 2008). Other common symptoms include severe dyspnea, perspiration, and lightheadedness. There may be gender differences in symptoms (Figure 5.4).

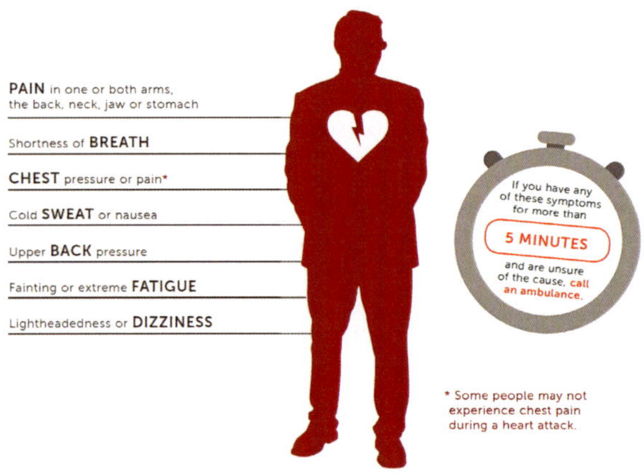

Figure 5.4. *Heart attack warning signs.*

Source: https://idf.org/media/uploads/2023/05/attachments-39.pdf.

5.1.2.3. Heart Failure

Heart failure happens when the heart muscle sustains enough damage to be unable to pump blood properly. Breathlessness, edema in the ankles or legs, exhaustion, and weakness are some symptoms. Treatment for heart failure must be started early and appropriately; it is not the same as treating a heart attack (Chait et al., 2005).

5.1.2.4. Sudden Coronary Death

An abrupt stoppage of the heart's blood pumping function can result in sudden death. Either a severe irregularity in the heartbeat rhythm or a massive heart attack could be the cause (Ferrarezi et al., 2007).

5.1.3. Peripheral Vascular Disease

Peripheral vascular disease (PVD) is a condition characterized by narrowing or blockage of the blood vessels outside of the heart and brain, primarily affecting the arteries that supply blood to the legs and feet. This condition, also known as peripheral artery disease (PAD), is a manifestation of atherosclerosis, a process where plaque buildup within the arteries restricts blood flow to tissues and organs. PVD commonly affects the lower extremities but can also occur in other peripheral arteries, such as those supplying the arms, kidneys, and intestines (Leahy, 2005).

The hallmark symptom of PVD is intermittent claudication, which presents as cramping pain or discomfort in the legs during physical activity, such as walking or climbing stairs, and typically resolves with rest. Other symptoms may include numbness, tingling, weakness, or a feeling of coldness in the legs or feet. In advanced stages, PVD can lead to critical limb ischemia, characterized by severe pain at rest, non-healing wounds or ulcers, and tissue necrosis, which may necessitate amputation if left untreated.

The risk factors for PVD are similar to those for other forms of cardiovascular disease and include smoking, diabetes, hypertension, dyslipidemia, obesity, physical inactivity, and advancing age. Smoking is considered the most significant modifiable risk factor for PVD, as it accelerates atherosclerosis and increases the risk of developing severe forms of the disease (Belke et al., 2002).

Diagnosis of PVD involves a combination of clinical evaluation, non-invasive vascular testing, and imaging studies. Ankle-brachial index (ABI) measurement, which compares blood pressure in the ankles to that in the arms, is a simple and reliable screening test for PVD. Additional tests, such as Doppler ultrasound, computed tomography angiography (CTA), magnetic resonance angiography (MRA), or conventional angiography, may be performed to assess the location and severity of arterial blockages (Schena et al., 2005).

Management of PVD aims to relieve symptoms, improve functional status, prevent disease progression, and reduce the risk of cardiovascular events. Lifestyle modifications, including smoking cessation, regular exercise, healthy diet, and weight management, are fundamental components of PVD management. Pharmacological interventions, such as antiplatelet agents (e.g., aspirin, clopidogrel), statins, antihypertensive medications, and medications to control blood sugar in diabetic patients, are prescribed to reduce cardiovascular risk factors and improve blood flow (Gesualdo et al., 1999). In cases of severe PVD or critical limb ischemia, revascularization procedures may be necessary to restore blood flow to the affected limb. These procedures may include endovascular interventions, such as balloon angioplasty with or without stenting, or surgical bypass grafting to create alternative routes for blood flow bypassing the blocked arteries (Wolf and Ziyadeh, 1997).

5.1.4. Risk Factors

The following risk factors raise the chance of a CVD event: high blood pressure, unhealthy diet, family history, overweight/obesity, diabetes, elevated low-density lipoproteins (LDL) or low high-density lipoproteins (HDL) cholesterol, current smoking, physical inactivity, and overweight/obesity (Figure 5.5) (Kannel, 1985).

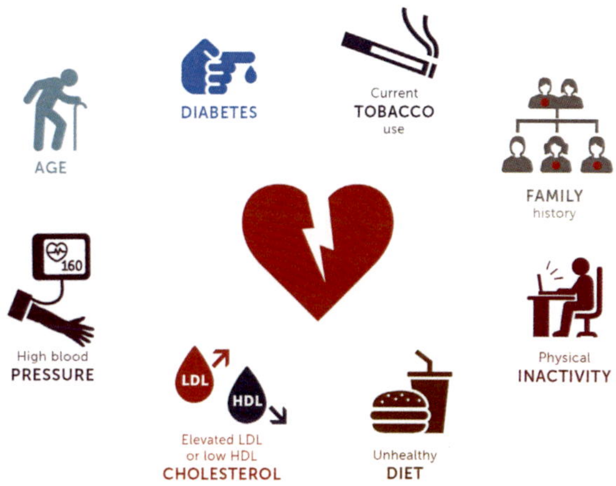

Figure 5.5. *Cardiovascular Disease (CVD) risk factors.*

Source: https://idf.org/media/uploads/2023/05/attachments-39.pdf.

5.2. CV RISK FACTORS AND CVD

5.2.1. Obesity

Patients with diabetes, especially those with type 2 diabetes, frequently have obesity, which is linked to a higher risk of CVD. Low-grade inflammation may be one mechanism that ties obesity and diabetes to later-onset cardiovascular disease (Taskinen, 2003). The overexpression of several cytokines by adipose tissue, such as tumor necrosis factor-α, interleukin (IL)-1, IL-6, leptin, resistin MCP-1, PAI-1, fibrinogen, and angiotensin, is linked to diabetes mellitus and insulin resistance. The overexpression of these cytokines can result in endothelial dysfunction, MI, and cardiomyopathy (CMP) by exacerbating inflammation and lipid accumulation, which are harmful to blood vessels. Moreover, elevated levels of C-reactive protein (CRP) have been observed in diabetic patients, which may be linked to endothelial dysfunction. (Shoelson et al., 2006) Numerous investigations have shown that CRP inhibits the production of prostacyclin and nitric oxide (NO) by endothelial cells, two processes essential for vessel compliance. Additionally, it has been demonstrated that CRP increases the uptake of oxidized low-density lipoprotein (LDL) in the walls of the coronary vasculature, which may be linked to the development of atherosclerotic plaques and endothelial dysfunction. Additionally, adiponectin production is reduced in DM patients, which may lead to a reduction in endothelial function. By raising NO production and decreasing adhesion molecule expression, adiponectin contributes to the limitation of endothelial dysfunction. By preventing LDL oxidation, adiponectin also provides protection against the atherosclerotic process. Individuals with diabetes may be more susceptible to myocardial infarction due to this rise in atherosclerotic plaque. Specifically, elevated levels of the inflammatory cytokine IL-1, observed in diabetes mellitus patients, may play a role in the instability of atheromatous plaques and consequent MI. In individuals with type 2 diabetes, insulin resistance is also linked to an increase in plasma free fatty acids, which raises muscle triglyceride stores, hepatic glucose synthesis, and insulin production. Insulin resistance has also been connected through contractile dysfunction and cardiomyocyte hypertrophy to CMP in diabetics (Krauss and Siri, 2004).

5.2.2. Hypertension

Patients with T1DM and T2DM are highly likely to have hypertension; the prevalence rates are 30% and 60%, respectively. Diabetic nephropathy (DN) is closely associated with hypertension in patients with diabetes. In diabetic kidney disease (DN), hyperglycemia stimulates renal cells, which results in the release of growth factors, cytokines, and humoral mediators. The production of these factors is frequently in charge of the structural changes that diabetic patients' glomeruli exhibit, such as increased collagen deposition of the extracellular matrix, hyaline arteriolosclerosis (mainly of the efferent arteriole), and increased permeability of the glomerular basement membrane. These structural alterations raise filtration pressure, which frequently results in microalbuminemia and the renin-angiotensin system's compensatory activation (RAAS) (Solano and Goldberg, 2006). Chronic RAAS activation frequently results in hypertension, which puts further strain on the glomeruli and damages diabetic patients' nephrons even more. If DN is not treated, it can develop into a nephrotic syndrome, which is characterized by hyperlipidemia, proteinuria, and a hypercoagulable state (because of the loss of ATIII). This condition may increase the risk of cardiovascular disease (CVD) in patients with diabetes who also have renal failure. (Gesualdo et al., 1991)

5.2.3. Dyslipidemia

Dyslipidemia is more likely to develop in diabetic patients. An explanation for this association could be the elevated release of free fatty acids found in fat cells resistant to insulin. Elevated free-fatty acid levels stimulate the synthesis of triglycerides, which in turn triggers the release of very low-density lipoprotein (VLDL) and apolipoprotein B (ApoB). Elevated levels of VLDL and ApoB have been linked to a higher risk of CVD. Hyperinsulinemia is linked to low levels of high-density lipoprotein (HDL) cholesterol in addition to elevated ApoB and VLDL. Additionally, lipoproteins (especially LDL and VLDL) may be adversely affected by hyperglycemia due to increased glycosylation and oxidation, which can reduce vascular compliance and hasten the onset of aggressive atherosclerosis. Increased stimulation of ApoB and VLDL cholesterol, decreased HDL levels, lipoprotein modification, high circulating FFA and triglycerides, and decreased HDL levels have all been observed in DM patients and are likely contributing factors to the high prevalence of CVD in this population (Chahil and Ginsberg, 2006).

5.2.4. Diabetic Cardiomyopathy

DM does not appear to be responsible for the development of CMP only through hypertension and coronary atherosclerosis. Numerous noninvasive studies have detailed this diabetic CMP, which includes modifications to the LV structure and cardiac function of diabetics. In particular, compared to people without diabetes, diabetics typically have larger hearts, especially the left ventricle (LV). This could be connected to an increase in the release of cytokines from adipocytes, such as resistin and leptin, which cause cardiomyocytes to become hypertrophied. Even after controlling for covariates, a multiethnic population study revealed that patients with T2DM had a higher probability of having an LV mass that is greater than the 75th%ile. In addition, DM patients typically exhibit a slightly reduced diastolic function in comparison to non-diabetics (Mooradian et al., 2007).

A plausible explanation could be that patients with diabetes mellitus have elevated myocardial triglyceride levels due to increased triglyceride synthesis. Elevated triglyceride accumulation in the heart is linked to lipotoxicity and modified calcium hemostasis in the heart, both of which have an adverse effect on diastolic function. This may contribute to the explanation of the observation that diastolic dysfunction affects 40–75% of people with diabetes mellitus (DM) who do not exhibit overt coronary artery disease (CAD). Doppler strain analysis of peak systolic velocity and tissue Doppler imaging have also revealed subtle abnormalities in systolic function in DM patients. Impaired contractile reserve and myocardial sympathetic innervation may be linked to this systolic dysfunction. Furthermore, patients with DM have been found to have interstitial fibrosis with increased collagen deposition, which may be detrimental to the reduced cardiac function that is characteristic of diabetics. Patients with diabetes are probably more susceptible to heart failure (HF) due to numerous mechanisms that lead to reductions in systolic and diastolic function. Compared to the general population (4%–6%), diabetic patients have a higher prevalence of heart failure and preserved ejection fraction (16%–31%). Traditional CV risk factors may contribute to some of the difference, but diabetes mellitus (DM) may also affect cardiac structure and function on its own by encouraging hypertrophy and fibrosis (Hamilton and Watts, 2013).

5.2.5. Cardiovascular Autonomic Neuropathy

Patients with diabetes mellitus frequently experience cardiovascular autonomic neuropathy (CAN), which is associated with a higher 5-year mortality rate from CVD. The following are the clinical signs and symptoms of CAN: increased QT interval, postural hypotension, exercise intolerance, resting tachycardia, and perioperative instability (Asghar et al., 2009). The clinical signs and symptoms of CAN are associated with a higher risk of renal disease, stroke, cardiovascular disease, and sudden death. The autonomic nervous system's (ANS) dysregulation, characterized by elevated inflammatory markers and increased sympathetic activity, is probably linked to the onset and progression of CAN. Arterial stiffness, left ventricular hypertrophy, and ventricular diastolic dysfunction can result from ANS dysfunction because the ANS regulates the sinus node's activity, end diastolic volume, end systolic volume, and systemic vascular resistance. Patients with diabetes mellitus have an increased risk of developing both CAN and CVD due to the increased incidence of CAN associated with aging and inadequate glycemic control (Vinik and Ziegler, 2007).

5.2.6. Myocardial Infarction and DM

Patients with diabetes have a higher incidence of MI than those without the disease, making diabetes a major risk factor for the development of CAD. Furthermore, diabetic patients experience greater rates of re-infarction, morbidity, and mortality after MIs than non-diabetics, with a one-year mortality rate of almost 50%. The most recent research suggests that the underlying atherosclerotic process is similar in patients with and without diabetes mellitus, despite the fact that the precise pathophysiology of CAD progression in these patients remains unknown. Increased coagulability is thought to be the cause of the higher incidence of myocardial infarction in DM patients. Numerous investigations have revealed that the glycoprotein IIB/IIIA receptors and vWF, which are in charge of platelet activation, are expressed more frequently in diabetics (Galderisi et al., 1991). Additionally, plasminogen activator inhibitor type 1 is elevated in DM patients, which may slow fibrinolysis, promote thrombus formation, and quicken plaque formation. Lastly, because diabetes causes proteinuria, diabetic patients also typically have lower levels of circulating anticoagulants like protein C and antithrombin III. These variables together put DM patients in a procoagulant and prothrombotic state, which could explain why diabetic patients have higher rates of MI (Santra et al., 2011).

The increased incidence of MI observed in patients with diabetes may also be attributed to silent myocardial ischemia. Angina that follows ischemia frequently acts as a warning flag for individuals who are developing obstructive CAD. Silent ischemia, on the other hand, is frequently asymptomatic and discovered later in the course of CAD, which is linked to increased rates of MI-related death and morbidity. Patients with diabetes mellitus (10%–20%) are far more likely to experience silent ischemia than patients without the disease (1%–4%). This discrepancy could account for the finding in certain angiographic investigations that diabetic patients typically had more advanced CAD at the time of diagnosis. One possibility for the higher frequency of silent ischemia in DM patients is diabetic neuropathy (Eguchi et al., 2008).

5.3. TREATMENT

Since CVD is the most common cause of death and morbidity among DM patients, effective treatment is essential to reducing the risk of CV events in the future, especially for MI, CAD, stroke, and congestive heart failure (CHF) in diabetics. Diabetic patients are more likely to experience CV complications due to many common CV risk factors, including dyslipidemia, obesity, hypertension, autonomic dysfunction, and suboptimal glycemic control. Although it can be difficult to achieve, therapy aimed at changing these risk factors can improve CV outcomes. The recommendations often change or vary depending on which organization publishes them, and the guidelines concerning these risk factors are usually different from the guidelines for patients who are not diabetic. Furthermore, there is occasionally ambiguity and contradiction in the research on the relationship between these various risk factors and the CV risk profile of diabetics. This section aims to give the most recent recommendations for treating hypertension, autonomic dysfunction, dyslipidemia, and glycemic control in diabetic patients. It also describes the research that has been done on each of these subjects (Patil et al., 2011).

5.4. GLYCEMIC CONTROL

Current treatment recommendations for patients

with DM place a strong emphasis on closely monitoring and controlling glycemic levels in an effort to improve cardiac outcomes, as numerous studies have linked poor glycemic control to worse CV outcomes. However, the precise glycemic level that diabetics should aim for is debatable and varies based on the organization developing the guidelines. For instance, the American Association of Clinical Endocrinologists' current guidelines encourage physicians to treat patients whose hemoglobin A1c (HbA1c) value is higher than 6% by combining pharmacological agents, weight loss, and lifestyle modification. The goal of the guidelines is to have an HbA1c of less than or equal to 6% (Brooks et al., 2008). For non-pregnant patients with T1DM or T2DM, the ACC/AHA has a somewhat more lenient A1c goal of less than 7% to lower the risk of microvascular or macrovascular complications. Furthermore, the ACC/AHA qualifies their recommendation by stating that patients with a history of severe hypoglycemia, a short life expectancy, advanced microvascular or macrovascular complications, numerous comorbidities, or long-term diabetes may benefit from an A1c goal of greater than 7. Additionally, the recommendation notes that some diabetic patient populations, such as those with a short duration of diabetes, a long life expectancy, and no cardiovascular disease (CVD), may benefit from an A1c goal lower than the general goal of less than 7%. For diabetic patients, the VA/DoD guidelines employ a more customized algorithm to determine an appropriate A1c goal. Depending on the patient's current health status, comorbid conditions, life expectancy, risk of hypoglycemia, and length of diabetes status, the recommended target A1c ranges from < 7 to < 9. (Pogach et al., 2011)

5.5. CV OUTCOMES

Numerous studies have looked into how treating hyperglycemia aggressively affects the outcomes of cardiovascular disease in diabetic patients. One of the first multi-center, randomized control trials to look into the impact of strict glycemic control in patients with newly diagnosed type 2 diabetes was the United Kingdom Prospective Diabetes Study (UKPDS) trial. Patients received ten years of follow-up after being randomly assigned to receive either "intensive" or "conventional" glycemia-lowering therapy. Compared to the group receiving conventional therapy, which did not significantly alter their HbA1c (median 7.9%), the intensive glycemic group experienced an 11% reduction in HbA1c over a ten-year period (median 7.0%). A 25% decrease in microvascular disease (mainly from decreased retinopathy) and a 12% reduction in all diabetes-related endpoints were the main outcomes observed in the group with stricter glycemic control. Furthermore, while not statistically significant, the intensive therapy group showed a trend towards a decline in macrovascular disease (Shivalkar et al., 2006).

The VADT trial was a sizable investigation that looked into the impact of strict glycemic control in T2DM patients. The majority of the participants in this study were adult men with poorly controlled type 2 diabetes (T2DM), with an average HbA1c of 9.4% and an average disease duration of 11.5 years. Their mean age was 60.44 years. The participants were monitored for five and a half years after being randomly assigned to receive either "intensive" or "conventional" glycemia-lowering therapy. Over the course of the trial, the group with tighter glycemic control did see a significantly greater decrease in A1c levels (6.9% vs. 8.4%); however, neither MI nor all cause mortality showed a significant decline in the "intensive" therapy group when compared to the "conventional" therapy group (Sharma et al., 2004).

In adults with type 2 diabetes, the advance trial focused on the vascular effects of intensive glycemic therapy. T2DM patients with a history of significant macrovascular or microvascular disease were enrolled in this extensive multi-center randomized control trial from 215 participating centers spread across 20 countries. Following a 5-year period, subjects were randomized to receive either a "intensive" or "standard" glycemia-lowering strategy. With an HbA1c of less than or equal to 6.5%, the intensive glycemic therapy group received treatment. The group that was randomly assigned to the stricter glycemic control did see a notable decrease in HbA1c (6.5% vs. 7.3%) and a 23% decrease in microvascular events, mainly nephropathy. The groups did not differ in terms of MI or all-cause mortality, although the group receiving "intensive" therapy saw a higher hospitalization rate for severe hypoglycemia (McGavock et al., 2007).

The primary focus of the accord trial, which ran alongside the Advance trial, was whether or not strict glycemic control decreased the risk of cardiovascular events. This multi-center randomized control trial examined whether standard glycemic control (HbA1c of 7%–7.9%) and extremely tight glycemic control (less than or equal to an HbA1c of 6%) had lower rates of nonfatal MI, nonfatal stroke, and CV death in older adults. The group with stricter glycemic control did, in fact, achieve a significantly lower HbA1c than those receiving standard treatment (7.3% vs. 6.5%) during the course of an average follow-up of 3.4 years. Although the intensive glycemic control group experienced slightly lower rates of nonfatal MI, the trial was terminated early at 3 years and 7 months due to increased rates of CV and all-cause mortality in the intensive treatment group. According to the Advance trial, there was a higher risk of hypoglycemia and weight gain in the group with strict glycemic control (Rijzewijk et al., 2008).

The long-term follow-up trial EDIC and the Diabetes Control and Complications Trial (DCCT) looked into the effects of rigorous glycemic control combined with intensive therapy on CV outcomes in T1DM patients. Young T1DM patients (ages 13 to 39) were randomly assigned to receive either "intensive" or "conventional" glycemic therapy in these trials, with the "intensive" treatment group having an HbA1c target of 7%. The main outcome of the DCCT trial was a 70% reduction in microvascular complications, specifically retinopathy, in the group with strict glycemic control after ten years of follow-up (Aasum et al., 2003). Furthermore, compared to the group receiving conventional glycemic therapy, those receiving intensive glycemic treatment experienced a 42% decrease in CV events, according to the long-term follow-up study EDIC (Fang et al., 2005).

Although there seems to be a connection between diabetic patients' CV outcomes and glycemic control, there have been contradictory results regarding the impact of strict glycemic control on CVD. Extensive glycemic control (HbA1c ≤ 6.5%) does not appear to significantly improve CV outcomes in patients with type 2 diabetes when compared to standard glycemic control targets (HbA1c of 7%–7.9%). Tighter glycemic control may lead to a slight decrease in microvascular events in T2D patients, but rates of all-cause and CV-specific mortality do not appear to significantly improve. Additionally, as the ACCORD trial demonstrated, extremely strict glycemic control (HbA1c ≤ 6%) may put patients at higher risk for hypoglycemia, weight gain, and all cause mortality. Tighter glycemic control does seem to help patients with type 1 diabetes. Intense glycemic therapy (target HbA1c ≥ 7%) may help lower the rates of microvascular and macrovascular disease in T1D patients, according to the DCCT and EDIC trials (Yu et al., 2002).

According to one possible interpretation of the studies conducted thus far, any benefit that intensive treatment of hyperglycemia may have in reducing risk may be outweighed by the concurrent CV risk factors that diabetics have. Therefore, the greatest benefit from more intensive therapy in terms of CV outcomes may come from diabetic patients who achieve tighter glycemic control earlier in the course of their disease and before the development of other CV risk factors. For this reason, rather than establishing a single A1c cutoff for all diabetic patients, many of the new guidelines aim to customize A1c goals to the specific patient. For instance, the glycemic goals set by the ACC/AHA and VA/DoD are modified in response to variables like age, duration of the illness, and cardiovascular risk. While more research is required to establish the ideal glycemic treatment objective for these various patient populations, diabetic patients may benefit from modifying their target A1c based on their current level of CVD risk (Ng et al., 2010).

5.5.1. Obesity

Obesity is associated with increased rates of CV morbidity and mortality and is a common comorbidity of diabetes, especially type 2 diabetes. Thus, to improve their CV risk profile and lower their risk of CVD, current treatment recommendations for overweight and obese patients with DM encourage weight loss. For diabetic patients who are overweight or obese, it is advised to lose 5% of their body weight over a four-year period. There is "moderate" evidence to support the hypothesis that diabetic patients who lose 5% of their body weight through lifestyle changes also have higher levels of HDL-c, lower triglycerides, and fewer newly prescribed lipid-lowering drugs. Furthermore, a "high" degree of evidence indicates that orlistat is linked to larger drops in fasting blood glucose and HbA1c and causes weight loss of 2-3 kg in overweight and obese diabetic patients at 1 and 2 years. Based on the consistency of the results, scientific methodology, and scientific strength, these recommendations were rated as high, moderate, or low (Jensen et al., 2014). Numerous studies have examined the effectiveness of weight loss in lowering the incidence and severity of DM, given that obesity is a significant risk factor for both T2DM and CVD. Reducing body weight in pre-diabetic patients has been the focus of some studies in an effort to lower the incidence of DM that follows. Notably, the diabetes prevention program (DPP) and the Finnish diabetes prevention studies assessed how behavior modification affected pre-diabetic adults' weight loss and subsequently increased their risk of developing diabetes. According to the similar findings of both studies, individuals assigned to the lifestyle intervention group lost significantly more weight and had a lower chance of developing diabetes than the control group. Other research has examined strategies for achieving weight loss and enhancing the cardiovascular risk profile of individuals with diabetes. Intensive lifestyle interventions, weight-loss drugs, and bariatric surgery were among the many strategies used to help diabetic patients lose weight and improve their CV risk profile by lowering their blood pressure, cholesterol, and glycemic control (Ng et al., 2009).

There is conflicting evidence regarding whether weight loss in diabetic patients truly lowers subsequent CV morbidity and mortality, despite the fact that numerous studies have demonstrated that weight loss is achievable in this population. There hasn't been enough data to determine whether mild weight loss lowers the CV risk in patients with diabetes mellitus. The Look AHEAD trial did not find that weight loss had any effect on hospitalization for angina, MI, stroke, or CV mortality after 9 and a half years of follow-up, although the SCOUT trial found that modest weight loss could improve 5-year CV mortality rates among diabetic patients (Ernande et al., 2010).

Currently, a goal weight loss of 5% is advised for patients with diabetes mellitus who are overweight or obese. Thus far, research has shown that a range of strategies, such as bariatric surgery, medication, and intensive behavioral modification therapy, can be used to achieve this goal in patients who are either pre-diabetic or already have diabetes. Furthermore, all of these weight-loss strategies seem to either improve the CV risk profile of diabetic patients or lower the rates of incident DM in pre-diabetic individuals. It is unclear, nevertheless, if diabetic patients who lose a little weight experience a decline in CVD (Scognamiglio et al., 1998).

It is possible that modest weight loss won't significantly improve CV outcomes in older adults with DM because their CV risk profile is too high. It may be more beneficial to target pre-diabetics with obesity before they experience diabetes mellitus. Weight loss can lower the incidence of incident diabetes, as programs like the DPP have shown. However, more research is required to ascertain whether even modest weight loss in pre-diabetic patients improves CV morbidity and mortality. It is also possible that even though patients with DM appear to benefit from modest weight loss in terms of their CV risk profile, more significant weight loss may be required to observe more noticeable increases in the rates of CV events. There may be a dose effect between weight loss and CV health, which could be further explored in studies on the impact of weight loss exceeding 5% on CVD in diabetic patients (Regan et al., 1977).

5.5.2. Hypertension

As a major risk factor for CVD and a common comorbidity of patients with diabetes mellitus, the current treatment guidelines strongly advise clinicians to lower blood pressure in patients with hypertension. Numerous research have looked into the impact of lowering blood pressure in diabetic patients on the results of cardiovascular disease. In patients with type 2 diabetes, the UKPDS 38 trial looked at the impact of strict blood pressure control (< 150/85) versus less strict control (< 180/105) on macrovascular and microvascular complications. The patients in the tightly controlled blood pressure group (144/82 mmHg) had a significantly lower mean blood pressure after a 9-year follow-up than the patients in the less tightly controlled group (154/87 mmHg). Furthermore, compared to the group with less tightly controlled blood pressure, the tighter control group had a 34% reduction in the risk of macrovascular disease (myocardial infarction, sudden death, stroke, and peripheral vascular disease) and a 37% reduction in the risk of microvascular disease (retinopathy requiring photocoagulation, vitreous hemorrhage, and fatal or non-fatal renal failure) (Tribouilloy et al., 2008).

Many studies have demonstrated that lowering blood pressure in diabetics does improve cardiovascular (CV) outcomes; however, the ACCORD-BP trial looked at the impact of intensive versus standard blood pressure control (systolic < 140 mmHg) on the risk of major CV events that could be fatal or nonfatal in patients with type 2 diabetes. Compared to the standard BP control group (1.87% vs. 2.09% per year), the group with intensive BP control did not experience a decrease in fatal and nonfatal major CV events after 4+7 years of follow-up. Furthermore, there were more adverse events, such as hypotension, syncope, bradycardia or arrhythmia, hyperkalemia, angioedema, and renal failure, in the intensive blood pressure group (Cushman et al., 2010).

According to new treatment guidelines based on the outcomes of these trials, individuals with diabetes who are between the ages of 18 and 60 should begin pharmacologic treatment at a SBP of > 140 mmHg or a DBP of > 90 mmHg. A SBP of less than 150 mmHg or a DBP of less than 90 mmHg is the cutoff point for patients over 60 to begin treatment (Magri et al., 2012). The general non-Black population and the Black population are recommended to use different types of pharmaceutical therapy. A thiazide-type diuretic, calcium channel blocker (CCB), angiotensin-converting enzyme (ACE) inhibitor, or angiotensin receptor blocker (ARB) should be the first line of treatment for non-Black patients with diabetes mellitus and hypertension. A thiazide-type diuretic or a CCB should be the first line of treatment for black patients with DM and hypertension. ARBs or ACE inhibitors should also be used to treat hypertensive patients with CKD and DM to enhance renal outcomes. Numerous studies—including the ALLHAT trial—have found no discernible variation in the risk of coronary heart disease, nonfatal myocardial infarction, overall mortality, or other clinical complications related to the initial antihypertensive drug therapy used to treat diabetic patients, despite the fact that different antihypertensive agents have different metabolic effects when used to treat hypertension. This would imply that variations in metabolism among the different antihypertensive medications do not significantly contribute to the development of CVD later on in DM patients (From et al., 2006). It should be noted that these recommendations have generated controversy. Based on earlier research assessing blood pressure control and the subsequent development of cardiovascular disease in African Americans, women, and the elderly, many authors have contended that the guidelines are excessively lax in the treatment of these at-risk groups. It is likely that there is a therapeutic blood pressure range that lowers the cardiovascular risk and shields diabetic patients from the negative effects of hypotension. It is unclear if the new recommendations fall within this therapeutic blood pressure range, especially given the higher systolic blood pressure threshold in adults over 60. Little research has been done to determine the appropriate treatment range for various age groups. Furthermore, the impact of hypertension on cardiovascular health may vary amongst racial subgroups. To determine the optimal blood pressure range for adults across various age and racial demographic groups, more research is required (Dei et al., 2015).

5.5.3. Dyslipidemia

Dyslipidemia is linked to a higher risk of CVD and is prevalent in DM patients. To help lower their risk of further CV events, healthcare professionals are urged to recognize and treat patients with dyslipidemia aggressively. The current recommendation for treating dyslipidemia in diabetic patients varies according to age and is consistent with the understanding that the clinical trial-validated approach is to treat patients with fixed-dose statins rather than to specific LDL target levels. Therefore, if a diabetic patient has clinical evidence of atherosclerotic CVD or an LDL-c greater than 189 mg/dL, it is advised that they take a high-intensity statin. This recommendation applies to patients under the age of 40. Starting statin therapy is advised for all diabetic patients over 40. Over-40-year-olds who have an estimated 10-year ASCVD risk of more than 7.5% are treated with high-intensity statins; those whose risk is less than 7.5% are treated with moderate-intensity statins (Rolim et al., 2008).

The impact of treating dyslipidemia in diabetic patients as a way to reduce CV risk has been the subject of numerous studies. The CARDS study was the first multicenter randomized controlled trial designed to assess statin therapy in T2DM patients prospectively. A placebo or 10 mg/d of atorvastatin was administered randomly to adult T2DM patients. The group treated with atorvastatin experienced an average reduction in total cholesterol of 26% and in LDL-c of 40% over the course of a follow-up period of 3.9 years. Furthermore, compared to the placebo-treated group, the statin therapy group experienced a reduction of 37% in cardiovascular events, 27% in all-cause mortality, and 48% in stroke. The substantial benefit of statin therapy led to the early termination of the CARDS trial (Prince et al., 2010).

Following the CARDS trial's conclusion that statin therapy significantly improved cardiovascular outcomes for patients with diabetes, the TNT trial looked at the impact of high-dose statins on mortality from CAD, MI that is not fatal, and stroke that is either fatal or nonfatal in patients with type 2 diabetes. The adult T2DM patients were followed for an average of 4.9 years after being randomly assigned to receive either a low dose (10 mg/d) or a high dose (80 mg/d) of statin. The high dose stain group outperformed the lower dose group in terms of reduction in combined CAD mortality, nonfatal MI, and fatal or nonfatal stroke (8.7% vs. 10.9%). They also achieved a greater reduction in LDL-c (77 mg/dL vs. 101 mg/dL). The higher dose group did, however, experience a higher incidence of side effects, such as myalgia, rhabdomyolysis, or a persistent increase in alanine aminotransferase or aspartate aminotransferase (Vinik and Ziegler, 2007).

As many studies had demonstrated that statins, particularly high-dose statins, had CV benefit in diabetic patients, the 4D study examined the effect of statins in diabetic patients receiving hemodialysis. In the 4D trial, diabetic patients receiving hemodialysis were randomly assigned either 20 mg of atorvastatin per day or a placebo (Kannel and McGee, 1979). The purpose of the study was to determine if a low-dose statin in diabetic patients with end stage renal disease lowered the rates of death from cardiac causes, nonfatal myocardial infarction, and stroke as compared to the placebo group. The group randomized to the statin therapy did have a significant reduction in their LDL-c compared to the placebo group (-42.0% *vs* -1.3%), but there was no significant difference between the groups in CV outcomes after 3.96 years of follow-up. In addition, there were significantly more cases of fatal stroke in the statin therapy group than those treated with a placebo (Fuller et al., 1983).

While the previous studies had focused on reducing cholesterol in diabetic patients using statin therapy, other research groups have investigated the effect of non-statin lipid-lowering therapies on CVD in diabetic patients. For example, the FIELD trial evaluated if lowering cholesterol *via* fenofibrate therapy could improve CV outcomes in patients with DM. In the FIELD trial, diabetic patients (mean age 62 years; 63% men) were randomized to either receive a fenofibrate (200 mg/d) or a placebo and then assessed for subsequent rates of fatal coronary heart disease (CHD) or nonfatal MIs. While the group randomized to the fenofibrate therapy did reduce their cholesterol compared to the placebo group at 4 mo (total cholesterol, LDL-cholesterol, and triglycerides by 11%, 12%, and 29%, respectively), the differences decreased between the groups as the trial continued due in a large part to patients starting additional cholesterol lowering therapies outside of the study. After a median of 5 years, the group randomized to the fenofibrate group had a combined 11% reduction in fatal CHD or nonfatal MIs, but this difference was non-significant (Haffner, 2000). The fenofibrate group did however have a statistically significant reduction (24%) in nonfatal MI's compared to the placebo group. In addition, since HDL has been identified in many large prospective studies to be associated with improved CV health, some research groups have investigated whether raising HDL through pharmaceutical agents reduces the risk of CV events. The HATS trial was the first to investigate the effect of increasing HDL with Niacin therapy and generated promising results on improving CV outcomes in adult patients (16% with DM). After 38 mo of follow-up, the group randomized to the niacin therapy did have a significant increase in HDL and patients with T2DM had a 13% decrease in absolute risk of CV disease. Recently however, the AIM-HIGH trial found no significant clinical benefit in adding Niacin therapy to patients with atherosclerotic CVD as compared to a placebo. The trial was stopped after 3 years due to lack of efficacy; the group randomized to the niacin therapy (34% with DM) did not have a significant reduction in composite coronary heart disease, nonfatal myocardial infarction, ischemic stroke, hospitalization for an acute coronary syndrome, or symptom-driven coronary or cerebral revascularization (16.4% *vs* 16.2%) despite significant improvements in HDL (25% *vs* 11.8%). These findings were similar between diabetics and nondiabetics (Williams et al., 2003).

A significant risk factor for CVD, dyslipidemia is common in diabetic patients. According to current treatment guidelines, physicians should primarily use statins to lower lipid levels in diabetic patients; the dosage of the medication should be determined by the patient's risk level. A combination of statins and other lipid-lowering treatments may provide additional CV benefit for patients with diabetes mellitus, according to certain trials (Vinik et al., 2001). For instance, in the IMPROVE-IT trial, it was discovered that ezetimibe, a cholesterol absorption inhibitor, plus simvastatin reduced the risk of cardiovascular events in patients with diabetes who had acute coronary syndrome, better than simvastatin alone. Based on available data, patients with diabetes mellitus may benefit from statin therapy for their cardiovascular health. Higher dosages and combined lipid-lowering treatments may also offer additional CV protection. Although some meta-analyses have indicated that statin therapy may be linked to a higher incidence of diabetes mellitus, the benefits of the medication in patients with diabetes far exceed the risks. Statins have shown to be more effective than other lipid-lowering medications in reducing cardiovascular events; fenofibrates are one such example. Pharmacological agents that increase HDL also seem to offer little to no benefit to the cardiovascular system. To fully comprehend HDL's role in CV health, more research is required (Vischer et al., 1998).

5.5.4. CAN

CAN is a frequent side effect of diabetes that raises the risk of CV-related morbidity and death in DM patients. Diabetes patients frequently have autonomic dysfunction, which is linked to a high risk of cardiac arrhythmias, sudden death, silent myocardial ischemia, diabetic cardiomyopathy, stroke, and both intraoperative and perioperative CV instability. Heart rate variability (variability in the instantaneous beat-to-beat intervals), orthostatic hypotension, exercise intolerance, resting tachycardia, and abnormal blood pressure regulation are some of the most prevalent clinical manifestations of CAN (Sobel et al., 1998).

The pathogenesis and complications of CAN can be slowed down by treating autonomic dysfunction early on. Tight glycemic control may be crucial in lowering the incidence of CAN in DM patients, according to certain studies. For instance, the DCCT showed that patients' risk of developing autonomic dysfunction was significantly lower in those with better glycemic control, as indicated by Hba1c, as indicated by a CAN index. Some trials, such as the Steno-2 study, found that reducing the prevalence of CAN in T2DM patients was possible by improving glucose control and other cardiovascular risk factors. However, the effect of glycemic control on CAN in patients with T2DM has not been as clear-cut. Autonomic dysfunction has been improved by lifestyle interventions aimed at promoting weight loss and increasing exercise endurance. Aldose reductase inhibitors, ACE inhibitors, and angiotensin receptor blockers are examples of pharmaceutical therapy that appears to help slow the progression of CAN. Furthermore, by reducing ventricular hypertrophy and restoring calcium homeostasis in diabetic cardiomyocytes, IGF-1, ACE inhibitors, and beta-blockers seem to be helpful in the treatment of diabetic cardiomyopathy. However, more research is required to confirm which pharmacological intervention is most effective for diabetic patients with CAN. (Gaede et al., 2003)

5.6. FUTURE DIRECTIONS IN THE TREATMENT OF DM

Even though many trials have contributed to our understanding of DM's relationship to CVD, more work is needed to accurately identify and measure CV risk in DM patients. Further investigation is required to determine the relationship between glycemic control and CVD. There is proof that patients with diabetes mellitus benefit from better glycemic control in terms of their cardiovascular health. According to one study, the degree of coronary artery disease can be independently predicted by a patient's HbA1c in those without diabetes. This finding implies that glucose control is essential for maintaining the health of the cardiovascular system in all patient populations. While large randomized control trials like ADVANCE and ACCORD have demonstrated that the effect of strict glycemic control on subsequent CVD is modest and largely attributable to coexisting traditional risk factors, this observational trial suggests an independent association between glycemic levels and CVD (Ceriello et al., 1990).

Inadequate measurement instruments could be one reason for the contradictory findings about the connection between glycemic control and CVD. For instance, fasting plasma glucose (FPG) is frequently used to determine glycemia; however, research has shown that diabetic patients' FPG levels vary daily within-person by 12 to 15%. Although there is evidence that biological variations and differences in RBC survival among patients cause HbA1c to not accurately reflect glycemic control, the day-to-day within-person variance for HbA1c is much better (< 2%). Setting clinically meaningful goals for patients with diabetes mellitus requires accurately measuring glycemia and relating it to CV risk, if glycemic control is important at all (Boras et al., 2010).

The severity and course of CVD may also be influenced by the length of time and the point at which improved glycemic control occurs. The UKPDS showed that in middle-aged adults (median 54 years) with recent DM diagnosis, strict glycemic control was linked to improved CV outcomes (Wackers et al., 2004). On the other hand, strict glycemic control may not prevent further cardiovascular disease (CVD) and may even be detrimental to patients who are slightly older and have had diabetes for a longer period of time, according to the findings of the ADVANCE and ACCORD trials. This may demonstrate that aggressively treating hyperglycemia in high-risk patients with long-standing diabetes mellitus is too late to produce a clinically meaningful effect, and that treating patients aggressively early on may be more advantageous for those diagnosed with the disease soon after. Further research is required to clarify the connection between glycemic control and the onset of CVD and to ascertain whether the timing of treatment onset and duration affects the incidence of CV events in DM patients (Fazzini et al., 1993).

The optimal course of action for reducing the incidence and severity of cardiomyopathy and CAN in DM patients will require more investigation. Numerous studies have shown that patients with diabetes mellitus (DM) are more likely to experience autonomic dysfunction and diabetic cardiomyopathy, two disease processes that increase the risk of future cardiovascular problems. It appears that pharmacological agents, stricter glycemic control, and lifestyle modification can slow the progression of diabetic cardiomyopathy and CAN. Few studies, however, have looked into the best specific therapies for treating these conditions and what can be done to stop these disease processes from ever developing (Koistinen, 1990).

To enhance our understanding of the monitoring and management of traditional CV risk factors in diabetic patients, such as blood pressure, obesity, and dyslipidemia, more research is required. For instance, combination therapy may be more effective than statin monotherapy in treating dyslipidemia, despite the current recommendation to the contrary. The best course of treatment for managing dyslipidemia in diabetic patients may be determined by further studies such as IMPROVE-IT. Furthermore, since HDL's impact on CV health is complex, more research is required to ascertain whether pharmaceuticals that raise HDL can benefit diabetic patients clinically. It is also not entirely clear how weight loss affects DM patients or how much weight loss is required to produce clinically meaningful improvements in CV outcomes. Diabetes patients with additional cardiovascular risk factors and comorbidities may find that a 5% weight loss is insufficient. To find out how much weight needs to be lost to benefit from CV, as well as the most effective way to get there, more research is required. Lastly, it will be important to continuously monitor the consequences of the new blood pressure guidelines in the future, especially for adults over 60 who now fall below the higher systolic blood pressure threshold (Ziegler et al., 1992).

A Closer Look

Cardiovascular Disease in Type 2 Diabetes Mellitus

Cardiovascular disease (CVD) is a leading cause of morbidity and mortality in individuals with type 2 diabetes mellitus (T2DM). Type 2 diabetes, characterized by insulin resistance and relative insulin deficiency, significantly increases the risk of developing a range of cardiovascular conditions, including coronary artery disease, heart failure, stroke, and peripheral arterial disease. This heightened risk is due to a combination of factors associated with diabetes, such as chronic hyperglycemia, dyslipidemia, hypertension, and pro-inflammatory and pro-thrombotic states.

One of the primary mechanisms linking T2DM to CVD is atherosclerosis, the buildup of fatty deposits or plaques within the arterial walls, which leads to narrowed and hardened arteries. Chronic hyperglycemia in T2DM accelerates the process of atherosclerosis by promoting endothelial dysfunction, oxidative stress, and inflammation. Endothelial dysfunction, in particular, reduces the availability of nitric oxide, a molecule essential for vascular relaxation and health, thereby contributing to vascular stiffness and increased blood pressure (O'Brien et al., 1986).

Dyslipidemia, commonly seen in T2DM, further exacerbates cardiovascular risk. Patients with T2DM often have elevated levels of triglycerides, low levels of high-density lipoprotein (HDL) cholesterol, and an abundance of small, dense low-density lipoprotein (LDL) particles. This lipid profile is particularly atherogenic, meaning it greatly enhances the potential for plaque formation and growth, leading to coronary artery disease and other vascular complications (Garber et al., 2013).

Hypertension, or high blood pressure, frequently coexists with T2DM and is a major contributor to cardiovascular complications. The combination of hypertension and diabetes significantly increases the strain on the cardiovascular system, promoting damage to the heart and blood vessels. This synergistic effect not only heightens the risk of coronary artery disease but also increases the likelihood of heart failure and stroke.

Moreover, the chronic inflammatory state associated with T2DM plays a crucial role in the development and progression of CVD. Elevated levels of inflammatory markers, such as C-reactive protein (CRP) and interleukin-6 (IL-6), are often observed in individuals with T2DM. Inflammation contributes to plaque instability, making plaques more prone to rupture and leading to acute cardiovascular events like myocardial infarction and ischemic stroke (Skyler et al., 2009).

Effective management of cardiovascular risk in T2DM involves a multifaceted approach targeting glycemic control, lipid levels, blood pressure, and lifestyle factors. Glycemic control, typically monitored through HbA1c levels, is essential to reduce microvascular complications and, to some extent, macrovascular complications. Statins are widely used to manage dyslipidemia and lower LDL cholesterol levels, thereby reducing the risk of atherosclerotic events. Antihypertensive medications, such as ACE inhibitors or angiotensin II receptor blockers (ARBs), are crucial for managing blood pressure and providing cardiovascular protection (King et al., 1999).

Lifestyle interventions, including a healthy diet, regular physical activity, weight management, and smoking cessation, are foundational to reducing cardiovascular risk in individuals with T2DM. These lifestyle changes help improve insulin sensitivity, lower blood pressure, and improve lipid profiles, thereby mitigating the risk of cardiovascular complications.

Summary

- Cardiovascular disease (CVD) is a class of diseases that involve the heart or blood vessels, and is tone of the most common causes of death and disability among people with diabetes. Diabetes is associated with high blood pressure and cholesterol levels, and these lead to increased risk of atherosclerosis (narrowing of the arteries). This can lead to symptoms such as angina pectoris or intermittent claudication. High blood glucose can make the blood coagulation system more active, increasing the risk of blood clots. Together these can lead to arteries being blocked completely, stopping the blood flow, resulting in conditions such as myocardial infarction, stroke and gangrene.
- The heart receives its blood supply from the coronary arteries. Coronary artery disease occurs when these arteries are narrowed or blocked. Coronary artery disease, also known as ischaemic heart disease, atherosclerotic heart disease or coronary heart disease is a group of diseases that includes angina pectoris, heart attack, heart failure and sudden coronary death.
- Obesity is common in patients with DM, particularly T2DM, and is associated with an increased risk of CVD. One possible mechanism linking DM and obesity with subsequent CVD is low-grade inflammation.
- Diabetic patients are at increased risk of developing dyslipidemia. One mechanism underlying this connection is increased free fatty-acid release present in insulin-resistant fat cells. High levels of free-fatty acids promote triglyceride production, which in turn stimulates the secretion of apolipoprotein B (ApoB) and very LDL (VLDL) cholesterol.
- Cardiovascular autonomic neuropathy (CAN) is common among patients with DM and is correlated with an increased 5-year mortality rate from CVD. The clinical manifestations of CAN are resting tachycardia, postural hypotension, exercise intolerance, abnormal coronary vasomotor regulation, increased QT interval, and perioperative instability.
- Diabetes Control and Complications Trial (DCCT) and the long-term follow-up trial EDIC investigated how strict glycemic control with intensive therapy affected CV outcomes in patients with T1DM. These trials randomized young (ages 13-39 years) patients with T1DM to either "intensive" or "conventional" glycemic therapy with an HbA1c goal of 7% in the group for those in the "intensive" treatment group.

References

1. Aasum, E., Hafstad, A. D., Severson, D. L., & Larsen, T. S. (2003). Age-dependent changes in metabolism, contractile function, and ischemic sensitivity in hearts from db/db mice. *Diabetes, 52*(2), 434–441.
2. Aguiree, F., Brown, A., Cho, N. H., Dahlquist, G., Dodd, S., Dunning, T., Hirst, M., Hwang, C., Magliano, D., & Patterson, C. (2013). *IDF Diabetes Atlas.*
3. American Diabetes Association. (2008). Economic costs of diabetes in the U.S. in 2007. *Diabetes Care, 31*(3), 596–615.

4. Asghar, O., Al-Sunni, A., Khavandi, K., Khavandi, A., Withers, S., Greenstein, A., Heagerty, A. M., & Malik, R. A. (2009). Diabetic cardiomyopathy. *Clinical Science, 116*(10), 741–760.

5. Ashraf, H., Boroumand, M. A., Amirzadegan, A., Talesh, S. A., & Davoodi, G. (2013). Hemoglobin A1C in non-diabetic patients: An independent predictor of coronary artery disease and its severity. *Diabetes Research and Clinical Practice, 102*(3), 225–232.

6. Bahia, L. R., Araujo, D. V., Schaan, B. D., Dib, S. A., Negrato, C. A., Leão, M. P., Ramos, A. J., Forti, A. C., Gomes, M. B., Foss, M. C., et al. (2011). The costs of type 2 diabetes mellitus outpatient care in the Brazilian public health system. *Value in Health, 14*(1), S137–S140.

7. Barouch, L. A., Berkowitz, D. E., Harrison, R. W., O'Donnell, C. P., & Hare, J. M. (2003). Disruption of leptin signaling contributes to cardiac hypertrophy independently of body weight in mice. *Circulation, 108*(6), 754–759.

8. Belke, D. D., Betuing, S., Tuttle, M. J., Graveleau, C., Young, M. E., Pham, M., Zhang, D., Cooksey, R. C., McClain, D. A., & Litwin, S. E. (2002). Insulin signaling coordinately regulates cardiac size, metabolism, and contractile protein isoform expression. *Journal of Clinical Investigation, 109*(5), 629–639.

9. Boden, W. E., Probstfield, J. L., Anderson, T., Chaitman, B. R., Desvignes-Nickens, P., Koprowicz, K., McBride, R., Teo, K., & Weintraub, W. (2011). Niacin in patients with low HDL cholesterol levels receiving intensive statin therapy. *New England Journal of Medicine, 365*(23), 2255–2267.

10. Boras, J., Brkljačić, N., Ljubičić, A., & Ljubić, S. (2010). Silent ischemia and diabetes mellitus. *Diabetologia Croatica, 39*(1), 57–65.

11. Brooks, B. A., Franjic, B., Ban, C. R., Swaraj, K., Yue, D. K., Celermajer, D. S., & Twigg, S. M. (2008). Diastolic dysfunction and abnormalities of the microcirculation in type 2 diabetes. *Diabetes, Obesity and Metabolism, 10*(9), 739–746.

12. Brown, B. G., Zhao, X. Q., Chait, A., Fisher, L. D., Cheung, M. C., Morse, J. S., Dowdy, A. A., Marino, E. K., Bolson, E. L., Alaupovic, P., et al. (2001). Simvastatin and niacin, antioxidant vitamins, or the combination for the prevention of coronary disease. *New England Journal of Medicine, 345*(22), 1583–1592.

13. Cannon, C. P., Blazing, M. A., Giugliano, R. P., McCagg, A., White, J. A., Theroux, P., Darius, H., Lewis, B. S., Ophuis, T. O., Jukema, J. W., et al. (2015). Ezetimibe added to statin therapy after acute coronary syndromes. *New England Journal of Medicine, 372*(25), 2387–2397.

14. Centers for Disease Control and Prevention. (2014). *National Diabetes Statistics Report: Estimates of Diabetes and its Burden in the United States, 2014*. U.S. Department of Health and Human Services.

15. Ceriello, A., Giugliano, D., Quatraro, A., Marchi, E., Barbanti, M., & Lefèbvre, P. (1990). Evidence for a hyperglycaemia-dependent decrease of antithrombin III-thrombin complex formation in humans. *Diabetologia, 33*(3), 163–167.

16. Chahil, T. J., & Ginsberg, H. N. (2006). Diabetic dyslipidemia. *Endocrinology and Metabolism Clinics of North America, 35*(3), 491–510.

17. Chait, A., Han, C. Y., Oram, J. F., & Heinecke, J. W. (2005). Lipoprotein-associated inflammatory proteins: Markers or mediators of cardiovascular disease? *Journal of Lipid Research, 46*(3), 389–403.

18. Colhoun, H. M., Betteridge, D. J., Durrington, P. N., Hitman, G. A., Neil, H. A., Livingstone,

S. J., Thomason, M. J., Mackness, M. I., Charlton-Menys, V., & Fuller, J. H. (2004). Primary prevention of cardiovascular disease with atorvastatin in type 2 diabetes in the Collaborative Atorvastatin Diabetes Study (CARDS): Multicenter randomized placebo-controlled trial. *Lancet, 364*(9435), 685–696.

19. Cushman, W. C., Evans, G. W., Byington, R. P., Goff, D. C., Grimm, R. H., Cutler, J. A., Simons-Morton, D. G., Basile, J. N., Corson, M. A., Probstfield, J. L., et al. (2010). Effects of intensive blood-pressure control in type 2 diabetes mellitus. *New England Journal of Medicine, 362*(17), 1575–1585.

20. Dei Cas, A., Khan, S. S., Butler, J., Mentz, R. J., Bonow, R. O., Avogaro, A., Tschoepe, D., Doehner, W., Greene, S. J., Senni, M., et al. (2015). Impact of diabetes on epidemiology, treatment, and outcomes of patients with heart failure. *Journal of the American College of Cardiology: Heart Failure, 3*(2), 136–145.

21. Duckworth, W. C., McCarren, M., & Abraira, C. (2001). Glucose control and cardiovascular complications: The VA Diabetes Trial. *Diabetes Care, 24*(6), 942–945.

22. Duncan, B. B., Schmidt, M. I., Pankow, J. S., Ballantyne, C. M., Couper, D., Vigo, A., Hoogeveen, R., Folsom, A. R., & Heiss, G. (2003). Low-grade systemic inflammation and the development of type 2 diabetes: The Atherosclerosis Risk in Communities study. *Diabetes, 52*(7), 1799–1805.

23. Eguchi, K., Boden-Albala, B., Jin, Z., Rundek, T., Sacco, R. L., Homma, S., & Di Tullio, M. R. (2008). Association between diabetes mellitus and left ventricular hypertrophy in a multiethnic population. *American Journal of Cardiology, 101*(12), 1787–1791.

24. Ernande, L., Rietzschel, E. R., Bergerot, C., De Buyzere, M. L., Schnell, F., Groisne, L., Ovize, M., Croisille, P., Moulin, P., Gillebert, T. C., et al. (2010). Impaired myocardial radial function in asymptomatic patients with type 2 diabetes mellitus: A speckle-tracking imaging study. *Journal of the American Society of Echocardiography, 23*(12), 1266–1272.

25. Fang, Z. Y., Schull-Meade, R., Leano, R., Mottram, P. M., Prins, J. B., & Marwick, T. H. (2005). Screening for heart disease in diabetic subjects. *American Heart Journal, 149*(2), 349–354.

26. Fazzini, P. F., Prati, P. L., Rovelli, F., Antoniucci, D., Menghini, F., Seccareccia, F., & Menotti, A. (1993). Epidemiology of silent myocardial ischemia in asymptomatic middle-aged men (the ECCIS Project). *American Journal of Cardiology, 72*(17), 1383–1388.

27. Ferrarezi, D. A., Cheurfa, N., Reis, A. F., Fumeron, F., & Velho, G. (2007). Adiponectin gene and cardiovascular risk in type 2 diabetic patients: A review of evidence. *Arquivos Brasileiros de Endocrinologia & Metabologia, 51*(2), 153–159.

28. From, A. M., Leibson, C. L., Bursi, F., Redfield, M. M., Weston, S. A., Jacobsen, S. J., Rodeheffer, R. J., & Roger, V. L. (2006). Diabetes in heart failure: Prevalence and impact on outcome in the population. *American Journal of Medicine, 119*(7), 591–599.

29. Fuller, J. H., Shipley, M. J., Rose, G., Jarrett, R. J., & Keen, H. (1983). Mortality from coronary heart disease and stroke in relation to degree of glycaemia: The Whitehall study. *British Medical Journal (Clinical Research Edition), 287*(6394), 867–870.

30. Gaede, P., Vedel, P., Larsen, N., Jensen, G. V., Parving, H. H., & Pedersen, O. (2003). Multifactorial intervention and cardiovascular disease in patients with type 2 diabetes. *New England Journal of Medicine, 348*(5), 383–393.

31. Galderisi, M., Anderson, K. M., Wilson, P. W., & Levy, D. (1991). Echocardiographic evidence for

the existence of a distinct diabetic cardiomyopathy (the Framingham Heart Study). *American Journal of Cardiology, 68*(1), 85–89.

32. Garber, A. J., Abrahamson, M. J., Barzilay, J. I., Blonde, L., Bloomgarden, Z. T., Bush, M. A., Dagogo-Jack, S., Davidson, M. B., Einhorn, D., Garvey, W. T., et al. (2013). American Association of Clinical Endocrinologists' comprehensive diabetes management algorithm 2013 consensus statement–executive summary. *Endocrine Practice, 19*(6), 536–557.

33. Gesualdo, L., Ranieri, E., Monno, R., Rossiello, M. R., Colucci, M., Semeraro, N., Grandaliano, G., Schena, F. P., Ursi, M., & Cerullo, G. (1999). Angiotensin IV stimulates plasminogen activator inhibitor-1 expression in proximal tubular epithelial cells. *Kidney International, 56*(2), 461–470.

34. Haffner, S. M. (2000). Coronary heart disease in patients with diabetes. *New England Journal of Medicine, 342*(15), 1040–1042.

35. Hamilton, S. J., & Watts, G. F. (2013). Endothelial dysfunction in diabetes: Pathogenesis, significance, and treatment. *Reviews in Diabetic Studies, 10*(2–3), 133–156.

36. James, P. A., Oparil, S., Carter, B. L., Cushman, W. C., Dennison-Himmelfarb, C., Handler, J., Lackland, D. T., LeFevre, M. L., MacKenzie, T. D., Ogedegbe, O., et al. (2014). 2014 evidence-based guideline for the management of high blood pressure in adults: Report from the panel members appointed to the Eighth Joint National Committee (JNC 8). *JAMA, 311*(5), 507–520.

37. James, W. P., Caterson, I. D., Coutinho, W., Finer, N., Van Gaal, L. F., Maggioni, A. P., Torp-Pedersen, C., Sharma, A. M., Shepherd, G. M., Rode, R. A., et al. (2010). Effect of sibutramine on cardiovascular outcomes in overweight and obese subjects. *New England Journal of Medicine, 363*(10), 905–917.

38. Jensen, M. D., Ryan, D. H., Apovian, C. M., Ard, J. D., Comuzzie, A. G., Donato, K. A., Hu, F. B., Hubbard, V. S., Jakicic, J. M., Kushner, R. F., et al. (2014). 2013 AHA/ACC/TOS guideline for the management of overweight and obesity in adults: A report of the American College of Cardiology/American Heart Association Task Force on Practice Guidelines and The Obesity Society. *Circulation, 129*(25 Suppl 2), S102–S138.

39. Kajstura, J., Fiordaliso, F., Andreoli, A. M., Li, B., Chimenti, S., Medow, M. S., Limana, F., Nadal-Ginard, B., Leri, A., & Anversa, P. (2001). IGF-1 overexpression inhibits the development of diabetic cardiomyopathy and angiotensin II-mediated oxidative stress. *Diabetes, 50*(6), 1414–1424.

40. Kannel, W. B. (1985). Lipids, diabetes, and coronary heart disease: Insights from the Framingham Study. *American Heart Journal, 110*(5), 1100–1107.

41. Kannel, W. B., & McGee, D. L. (1979). Diabetes and cardiovascular disease: The Framingham study. *JAMA, 241*(19), 2035–2038.

42. Keech, A., Simes, R. J., Barter, P., Best, J., Scott, R., Taskinen, M. R., Forder, P., Pillai, A., Davis, T., Glasziou, P., et al. (2005). Effects of long-term fenofibrate therapy on cardiovascular events in 9795 people with type 2 diabetes mellitus (the FIELD study): Randomized controlled trial. *Lancet, 366*(9500), 1849–1861.

43. Kim, M., Oh, J. K., Sakata, S., Liang, I., Park, W., Hajjar, R. J., & Lebeche, D. (2008). Role of resistin in cardiac contractility and hypertrophy. *Journal of Molecular and Cellular Cardiology, 45*(2), 270–280.

44. King, P., Peacock, I., & Donnelly, R. (1999). The UK prospective diabetes study (UKPDS): Clinical and therapeutic implications for type 2 diabetes. *British Journal of Clinical Pharmacology, 48*(5), 643–648.

45. Knowler, W. C., Barrett-Connor, E., Fowler, S. E., Hamman, R. F., Lachin, J. M., Walker, E. A., & Nathan, D. M. (2002). Reduction in the incidence of type 2 diabetes with lifestyle intervention or metformin. *New England Journal of Medicine, 346*(6), 393–403.

46. Koistinen, M. J. (1990). Prevalence of asymptomatic myocardial ischaemia in diabetic subjects. *BMJ, 301*(6745), 92–95.

47. Krakoff, L. R., Gillespie, R. L., Ferdinand, K. C., Fergus, I. V., Akinboboye, O., Williams, K. A., Walsh, M. N., Bairey Merz, C. N., & Pepine, C. J. (2014). 2014 hypertension recommendations from the eighth joint national committee panel members raise concerns for elderly black and female populations. *Journal of the American College of Cardiology, 64*(4), 394–402.

48. Krauss, R. M., & Siri, P. W. (2004). Dyslipidemia in type 2 diabetes. *Medical Clinics of North America, 88*(4), 897–909.

49. LaRosa, J. C., Grundy, S. M., Waters, D. D., Shear, C., Barter, P., Fruchart, J. C., Gotto, A. M., Greten, H., Kastelein, J. J., Shepherd, J., et al. (2005). Intensive lipid lowering with atorvastatin in patients with stable coronary disease. *New England Journal of Medicine, 352*(14), 1425–1435.

50. Leahy, J. L. (2005). Pathogenesis of type 2 diabetes mellitus. *Archives of Medical Research, 36*(3), 197–209.

51. Leri, A., Liu, Y., Wang, X., Kajstura, J., Malhotra, A., Meggs, L. G., & Anversa, P. (1999). Overexpression of insulin-like growth factor-1 attenuates the myocyte renin-angiotensin system in transgenic mice. *Circulation Research, 84*(7), 752–762.

52. Li, Y. W., & Aronow, W. S. (2011). Diabetes mellitus and cardiovascular disease. *Journal of Clinical & Experimental Cardiology, 2*(2).

53. Magri, C. J., Cassar, A., Fava, S., & Felice, H. (2012). Heart failure with preserved ejection fraction and diabetes mellitus. *Journal of Diabetes Research & Clinical Metabolism, 1*(1), 2.

54. Matheus, A. S., Cobas, R. A., & Gomes, M. B. (2008). Dyslipidemias in type 1 diabetes: A current approach. *Arquivos Brasileiros de Endocrinologia & Metabologia, 52*(2), 334–339.

55. Matheus, A. S., Tannus, L. R., Cobas, R. A., Palma, C. C., Negrato, C. A., & Gomes, M. B. (2013). Impact of diabetes on cardiovascular disease: An update. *International Journal of Hypertension, 2013*, 653789.

56. McGavock, J. M., Lingvay, I., Zib, I., Tillery, T., Salas, N., Unger, R., Levine, B. D., Raskin, P., Victor, R. G., & Szczepaniak, L. S. (2007). Cardiac steatosis in diabetes mellitus: A 1H-magnetic resonance spectroscopy study. *Circulation, 116*(10), 1170–1175.

57. Mooradian, A. D., Albert, S. G., & Haas, M. J. (2007). Low serum high-density lipoprotein cholesterol in obese subjects with normal serum triglycerides: The role of insulin resistance and inflammatory cytokines. *Diabetes, Obesity and Metabolism, 9*(4), 441–443.

58. Ng, A. C., Delgado, V., Bertini, M., van der Meer, R. W., Rijzewijk, L. J., Hooi Ewe, S., Siebelink, H. M., Smit, J. W., Diamant, M., Romijn, J. A., et al. (2010). Myocardial steatosis and biventricular strain and strain rate imaging in patients with type 2 diabetes mellitus. *Circulation, 122*(25), 2538–2544.

59. Ng, A. C., Delgado, V., Bertini, M., van der Meer, R. W., Rijzewijk, L. J., Shanks, M., Nucifora, G., Smit, J. W., Diamant, M., Romijn, J. A., et al. (2009). Findings from left ventricular strain and strain rate imaging in asymptomatic patients with type 2 diabetes mellitus. *American Journal of Cardiology, 104*(10), 1398–1401.

60. Norby, F. L., Wold, L. E., Duan, J., Hintz, K. K., & Ren, J. (2002). IGF-I attenuates diabetes-induced cardiac contractile dysfunction in ventricular myocytes. *American Journal of Physiology-Endocrinology and Metabolism, 283*(4), E658–E666.

61. O'Brien, I. A., O'Hare, P., Lewin, I. G., & Corrall, R. J. (1986). The prevalence of autonomic neuropathy in insulin-dependent diabetes mellitus: A controlled study based on heart rate variability. *Quarterly Journal of Medicine, 61*(238), 957–967.

62. O'Neil, P. M., Smith, S. R., Weissman, N. J., Fidler, M. C., Sanchez, M., Zhang, J., Raether, B., Anderson, C. M., & Shanahan, W. R. (2012). Randomized placebo-controlled clinical trial of lorcaserin for weight loss in type 2 diabetes mellitus: The BLOOM-DM study. *Obesity (Silver Spring), 20*(7), 1426–1436.

63. Ollerton, R. L., Playle, R., Ahmed, K., Dunstan, F. D., Luzio, S. D., & Owens, D. R. (1999). Day-to-day variability of fasting plasma glucose in newly diagnosed type 2 diabetic subjects. *Diabetes Care, 22*(3), 394–398.

64. Patel, A., MacMahon, S., Chalmers, J., Neal, B., Billot, L., Woodward, M., Marre, M., Cooper, M., Glasziou, P., Grobbee, D., et al. (2008). Intensive blood glucose control and vascular outcomes in patients with type 2 diabetes. *New England Journal of Medicine, 358*(24), 2560–2572.

65. Patil, V. C., Patil, H. V., Shah, K. B., Vasani, J. D., & Shetty, P. (2011). Diastolic dysfunction in asymptomatic type 2 diabetes mellitus with normal systolic function. *Journal of Cardiovascular Disease Research, 2*(4), 213–222.

66. Petersen, P. H., Jørgensen, L. G., Brandslund, I., De Fine Olivarius, N., & Stahl, M. (2005). Consequences of bias and imprecision in measurements of glucose and HbA1c for the diagnosis and prognosis of diabetes mellitus. *Scandinavian Journal of Clinical and Laboratory Investigation, 240*, 51–60.

67. Pogach, L., Conlin, P. R., Hobbs, C., & Vigersky, R. A. (2011). VA-DoD update of diabetes guidelines: What clinicians need to know about absolute risk of benefits and harms and A1c laboratory accuracy. *Federal Practitioner.*

68. Pop-Busui, R. (2010). Cardiac autonomic neuropathy in diabetes: A clinical perspective. *Diabetes Care, 33*(2), 434–441.

69. Prince, C. T., Secrest, A. M., Mackey, R. H., Arena, V. C., Kingsley, L. A., & Orchard, T. J. (2010). Cardiovascular autonomic neuropathy, HDL cholesterol, and smoking correlate with arterial stiffness markers determined 18 years later in type 1 diabetes. *Diabetes Care, 33*(3), 652–657.

70. Regan, T. J., Lyons, M. M., Ahmed, S. S., Levinson, G. E., Oldewurtel, H. A., Ahmad, M. R., & Haider, B. (1977). Evidence for cardiomyopathy in familial diabetes mellitus. *Journal of Clinical Investigation, 60*(4), 884–899.

71. Ren, J., Samson, W. K., & Sowers, J. R. (1999). Insulin-like growth factor I as a cardiac hormone: Physiological and pathophysiological implications in heart disease. *Journal of Molecular and Cellular Cardiology, 31*(11), 2049–2061.

72. Riddle, M. C. (2010). Effects of intensive glucose lowering in the management of patients with type 2 diabetes mellitus in the Action to Control Cardiovascular Risk in Diabetes (ACCORD) trial. *Circulation, 122*(8), 844–846.

73. Rijzewijk, L. J., van der Meer, R. W., Smit, J. W., Diamant, M., Bax, J. J., Hammer, S., Romijn, J. A., de Roos, A., & Lamb, H. J. (2008). Myocardial steatosis is an independent predictor of diastolic dysfunction in type 2 diabetes mellitus. *Journal of the American College of Cardiology, 52*(22), 1793–1799.

74. Rivellese, A. A., Riccardi, G., & Vaccaro, O. (2010). Cardiovascular risk in women with diabetes. *Nutrition, Metabolism, and Cardiovascular Diseases, 20*(6), 474–480.

75. Rolim, L. C., Sá, J. R., Chacra, A. R., & Dib, S. A. (2008). Diabetic cardiovascular autonomic neuropathy: Risk factors, clinical impact and early diagnosis. *Arquivos Brasileiros de Cardiologia, 90*(4), e24–e31.

76. Rolim, L. C., Sá, J. R., Chacra, A. R., & Dib, S. A. (2008). Neuropatia autonômica cardiovascular diabética: Fatores de risco, impacto clínico e diagnóstico precoce. *Arquivos Brasileiros de Cardiologia, 90*(4), e24–e32.

77. Sacks, D. B., Arnold, M., Bakris, G. L., Bruns, D. E., Horvath, A. R., Kirkman, M. S., Lernmark, A., Metzger, B. E., & Nathan, D. M. (2011). Guidelines and recommendations for laboratory analysis in the diagnosis and management of diabetes mellitus. *Diabetes Care, 34*(6), e61–e99.

78. Santra, S., Basu, A. K., Roychowdhury, P., Banerjee, R., Singhania, P., Singh, S., & Datta, U. K. (2011). Comparison of left ventricular mass in normotensive type 2 diabetes mellitus patients with that in the nondiabetic population. *Journal of Cardiovascular Disease Research, 2*(1), 50–56.

79. Schena, F. P., & Gesualdo, L. (2005). Pathogenetic mechanisms of diabetic nephropathy. *Journal of the American Society of Nephrology, 16*(Suppl. 1), S30–S33.

80. Scognamiglio, R., Avogaro, A., Casara, D., Crepaldi, C., Marin, M., Palisi, M., Mingardi, R., Erle, G., Fasoli, G., & Dalla Volta, S. (1998). Myocardial dysfunction and adrenergic cardiac innervation in patients with insulin-dependent diabetes mellitus. *Journal of the American College of Cardiology, 31*(2), 404–412.

81. Shah, R. V., & Goldfine, A. B. (2012). Statins and risk of new-onset diabetes mellitus. *Circulation, 126*(21), e282–e284.

82. Sharma, S., Adrogue, J. V., Golfman, L., Uray, I., Lemm, J., Youker, K., Noon, G. P., Frazier, O. H., & Taegtmeyer, H. (2004). Intramyocardial lipid accumulation in the failing human heart resembles the lipotoxic rat heart. *FASEB Journal, 18*(14), 1692–1700.

83. Shivalkar, B., Dhondt, D., Goovaerts, I., Van Gaal, L., Bartunek, J., Van Crombrugge, P., & Vrints, C. (2006). Flow mediated dilatation and cardiac function in type 1 diabetes mellitus. *American Journal of Cardiology, 97*(1), 77–82.

84. Shoelson, S. E., Lee, J., & Goldfine, A. B. (2006). Inflammation and insulin resistance. *Journal of Clinical Investigation, 116*(7), 1793–1801.

85. Sjöström, L., Lindroos, A. K., Peltonen, M., Torgerson, J., Bouchard, C., Carlsson, B., Dahlgren, S., Larsson, B., Narbro, K., Sjöström, C. D., et al. (2004). Lifestyle, diabetes, and cardiovascular risk factors 10 years after bariatric surgery. *New England Journal of Medicine, 351*(26), 2683–2693.

86. Skyler, J. S., Bergenstal, R., Bonow, R. O., Buse, J., Deedwania, P., Gale, E. A., Howard, B. V., Kirkman, M. S., Kosiborod, M., Reaven, P., et al. (2009). Intensive glycemic control and the prevention of cardiovascular events: Implications of the ACCORD, ADVANCE, and VA diabetes trials: A position statement of the American Diabetes Association and a scientific statement of the American College of Cardiology Foundation and the American Heart Association. *Circulation, 119*(2), 351–357.

87. Sobel, B. E., Woodcock-Mitchell, J., Schneider, D. J., Holt, R. E., Marutsuka, K., & Gold, H. (1998). Increased plasminogen activator inhibitor type 1 in coronary artery atherectomy specimens from type 2 diabetic compared with nondiabetic patients: A potential factor predisposing to thrombosis and its persistence. *Circulation, 97*(22), 2213–2221.

88. Solano, M. P., & Goldberg, R. B. (2006). Management of dyslipidemia in diabetes. *Cardiology in Review, 14*(3), 125–135.

89. Stone, N. J., Robinson, J. G., Lichtenstein, A. H., Bairey Merz, C. N., Blum, C. B., Eckel, R. H., Goldberg, A. C., Gordon, D., Levy, D., Lloyd-Jones, D. M., et al. (2014). 2013 ACC/AHA guideline on the treatment of blood cholesterol to reduce atherosclerotic cardiovascular risk in adults: A report of the American College of Cardiology/American Heart Association Task Force on Practice Guidelines. *Circulation, 129*(25 Suppl 2), S1–S45.

90. Taskinen, M. R. (2003). Diabetic dyslipidaemia: From basic research to clinical practice. *Diabetologia, 46*(6), 733–749.

91. The Diabetes Control and Complications Trial Research Group. (1993). The effect of intensive treatment of diabetes on the development and progression of long-term complications in insulin-dependent diabetes mellitus. *The New England Journal of Medicine, 329*(14), 977–986.

92. The effect of intensive diabetes therapy on measures of autonomic nervous system function in the Diabetes Control and Complications Trial (DCCT). (1998). *Diabetologia, 41*(4), 416–423.

93. Tight blood pressure control and risk of macrovascular and microvascular complications in type 2 diabetes: UKPDS 38. (1998). *UK Prospective Diabetes Study Group. BMJ, 317*(7160), 703–713.

94. Tribouilloy, C., Rusinaru, D., Mahjoub, H., Tartière, J. M., Kesri-Tartière, L., Godard, S., & Peltier, M. (2008). Prognostic impact of diabetes mellitus in patients with heart failure and preserved ejection fraction: A prospective five-year study. *Heart, 94*(12), 1450–1455.

95. Tuomilehto, J., Lindström, J., Eriksson, J. G., Valle, T. T., Hämäläinen, H., Ilanne-Parikka, P., Keinänen-Kiukaanniemi, S., Laakso, M., Louheranta, A., Rastas, M., et al. (2001). Prevention of type 2 diabetes mellitus by changes in lifestyle among subjects with impaired glucose tolerance. *New England Journal of Medicine, 344*(18), 1343–1350.

96. Turnbull, F., Neal, B., Algert, C., Chalmers, J., Chapman, N., Cutler, J., Woodward, M., & MacMahon, S. (2005). Effects of different blood pressure-lowering regimens on major cardiovascular events in individuals with and without diabetes mellitus: Results of prospectively designed overviews of randomized trials. *Archives of Internal Medicine, 165*(12), 1410–1419.

97. Vicenová, B., Vopálenský, V., Burýsek, L., & Pospísek, M. (2009). Emerging role of interleukin-1 in cardiovascular diseases. *Physiological Research, 58*(4), 481–498.

98. Vinik, A. I., & Ziegler, D. (2007). Diabetic cardiovascular autonomic neuropathy. *Circulation, 115*(3), 387–397.

99. Vinik, A. I., Erbas, T., Park, T. S., Nolan, R., & Pittenger, G. L. (2001). Platelet dysfunction in type 2 diabetes. *Diabetes Care, 24*(9), 1476–1485.

100. Vischer, U. M., Emeis, J. J., Bilo, H. J., Stehouwer, C. D., Thomsen, C., Rasmussen, O., Hermansen, K., Wollheim, C. B., & Ingerslev, J. (1998). von Willebrand factor (vWf) as a plasma marker of endothelial activation in diabetes: Improved reliability with parallel determination of the vWf propeptide (vWf: AgII). *Thrombosis and Haemostasis, 80*(6), 1002–1007.

101. Wackers, F. J., Young, L. H., Inzucchi, S. E., Chyun, D. A., Davey, J. A., Barrett, E. J., Taillefer, R., Wittlin, S. D., Heller, G. V., Filipchuk, N., et al. (2004). Detection of silent myocardial ischemia in asymptomatic diabetic subjects: The DIAD study. *Diabetes Care, 27*(8), 1954–1961.

102. Wanner, C., Krane, V., März, W., Olschewski, M., Mann, J. F., Ruf, G., & Ritz, E. (2005). Atorvastatin in patients with type 2 diabetes mellitus undergoing hemodialysis. *New England Journal of Medicine, 353*(3), 238–248.

103. Watts, G. F., & Playford, D. A. (1998). Dyslipoproteinaemia and hyperoxidative stress in the pathogenesis of endothelial dysfunction in non-insulin dependent diabetes mellitus: An hypothesis. *Atherosclerosis, 141*(1), 17–30.

104. Whelton, P. K., Barzilay, J., Cushman, W. C., Davis, B. R., Iiamathi, E., Kostis, J. B., Leenen, F. H., Louis, G. T., Margolis, K. L., Mathis, D. E., et al. (2005). Clinical outcomes in antihypertensive treatment of type 2 diabetes, impaired fasting glucose concentration, and normoglycemia: Antihypertensive and Lipid-Lowering Treatment to Prevent Heart Attack Trial (ALLHAT). *Archives of Internal Medicine, 165*(12), 1401–1409.

105. Wild, S., Roglic, G., Green, A., Sicree, R., & King, H. (2004). Global prevalence of diabetes: Estimates for the year 2000 and projections for 2030. *Diabetes Care, 27*(5), 1047–1053.

106. Williams, I. L., Noronha, B., & Zaman, A. G. (2003). Review: The management of acute myocardial infarction in patients with diabetes mellitus. *British Journal of Diabetes & Vascular Disease, 3*(6), 319–324.

107. Wing, R. R. (2010). Long-term effects of a lifestyle intervention on weight and cardiovascular risk factors in individuals with type 2 diabetes mellitus: Four-year results of the Look AHEAD trial. *Archives of Internal Medicine, 170*(17), 1566–1575.

108. Wing, R. R., Bolin, P., Brancati, F. L., Bray, G. A., Clark, J. M., Coday, M., Crow, R. S., Curtis, J. M., Egan, C. M., Espeland, M. A., et al. (2013). Cardiovascular effects of intensive lifestyle intervention in type 2 diabetes. *New England Journal of Medicine, 369*(2), 145–154.

109. Wolf, G., & Ziyadeh, F. N. (1997). The role of angiotensin II in diabetic nephropathy: Emphasis on nonhemodynamic mechanisms. *American Journal of Kidney Diseases, 29*(1), 153–163.

110. Writing Team for the Diabetes Control and Complications Trial/Epidemiology of Diabetes Interventions and Complications Research Group. (2003). Sustained effect of intensive treatment of type 1 diabetes mellitus on development and progression of diabetic nephropathy: The Epidemiology of Diabetes Interventions and Complications (EDIC) study. *JAMA, 290*(16), 2159–2167.

111. Yu, C. M., Chau, E., Sanderson, J. E., Fan, K., Tang, M. O., Fung, W. H., Lin, H., Kong, S. L., Lam, Y. M., Hill, M. R., et al. (2002). Tissue Doppler echocardiographic evidence of reverse remodeling and improved synchronicity by simultaneously delaying regional contraction after biventricular pacing therapy in heart failure. *Circulation, 105*(4), 438–445.

112. Zhang, X., & Chen, C. (2012). A new insight of mechanisms, diagnosis and treatment of diabetic cardiomyopathy. *Endocrine, 41*(3), 398–409.

113. Ziegler, D., Gries, F. A., Spüler, M., & Lessmann, F. (1992). The epidemiology of diabetic neuropathy. *Diabetic Cardiovascular Autonomic Neuropathy Multicenter Study Group. Journal of Diabetes Complications,* 6(1), 49–57.

Chapter

HYPERTENSION, DIABETES, AND THE EYE

6

Contents

INTRODUCTION

It is been said that the eyes serve as the soul's window. The eyes can sometimes be the first to show symptoms of systemic diseases because they mirror what is happening in the rest of the body. Globally, the two most common non-communicable diseases are diabetes mellitus and hypertension. Twenty-seven million people are thought to have diabetes, and twenty-eight million to have hypertension.

Both of them have eye conditions that, if left untreated, could result in blindness. Diabetes is the most common cause of blindness in individuals between the ages of 15 and 64. Diabetic retinopathy is responsible for 5% of blindness worldwide (Ahn et al., 2014).

Diabetes mellitus (DM) is a disorder characterized by impaired glucose metabolism that results in persistent hyperglycemia because of impairments in the synthesis or operation of insulin. It causes long-term harm and malfunction to numerous body organs, including the heart, blood vessels, kidneys, eyes, and nerves. Individuals who have diabetes frequently experience visual complications (Aiello et al., 1994).

A persistently high blood pressure is known as hypertension, and it increases the risk of target organ damage in the blood vessels, heart, brain, retina, and kidneys. When a person is not taking anti-hypertensive medication, the cutoff is arbitrarily set at a systolic blood pressure of 130 mmHg and a diastolic blood pressure of 90 mmHg. It is possible that a patient's eye symptoms will manifest hypertension for the first time (Baker et al., 2019).

Reducing risk factors is the most crucial treatment for diabetic and hypertensive retinopathy. Strict blood pressure and glucose management, weight loss, abstinence from alcohol and tobacco, low-fat diet, and exercise are all part of this (Baker et al., 2010).

Individuals with diabetes and hypertension need to take their medications as prescribed and notify their doctors of any changes in their vision. It is advised to have annual eye exams to detect these ocular complications because vision changes may not be apparent until the retina is seriously damaged. As vision loss may be the initial complaint, regular blood pressure checks and diabetes screenings are crucial (Baker et al., 2008).

Orientation and Directional Terms

Term	Definition	Illustration
Retinopathy	Retinopathy is a disease of the retina, or light-sensitive tissue at the back of the eye, that can cause vision impairment.	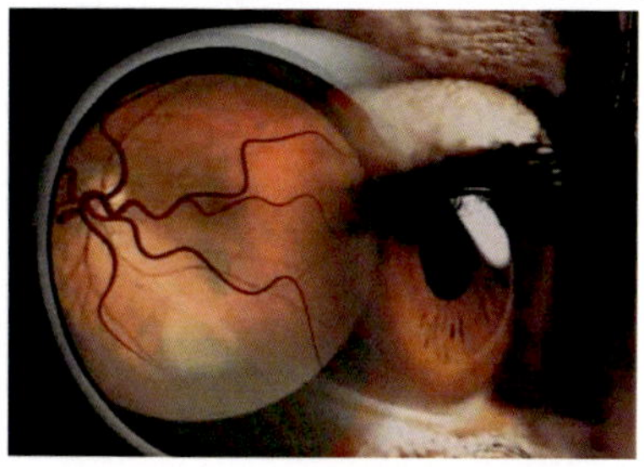
Optic neuropathy	Optic neuropathy is damage to the optic nerve, which is a bundle of nerve fibers in the retina that sends visual signals to the brain.	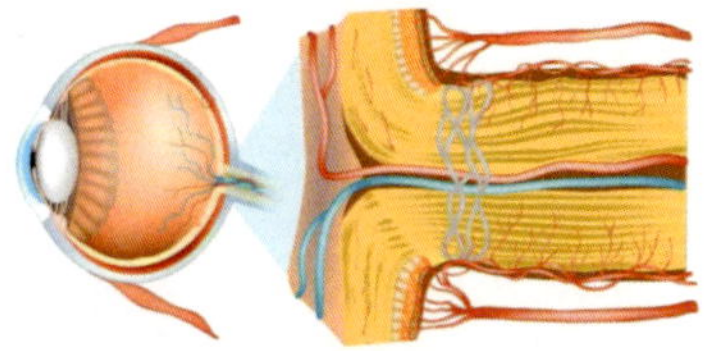
Choroidopathy	Choroidopathy, also known as central serous chorioretinopathy (CSC), is a disease that causes fluid to build up under the retina, the back part of the inner eye that sends sight information to the brain.	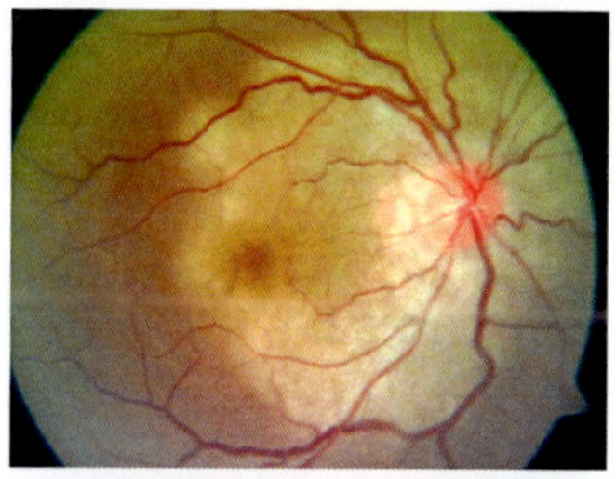
Hyperaldosteronism	Hyperaldosteronism is a condition that occurs when the adrenal glands produce too much aldosterone, a mineralocorticoid that regulates electrolytes and extracellular volume.	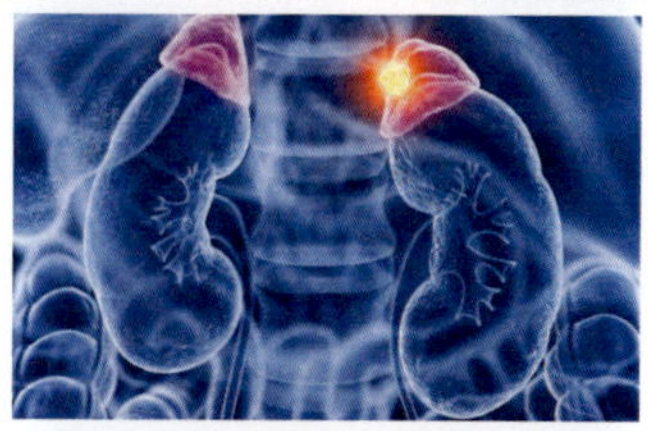
Retinal edema	Retinal edema, also known as macular edema, is a condition that occurs when fluid builds up in the retina, causing swelling.	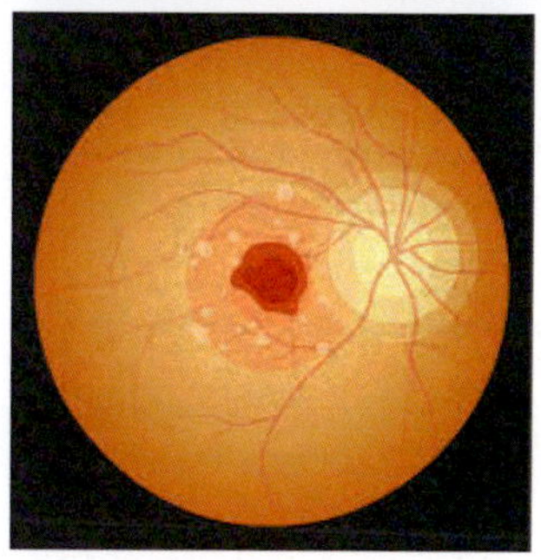

6.1. HYPERTENSIVE RETINOPATHY

One risk factor for systemic diseases that can harm target organs is hypertension. In particular, hypertension can have many detrimental effects on the eyes, including retinopathy, optic neuropathy, and choroidopathy. Major retinal vessels, including the branch retinal vein, central retinal vein, and central retinal artery, can also become occluded by hypertension (Bourke et al., 2004).

6.1.1. Disease Entity

6.1.1.1. Disease

Hypertensive retinopathy's arteriosclerotic alterations are brought on by persistently high blood pressure. In 2017, the American Heart Association/American College of Cardiology (ACC/AHA) proposed the following definitions of high blood pressure (Table 6.1) (ACC, 2017).

Table 6.1. *Blood Pressure Categories*

Category	Systolic (SBP)	Diastolic (DBP)
Elevated blood pressure	120-129 mmHg	< 80 mmHg
Stage 1 hypertension	130-139 mmHg	80-89 mmHg
Stage 2 hypertension	≥ 140 mmHg	≥ 90 mmHg

Source: https://eyewiki.org/Hypertensive_Retinopathy#:~:text=Etiology-,The%20arteriosclerotic%20changes%20of%20hypertensive%20retinopathy%20are%20caused%20by%20chronically,secondary%20to%20another%20disease%20process.

There are two disease processes involved in hypertensive retinopathy. Vasospasm to autoregulate perfusion is the cause of the acute effects of systemic arterial hypertension. Patients with long-term hypertension are at risk for visual loss due to complications from vascular occlusions or macroaneurysms, which are brought on by arteriosclerosis (Brown et al., 2022).

6.1.2. Epidemiology

Merely 52% of adults in the US have controlled blood pressure, while 33% have hypertension. In non-diabetic patients, hypertensive retinopathy can affect 2–17% of the population, although the prevalence varies by demographic category. Chinese and African Americans are more likely to suffer from hypertensive retinopathy. Furthermore, blood pressure incidence rises with age. Age groups under 45 years old are more affected by men than by women, while age groups over 65 years old are more affected by women (Brown et al., 2013).

6.1.3. Etiology

Hypertensive retinopathy, or SBP > 140 mmHg and DBP > 90 mmHg, is characterized by persistently high blood pressure, which leads to the arteriosclerotic alterations in the retina. Usually, primary hypertension is not a side effect of another illness process; rather, it is essential. Essential hypertension can be caused by a variety of environmental factors that can be changed, making it a polygenic disease. However, pheochromocytoma, primary hyperaldosteronism, Cushing's syndrome, renal parenchymal disease, renal vascular disease, coarctation of the aorta, obstructive sleep apnea, hyperparathyroidism, and hyperthyroidism can all lead to the development of secondary hypertension. In fact, bilateral vision loss from exudative retinal detachment, bilateral optic disc edema, and serous macular detachment can be seen in many young patients with secondary hypertension when they visit an ophthalmologist. Furthermore, it has been discovered that a higher risk of hypertensive retinopathy is linked to genetic factors (Davis et al., 1998).

6.1.4. Risk Factors

High salt diets, obesity, alcohol consumption, tobacco use, family history, stress, and ethnic background are risk factors for essential hypertension. The length of time that high blood pressure persists is the main risk factor for arteriosclerotic hypertensive retinopathy. The degree of blood pressure elevation over normal is the primary risk factor for malignant hypertension (De Silva et al., 2011).

Retinal vascular caliber may be influenced by genetics, according to certain research. Four novel loci (19q13, 6q24, 12q24, and 5q14) were found to be significantly correlated with retinal venular caliber in a 2010 population-based study. Moreover, locus 12q24 has been linked to both coronary heart disease and hypertension (DiMeglio et al., 2018).

6.1.5. Pathophysiology

Hypertensive retinopathy goes through vasoconstrictive, sclerotic, and exudative phases based upon the extent of hypertension control (Do et al., 2012).

6.1.5.1. Vasoconstrictive Phase

Because of the increased luminal pressures during the vasoconstrictive phase, retinal arteriole narrowing and vasospasm decrease flow via local autoregulatory mechanisms (Elliott and Varon, 2020).

6.1.5.2. Sclerotic Phase

In the sclerotic phase, the layers of the endothelial wall undergo changes such as intimal thickening, medial hyperplasia, and hyaline degradation in the arteriolar worsening arteriolar narrowing, AV crossing changes, and silver and copper wiring.

6.1.5.3. Exudative Phase

The blood-brain barrier is disrupted during the exudative phase, allowing plasma and blood to leak out and resulting in retinal hemorrhages, hard exudates, retinal ischemia, and necrosis of smooth muscle.

Necrotic vessels can bleed into the inner retina (dot blot hemorrhage) or the superficial retina (nerve fiber layer) to cause retinal hemorrhages. Ischemia to the nerve fiber layer as a result of fibrinous necrosis and luminal narrowing is the cause of cotton wool spots. Reduced axoplasmic flow, nerve swelling, and fluffy opacification are the results of neuronal ischemia. Exudates are produced later in the disease process as a result of lipid buildup around bleeding areas. Papilledema, which results from both ischemia and leakage of the arterioles supplying the optic disc that undergo fibrinous necrosis, can be brought on by malignant hypertension. Optic nerve edema is caused by ischemia, whereas hemorrhage and disc edema are caused by leakage (Engerman and Bloodworth, 1965).

Notably, changes in renal function correlate with the severity and degree of malignant hypertension, emphasizing the multi-organ damage brought on by systemic microvascular dysfunction.

6.1.6. Primary Prevention

The development of hypertensive retinopathy can be avoided with routine blood pressure monitoring and treatment.

6.1.7. Diagnosis

Based on coexisting hypertension and the clinical appearance of the condition on a dilated fundoscopic examination, hypertensive retinopathy is diagnosed.

6.1.7.1. Medical History

The history should concentrate on the signs and symptoms of hypertension, as well as the development of its complications. Patients should be questioned about the severity and duration of their hypertension, the medications they take, and their compliance with them to determine the severity of their hypertension disease. Asking about headaches, eye pain, decreased vision acuity, focal neurological deficits, chest pain, dyspnea on exertion, paroxysmal nocturnal dyspnea, orthopnea, and palpitations are some signs of hypertension. It is important to enquire about the complications associated with hypertension from patients, such as any history of heart failure, peripheral vascular disease, stroke, or transient ischemic attack. Asymptomatic patients might be the majority (Flynn et al., 1992).

6.1.7.2. Physical Examination

A patient with hypertension undergoes a physical examination that includes a dilated fundoscopy, neurological examination, cardiovascular examination, and pulmonary examination. Blood pressure should obviously be the main focus of vital signs. Peripheral pulses, carotid or renal bruits, and heart sounds (murmurs or gallops) are important components of the cardiovascular exam. If rales are evident, a pulmonary exam can pick up on heart failure symptoms. A thorough neurological examination can identify signs of cerebral ischemia. (Katakam, et al., 2008). Lastly, a dilated fundus examination is required to stage hypertensive retinopathy (Figure 6.1).

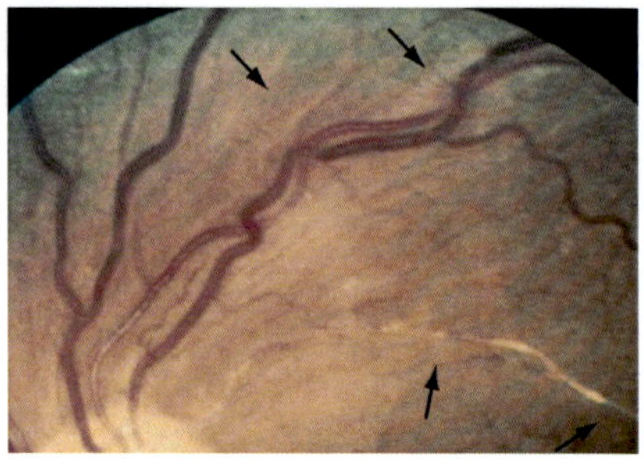

Figure 6.1. *Copper-wiring, arteriovenous nicking and silver-wiring seen in a patient with hypertensive retinopathy.*

Source: https://eyewiki.aao.org/w/images/1/thumb/3/33/HTN_RET_VESSELS.jpg/450px-HTN_RET_VESSELS.jpg,

6.1.7.3. Signs

Constricted and tortuous arterioles, retinal hemorrhage, hard exudates, cotton wool spots, retinal edema, and papilledema are among the symptoms of hypertensive retinopathy. Widening of the arteriole reflex, arteriovenous crossing signs, and copper or silver wire arterioles (copper or silver colored arteriole light reflex) are indicators of chronic arterial hypertension in the retina (Garner et al., 1979). Choroidopathy can also be brought on by malignant hypertension. Segmental infarction of the choriocapillaris is caused by fibrinoid necrosis of the choroidal arterioles. Elschnig spots, which are hyperpigmented patches in the choroid encircled by a ring of hypopigmentation, and Siegrist streaks, which are linear hyperpigmented lesions over choroidal arteries, are caused by inadequate perfusion of the choriocapillaris. Exudative retinal detachment can result from a focal pigment epithelium detachment brought on by hypertensive choroidopathy. Malignant hypertension typically affects younger patients with hypertensive choroidopathy (Gunn, 1892). Optic neuropathy can result from hypertension, particularly leading to swollen optic disks. Symptoms of hypertensive optic neuropathy include hemorrhages in a flame-like shape near the edge of the disk, blurred disk margins, congested retinal veins, papilledema, and macular exudates. In some cases, hard exudates can accumulate in the macula, forming a macular star. Patients with long-term high blood pressure may also exhibit optic nerve pallor (Harjasouliha et al., 2017).

6.1.7.4. Symptoms

1. Malignant Hypertension

Patients with acute malignant hypertension may experience headaches, blurred vision, or eye pain. (Lang, 2007). However, patients will present with the usual symptoms of macroaneurysms or vascular occlusions due to the complications of arteriosclerotic hypertensive changes.

2. Chronic Hypertension

Patients with chronic hypertension-related arteriosclerotic changes typically have decreased vision, but no other symptoms are present (Hayreh et al., 1994).

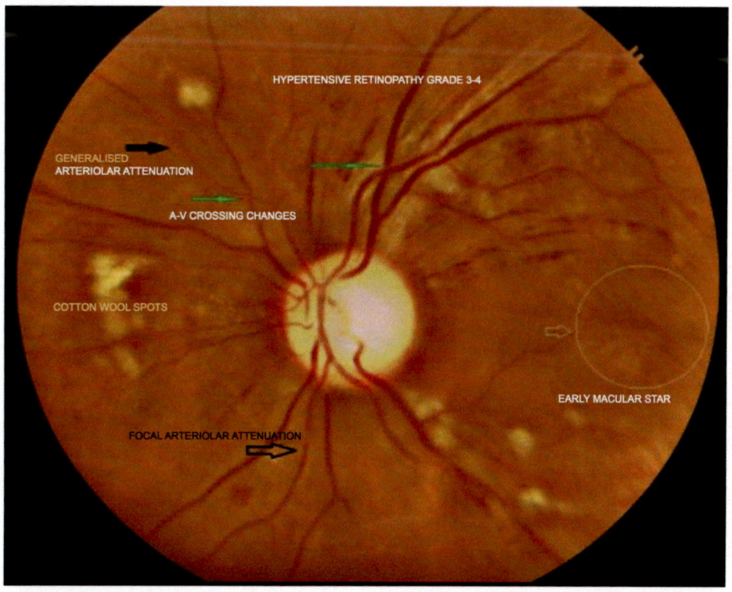

Figure 6.2. *Grade 3-4 Hypertensive retinopathy. A 56-year old patient presented with acute onset vision loss. Fundus examination revealed grade 3-4 hypertensive retinopathy changes including arterio-venous crossing changes, macular star and cotton wool spots.*

Source: https://eyewiki.aao.org/w/images/1/thumb/9/9d/HTN_RET_Findings.jpg/450px-HTN_RET_Findings.jpg.

The retinopathic alterations observed in both acute, malignant hypertension and chronic, systemic hypertension are explored in detail in the Scheie Classification below in Figure 6.2.

6.1.7.5. Clinical Diagnosis

The signs of malignant hypertension are well summarized by the Modified Scheie Classification of Hypertensive Retinopathy:

- **Grade 0:** No changes;
- **Grade 1:** Barely detectable arterial narrowing;
- **Grade 2:** Obvious arterial narrowing with focal irregularities;
- **Grade 3:** Grade 2 plus retinal hemorrhages, exudates, cotton wool spots, or retinal edema;
- **Grade 4:** Grade 3 plus papilledema.

The signs of chronic arteriosclerotic hypertension are also summarized by the Scheie Classification:

- **Stage 1:** Widening of the arteriole light reflex;
- **Stage 2:** Stage 1 + Arteriovenous crossing sign ;
- **Stage 3:** Copper wiring of arterioles (copper-colored arteriole light reflex);
- **Stage 4:** Silver wiring of arterioles (silver-colored arteriole light reflex).

Another classification schema is the Keith-Wagner-Barker classification proposed in 1939 are:

- **Grade 1:** Mild, generalized constriction of retinal arterioles;
- **Grade 2:** Definite focal narrowing of retinal arterioles + AV nicking;
- **Grade 3:** Grade 2 + flame-shaped hemorrhages + cotton-wool spots + hard exudates;
- **Grade 4:** Severe Grade 3 retinopathy + papilledema or retinal edema.

Of specific interest is the classification of hypertensive retinopathy by Wong and Mitchell (2004) in which the worsening grades of retinopathy were more strongly associated with systemic issues. The classification is as follows:

- **None:** No detectable signs;
- **Mild:** One or more of the following: generalized arteriolar narrowing, focal arteriolar narrowing, arteriovenous nicking, opacity ("copper wiring") of the arteriolar wall;
- **Moderate:** One or more of the following: retinal hemorrhage (blot, dot, or flame-shaped), microaneurysm, cotton-wool spot, hard exudate, or a combination of these signs;
- **Severe:** Moderate retinopathy plus swelling of the optic disc.

Subretinal fluid (SRF), one of the features of optical coherence tomography (OCT), has led to the proposal of a new classification as recently as 2014. When the OCT-based grading system was compared to the Keith-Wagner-Barker grading system, the study discovered a significant correlation between the following classification and final best-corrected visual acuity (Hayreh et al., 2009).

- Mild-Moderate Retinopathy;
- Malignant Retinopathy w/o SRF;
- Malignant Retinopathy w/ SRF.

6.1.7.6. Diagnostic Procedures

During acute malignant hypertension, fluorescein angiography (FA) will reveal retinal capillary nonperfusion, microaneurysm formation, and a dendritic pattern of choroidal filling in the initial phase. In the late phase, diffuse leakage will be observed. Meanwhile, Indocyanine green angiography will display a moth-eaten appearance of the choriocapillaris. FA can also detect hypertensive choroidopathy, showing focal choroidal hypoperfusion in the early stages and subretinal leakage in the later stages (Figure 6.3) (AAO, 2006).

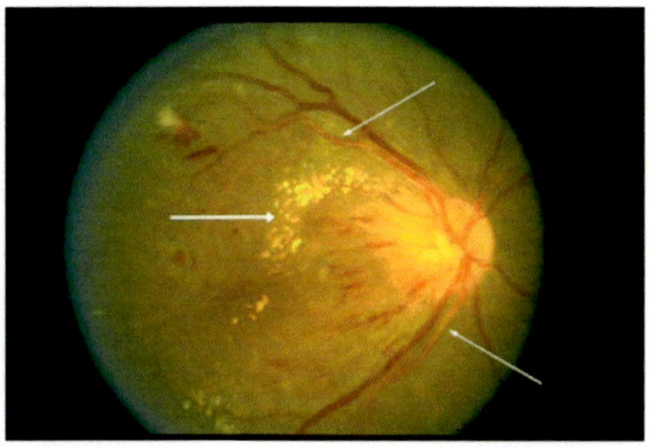

Figure 6.3. *Common hypertensive retinal changes are flame-shaped hemorrhages in the superficial layers of the retina and cotton-wool patches caused by occlusion of the precapillary arterioles with ischemic infarction of the inner retina. Long-standing hypertension can produce arteriolar sclerotic vascular changes, such as copper or silver wiring of the arterioles, as shown by the two arrows on the right, or arteriorvenous nicking. Another sign of chronic hypertension is lipid exudates resulting from abnormal vascular permeability, as shown by the arrow at left. More ominous in this photograph is swelling of the optic disc, seen here by the blurring of the temporal disc margins. This is the hallmark of malignant hypertension, which carries a poor prognosis for the patient's health if left untreated. BP must be emergently controlled to decrease the risk of developing heart and renal failure and hypertensive encephalopathy as well as stroke and permanent vision loss.*

Source: https://eyewiki.aao.org/w/images/1/thumb/3/33/Malignant_HTN_RET.jpg/450px-Malignant_HTN_RET.jpg.

6.1.8. Differential Diagnosis

Diabetic retinopathy is the most common differential diagnosis for hypertensive retinopathy accompanied by cotton wool spots, hard exudates, and diffuse retinal hemorrhage. By evaluating each of the individual systemic diseases, diabetic retinopathy can be differentiated from hypertensive retinopathy. Many illnesses, such as radiation retinopathy, anemia and other blood dyscrasias, ocular ischemic syndrome, and retinal vein occlusion, can cause diffuse retinal hemorrhage and mimic hypertensive retinopathy. Neuroretinitis, diabetic papillopathy, and anterior ischemic optic neuropathy are conditions that are associated with optic disc edema (Henderson et al., 2011).

6.1.9. Management

The main goal of treatment for hypertensive retinopathy is blood pressure reduction. To minimize ocular and systemic damage, it is critical to collaborate with the patient's primary care physician to ensure prompt evaluation and management. To treat hypertensive retinopathy appropriately and promptly and avoid vision-threatening complications, a thorough history is essential (Jacsobson et al., 1997).

6.1.9.1. General Treatment

Reducing the mean arterial pressure by 10-15% within the first hour is the treatment for moderate to severe hypertensive retinopathy. Notably, by the end of the first day of treatment, blood pressure should be reduced in a controlled manner and by no more than 25% relative to baseline to prevent additional ischemia damage to the target end organs. Parenteral antihypertensive medications are frequently needed for initial treatment before switching to oral medications. During the next two to three months, goal-oriented hypertension treatment seeks to reduce diastolic and systolic blood pressure to less than 80 mm Hg and less than 130 mm Hg, respectively (Jhaveri et al., 2022).

6.1.9.2. Medical Therapy

Medication used to lower blood pressure in

outpatient settings includes calcium channel blockers, diuretics, and angiotensin converting enzyme inhibitors. Central α2-adrenergic agonists, direct vasodilators, and α-adrenergic blockers are some other less frequently used drugs. For the purpose of managing hypertension, the patient should be closely monitored by his primary care physician. The patient should be referred to an emergency room for immediate blood pressure management if he is experiencing a hypertensive crisis (Keith et al., 1974).

Research on intravitreal antibody therapy (bevacizumab) against vascular endothelial growth factor for acute hypertensive retinopathy has demonstrated a decrease in retinal hemorrhage and macular edema. Furthermore, a different study revealed that patients with malignant hypertensive retinopathy recovered quickly after receiving bevacizumab. But the use of these agents is still relatively new and not widely accepted (Kim et al., 2012).

6.1.9.3. Medical Follow Up

The extent of hypertensive retinopathy and the state of hypertension determine the need for follow-up. For consistent, patient-specific follow-up, close communication between the ophthalmologist and primary care physician is essential.

6.1.9.4. Surgery

Essential hypertension and its ocular complications are not treatable surgically. Surgical intervention may be beneficial in treating secondary hypertension, contingent on the underlying cause.

6.1.9.5. Complications

Patients with hypertension are at risk for a variety of additional retinal vascular conditions, such as retinal macroaneurysms, central or branch retinal vein occlusion, and central or branch retinal artery occlusion. The formation of epiretinal membranes, tractional retinal detachment, vitreous hemorrhage, and neovascularization can all result from ischemia caused by vascular occlusions. Additionally, hypertension promotes a more advanced course of diabetic retinopathy. Chronic papilledema brought on by hypertensive optic neuropathy can result in optic nerve atrophy and a marked loss of visual acuity. It might also put glaucoma patients at risk. Proliferative hypertensive retinopathy is a term that was recently coined (Kim et al., 1999).

6.1.9.6. Prognosis

Individuals who have arteriosclerotic alterations and severe hypertensive retinopathy are more vulnerable to peripheral vascular disease, coronary heart disease, and stroke. Patients with untreated malignant hypertension had a 50% death rate after two months and a 90% death rate after a year. These patients continue to be at risk for retinal artery occlusions, retinal vein occlusions, and retinal macroaneurysms because the arteriosclerotic changes in the retina do not go away. Once blood pressure is under control, the majority of retinal abnormalities caused by malignant hypertension will improve; however, AV changes and arteriolar narrowing will persist. However, long-term declines in visual acuity could result from damage to the optic nerve and macula (Kishi et al., 1985).

6.2. DIABETIC RETINOPATHY

One of the most common consequences of diabetes is diabetic retinopathy, which typically affects both eyes and can occur in people with type 1 or type 2 diabetes. When you have diabetes, it is crucial to have regular eye exams because the condition develops gradually over many years. Maintaining strict blood sugar control can be used to either prevent retinopathy or slow down its progression. The thin inner light-sensitive layer in the back of the eyes is called the retina, and retinal disease is essentially damaged blood vessels in the retina (Figure 6.4) (Klein et al., 1998).

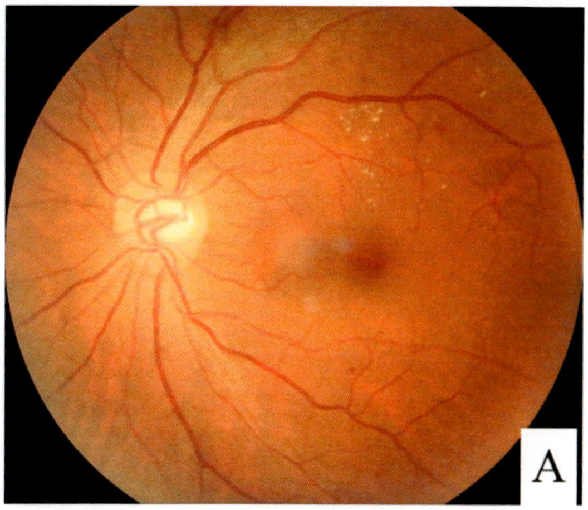

Figure 6.4. *Diabetic retinopathy.*

Source: By Shaofeng Hao, Changyan Liu, Na Li, Yanrong Wu, Dongdong Li, Qingyue Gao, Ziyou Yuan, Guanyan Li, Huilin Li, Jianzhou Yang, and Shengfu Fan. – (2022). "Clinical evaluation of AI-assisted screening for diabetic retinopathy in rural areas of midwest China." PLoS One 17 (10): e0275983. DOI:10.1371/journal.pone.0275983. PMID 36227905. PMC: 9560484. Figure 6.1, panel A, CC BY 4.0, https://commons.wikimedia.org/w/index.php?curid=124683504.

6.2.1. Key Facts about Diabetic Retinopathy

- There are millions of individuals worldwide living with diabetes, and about 80% of diabetic patients are likely to develop some stage of diabetic retinopathy. The longer people suffer from diabetes, the more likely they are to have diabetic retinopathy eventually.
- Diabetic retinopathy is one of the complications of diabetes which can lead to vision loss and sometimes even blindness. If not treated at the right time, even the best eye hospital will not be of any help to the patient.
- There are predictably no early symptoms associated with early stages of the condition, allowing the disease to advance until the point where it affects vision.
- Symptoms of advanced stages of retinopathy include:
  - Halo's around lights;
  - Blurry vision;
  - Loss of color and central vision;
  - Floaters;
- Early detection of the disease is vital; therefore, it is recommended that diabetic patients undergo an annual retinal exam with an optometrist or ophthalmologist. A high percentage of vision loss cases are avertable with early discovery and treatment.
- There is a group of eye diseases that can affect patients suffering from diabetes. Diabetes is an intricate metabolic disease in which your body can either:
  - Not produce insulin;
  - Produce insufficient insulin;
  - Can't use insulin efficiently.

For energy, the body's cells require sugar, or glucose, which is broken down and transported throughout the body by insulin. Insufficient insulin production causes blood sugar levels to rise, which can have detrimental effects on all bodily organs, including the eyes. Diabetes-related retinal disorders are referred to as diabetic retinopathy (Klein et al., 2009).

6.2.2. Disease Entity

As early as 250–300 BC, diabetes mellitus was recognized as a disease and was distinguished by the sweet taste of urine. When Mering and Minkowski removed the pancreas from a dog in 1889, the animal developed a severe and deadly form of diabetes, which led to the discovery of the pancreas' significance in this disease process. Since then, developments in medicine have produced many novel drug treatments and methods for the management of diabetes mellitus (Konstantinidis and Guex-Crosier, 2016).

Nevertheless, diabetes continues to rank among the world's ten most common and significant non-infectious causes of morbidity and death. An estimated 34,01 million Americans are over the age of 18, or 13,0% of the total U.S. population. S. 2018 saw adults with diabetes. This prevalence should reinforce the significance of understanding the diabetes disease process, as should the related illnesses that typically coexist with or follow diabetes (Lewis et al., 1976).

6.2.2.1. Disease

Diabetes-related microvascular end-organ damage is known as diabetic retinopathy. It spans the spectrum from proliferative diabetic retinopathy (PDR) to non-proliferative diabetic retinopathy (NPDR) and its stages. Associated diabetic macular edema (DME) may also show symptoms as the disease worsens (Liang and Goldberg, 1980).

Diabetic retinopathy is the most common cause of vision loss in patients aged 25–74 worldwide. It is projected that 191 million individuals worldwide will suffer from diabetic retinopathy by 2030, with 56 million of those cases being vision-threatening. According to the Wisconsin Epidemiologic Study of Diabetic Retinopathy (WESDR) Cohort, 60% of patients with type 2 diabetes and 99% of patients with type 1 diabetes exhibit some degree of retinopathy after 20 years of diabetes mellitus. Beyond the number of years since diagnosis and type of diabetes, there are many additional important risk factors for the development of diabetic retinopathy. Elevated blood pressure and hemoglobin A1c (HbA1c) levels are also linked to a higher risk of diabetic retinopathy (Lindley et al., 2009).

6.2.2.2. Etiology

Type 1 diabetes mellitus (T1DM) is typified by an autoimmune process that destroys beta cells in the pancreas, while type 2 diabetes mellitus (T2DM) is linked to a combination of genetics and lifestyle factors. Since retinal disease is an end-organ manifestation of the primary disease, the etiology of these two subtypes describes the etiology of diabetic retinopathy.

Compared to T1DM, T2DM has a stronger genetic correlation. Several genetic factors, such as TCF7L2, NOTCH2, KCNQ1, JAZF1, and MODY (a heterogeneous disorder with autosomal dominant transmission), have been implicated in the development of type 2 diabetes. A poor lifestyle combined with genetic predispositions raises the risk of type 2 diabetes.

Measurable antibodies against specific pancreatic β-cell proteins (insulin, islet antigen 2, zinc transporter 8, etc.) are present in more than 90% of individuals receiving a new diagnosis of T1DM.). The progressive loss of β-cells, reduced insulin release, and identifiable diabetes are all caused by these antibodies.

6.2.2.3. Risk Factors

- Diabetes duration;
- Uncontrolled glucose or blood pressure levels are associated with increased risk (see NHANES, UKDPS, WESDR references below);

- Hypertension;
- Dyslipidemia;
- Ethnicity;
- Pregnancy;
- Smoking.

6.2.2.4. General Pathology

Non-proliferative diabetic retinopathy (NPDR) and proliferative diabetic retinopathy (PDR) are the two main forms of diabetic retinopathy. The presence (proliferative) or absence (non-proliferative) of aberrant new blood vessels (retinal, optic disc, or iris/angle neovascularization) is what separates these two groups.

The primary factors that contribute to visual impairment in this patient population are of great concern. The basis of this disease process consists of the three items listed below, and the presence of them is correlated with the severity of the disease.

- Capillary leakage (DME);
- Capillary occlusion;
- Sequelae of retinal ischemia (retinal neovascularization, vitreous hemorrhage, tractional retinal detachment, neovascular glaucoma).

6.2.2.5. Pathophysiology

Retinal ischemia causes the release of VEGF, or vascular endothelial growth factor. VEGF causes two things: 1) angiogenesis, or the formation of new blood vessels; and 2) increased vascular permeability, which causes retinal swelling or edema.

6.2.3. Primary Prevention

Blood pressure and glucose regulation. A reduction in risk of 21% for any diabetes-related end-point (95% confidence interval: 17% to 24%, P<0.0001), 21% for diabetes-related deaths (15% to 27%, P<0.0001), 14% for myocardial infarction (8% to 21%, P<0.0001), and 37% for microvascular complications (33% to 41%, P<0.0001) was linked to every 1% decrease in updated mean HbA1c. (Report 35 of UKDPS) (Marcucci et al., 2011).

6.2.4. Diagnosis

6.2.4.1. History

Signs of floaters (vitreous hemorrhage), diminished or erratic vision (lens or macular edema), or abnormalities of the visual field (tractional detachment). Finding out the patient's hemoglobin A1c and whether or not their blood pressure is under control are crucial.

6.2.4.2. Physical Examination and Signs

It is necessary to do a dilated fundus examination and slit lamp examination. A patient with diabetes may have cataracts, aberrant blood vessels on the iris (called neovascularization of the iris, or rubeosis), and blood in the vitreous (or pigmented cells if there is a retinal detachment with hole formation). Checking the intraocular pressure (IOP) is important, particularly if NVI is observed. A macular examination (contact or non-contact lens) should be part of the dilated fundus examination to check for retinal swelling (DME), cotton wool spots, hard exudates, hemorrhage, and microaneurysms.

It is important to look for abnormal new blood vessels (also known as NVD, or neovascularization of the disc), optic nerve head pallor, and glaucomatous changes in the optic disc and surrounding area (up to one disc diameter). It is also important to look for any abnormal new blood vessels (also known as neovascularization elsewhere, or NVE) in the remaining retina (Matthews et al., 2004).

6.2.5. Symptoms

6.2.5.1. Clinical Diagnosis

The "macular area" is the region of the central retina that lies in the eye between the major branches (superior and inferior arcades) of the central retinal vessels (central retinal vein and central retinal artery). Beyond this, the retina is referred to as the "peripheral retina." In diabetic retinopathy, anomalous findings may appear in the central retinal area. Both the proliferative and non-proliferative forms of the illness may exhibit these findings. These macula-related abnormalities include yellow lipid and protein deposits (hard exudates), retinal bleeding (retinal hemorrhages), and abnormally dilated small vessel outpouchings (called microaneurysms). Macular edema is the term for when the macula thickens more than usual (Modi and Arsiwalla, 2020).

6.2.6. Classification of Non-proliferative Diabetic Retinopathy

Based on abnormal vascular findings (intraretinal microvascular anomalies, or IRMA), abnormal beading of the venous wall, and the presence or absence of retinal bleeding, non-proliferative diabetic retinopathy can be categorized into mild, moderate, or severe stages (Nguyen et al., 2009).

- **Mild**: few microaneurysms
- **Moderate**: increased number of microaneurysms and dot-blot hemorrhages. Cotton wool spots and hard exudates may be present.
- **Severe**: "4-2-1 rule" -- 4 quadrants of diffuse retinal hemorrhages and microaneurysms, 2 or more quadrants of venous beading, or 1 or more quadrants of IRMA

Although there is evidence that anti-vascular endothelial growth factor (VEGF) injections may help lessen the severity of retinopathy and lower the risk of vision complications, no treatment is typically administered at this stage (Ning et al., 2010).

6.2.7. Proliferative Diabetic Retinopathy

6.2.7.1. High-Risk Characteristics

- NVD > 1/4 to 1/3 disc area;
- Any NVD associated with vitreous or preretinal hemorrhage;
- Any NVE associated with vitreous or preretinal hemorrhage.

This is a progressive condition that frequently needs to be treated, particularly in patients who fit the high-risk criteria, to stop bleeding and the formation of scar tissue.

6.2.7.2. Diagnostic Procedures

When assessing the extent of retinal vascular abnormalities or ischemia, fluorescein angiography (FA) can be performed. The microaneurysm areas show up as hyperfluorescent spots and can leak on the late frames, which can lead to clinically significant areas of retinal edema. Leakage on the FA is also visible in the NVD/NVE areas. Hypofluorescent areas are those where capillary dropout and non-perfusion occur (Panton et al., 1990).

Retinal thickness measurements and the presence and location of intraretinal and/or subretinal fluid can both be ascertained with optical coherence tomography (OCT). To find out if the macular edema is improving with treatment, the OCT can be acquired one after the other.

6.2.7.3. Laboratory Test

Hemoglobin A1c measures glycemic control over the previous three months. An ideal target range is 5.5% – 6.0%, but this can be challenging to attain for some individuals. The general goal is to keep HbA1c levels ≤ 7, although for older patients (≥70 years), healthcare providers may aim for a slightly higher HbA1c due to lower levels being linked to higher morbidity in this age group.

6.2.8. Differential Diagnosis

6.2.8.1. Macular Edema with Retinal Hemorrhages

- Radiation retinopathy (history of radiation);
- Vein occlusion (occluded vessel seen, telangiectasia present);
- Parafoveal telangiectasia (telangiectatic vessels seen).

6.2.8.2. Retinal Neovascularization

- Vein occlusion;
- Retinal vasculitis;
- Sarcoidosis;
- Ocular ischemic syndrome;
- Sickle cell retinopathy (primarily peripheral neovascularization).

6.2.8.3. Iris Neovascularization

- Vein occlusion;
- Ocular ischemic syndrome.

6.2.9. Management

6.2.9.1. General Treatment

It is essential to have systemic control over diabetes, hypertension, hyperlipidemia, hypercholesterolemia, nephropathy, and other diseases.

6.2.9.2. Diabetic Macular Edema

In most cases, treating macular edema is necessary to try to improve or avoid vision loss. Treatment options include laser therapy or drug injections (corticosteroids or anti-VEGF therapies) to reduce macular edema and retinal swelling. After receiving an injection, patients may be seen every three months for macular edema or once a month initially. (Studies on DRCR, RIDE, RISE, DAVINCI, and ETDRS). Anti-VEGF medications are more effective than focal lasers, according to several studies (DRCR, READ2, RIDE, RISE, DAVINCI). In eyes with better vision (20/32 to 20/40), all three medications—bevacizumab, ranibizumab, and aflibercept—are effective for treating macular edema, according to a study by the DRCR network (Protocol T). Aflibercept exhibited better visual results than bevacizumab (at year 1 and year 2) and ranibizumab (at year 1 only) if visual acuity was 20/50 or lower (Pontremoli et al., 1996). A supplementary study conducted by the DRCR (Protocol AC) investigated step therapy by comparing initial treatment with bevacizumab followed by a switch to aflibercept if certain improvement criteria were not met, versus starting aflibercept immediately in eyes with visual acuity of 20/50 or worse. Both treatment approaches showed no significant difference in visual outcomes. Another study by the DRCR (Protocol V) revealed that for eyes with excellent visual acuity (20/25 or better), watchful observation was comparable to immediate anti-VEGF therapy. In cases where sustained visual acuity decline was observed, prompt treatment with anti-VEGF led to positive outcomes. In 2022, two new drugs (brolucizumab and faricimab) received FDA approval for DME treatment, demonstrating similar visual acuity outcomes as aflibercept with potential for longer dosing intervals. The FDA also approved a higher dose version of aflibercept (8 mg) in 2023 for treating DME, showing increased durability (Puklin et al., 1982).

6.2.9.3. Proliferative Diabetic Retinopathy

The main treatment for PDR is laser photocoagulation of the peripheral retina, called panretinal photocoagulation (PRP). This involves using a laser to remove some of the ischemic peripheral retina to reduce VEGF release and encourage regression of neovascularization. Successful treatment can help prevent vitreous hemorrhage and tractional retinal detachment. In more severe cases where the eye is filled with blood or scar tissue is causing issues, surgery such as vitrectomy may be required (Sapra et al., 2020).

In certain instances, anti-VEGF injections may be used to regress neovascularization in the eye. The DRCR protocol S found that the anti-VEGF drug ranibizumab was just as effective as PRP in treating patients with PDR. If PRP is not feasible due to issues like vitreous hemorrhage, anti-VEGF injections could aid in clearing the hemorrhage. It is important to monitor patients receiving only anti-VEGF injections since this treatment may not have long-term effects on neovascularization after treatment stops, unlike PRP. For patients who may not follow-up as necessary, PRP is preferred over anti-VEGF injections. However, a large case-control study showed no significant difference in the chances of TRD between injections alone and PRP alone (Scott et al., 2009).

When neovascular glaucoma and rubeosis coexist, anti-VEGF injections may occasionally be administered in addition to PRP. Another typical scenario involves first treating eyes with vitreous hemorrhage that is too dense for PRP with anti-VEGF injections, and then after the hemorrhage has sufficiently cleared, using a laser. In some circumstances, anti-VEGF injections are also administered before vitrectomy surgery in an effort to reduce the risk of intraoperative bleeding (Shantsila and Lip, 2017).

6.2.9.4. Surgery and Surgical Follow-up

The purpose of surgery is to remove scar tissue and blood from the surface of the retina and to apply laser treatment where necessary. It might be necessary to use silicone oil or intraocular gas during surgery to preserve the retina's reattachment to the eyewall and underlying layers (Sharp et al., 1995).

6.2.9.5. Complications

Injecting drugs into the eye or undergoing eye surgery carries a low but real risk of infection in the eyeball (endophthalmitis). Additionally, there is a risk of cataract progression with retinal surgery, as vitrectomy can speed up the formation of cataracts.

6.2.9.6. Prognosis

Research from the ETDRS indicates a correlation between the stage of retinopathy and the development of more advanced stages of retinopathy as well as visual loss.

6.3. DIABETES AND THE EYE

Diabetes is the main cause of new cases of blindness in adults aged 20-74 in the USA. This disease affects young adults in their prime working years and can result in high economic and social costs. Patients with diabetes who experience visual issues such as distortion, blurry vision, or floaters should seek immediate medical attention as it could potentially lead to irreversible blindness. Additionally, diabetic eye disease is linked to other serious health issues like chronic renal insufficiency, peripheral neuropathy, and coronary artery disease (Sinclair et al., 1999).

6.3.1. Anterior Segment Manifestations

Chronic hyperglycemia-induced autonomic

neuropathy may impair corneal sensation (CN V), which lowers the amount of aqueous tear film that must be produced to compensate, decreasing the tear film's effectiveness as it coats the cornea. This could present as a complaint of punctate epithelial keratitis (tiny erosions), keratitis sicca (extremely dry eyes), foreign-body sensation from "dry eyes (syndrome)," or eye fatigue from prolonged reading. The goal of treatment is to replace the watery part of tears (i.e., synthetic tears, q. I. PRN or d) or, in more complex situations, gel lubricants (i.e., puralube) or cyclosporine A (Restasis) applied topically (i.d.) Silicone punctual plugs used in punctual occlusion may be used to treat more resistant cases (Sladek et al., 2007).

Changes in the human crystalline lens can occur with rapid changes in blood sugar levels, leading to blurred vision which is a common symptom of Type 1 diabetes. The swelling and change in power of the lens caused by high blood sugar can result in a near-sighted shift in vision. The specific visual disturbances experienced depend on the patient's original refractive state. Tight control of blood sugar levels for a few months typically reverses these changes, requiring a temporary adjustment in eyeglass prescription (Stratton et al., 2000).

Osmotic shifts can have a transient or long-term impact on the lens's cortex and nucleus, which can lead to oxidative damage to the lens's constituent crystalline proteins (a and b). The posterior capsule of the lens experiences the "Classic" changes to the crystalline lens over an extended period of time (posterior subcapsular cataract, or PSC). PSC is typically irreversible when long-term, poorly managed diabetes is present. Cataract which persists after 3–4 months of "fairly good" glycemic control (i.e., FBS) (Stratton et al., 2001).

Long-term diabetics typically develop accelerated presbyopia, or the inability to read at the standard distance of 14 inches. without adding an optical reading to their prescription for glasses. People who are farsighted, or hyperopic, will need to have a reading addition added to their prescription sooner than people who are nearsighted, or myopic. Reduced accommodative amplitudes of the ciliary body as a result of autonomic neuropathy affecting CN III is thought to be the cause of accelerated presbyopia. The crystalline lens's early "hardening" as a result of hyperglycemia (oxidation of the crystalline lens proteins alpha- and beta-crystallins) may have played a role. Between the ages of 50 and 75, this shows up clinically as an increased near-prescription requirement (Stryjewski et al., 2016).

Diabetes-related double vision, or diplopia, can be caused by either true strabismus (an esotropia outward (CN III) or subacute or chronic posterior subcapsular cataract (PSC) formation) or by significant posterior subcapsular cataract (PSC) formation. Acute neuro-paresis (eye deviated in with CN VI palsy or eye deviated out with CN III palsy) is an infrequent side effect of long-term diabetes. This is an additional instance of autonomic neuropathy's eye manifestation. If the cause is solely diabetes, however, it is imperative to seek immediate ophthalmic and neurologic consultation. An anterior communicating artery macroaneurysm of the brain (compressing CN III) is one possibility to rule out in the differential diagnosis of recent onset exotropia (deviation of the eyes outward), which, if left untreated, can result in a massive subarachnoid hemorrhagic stroke and death (Nwanko et al., 2013).

It is interesting to note that both conditions can cause headaches and eye pain. This case of autonomic neuropathy is microvascular in nature, and systemic hypertension exacerbates it. Significantly, in diabetic CN III paresis, the nerve fibers responsible for iris pupil constriction are spared; instead, they are impacted in CN III exo-deviations linked to aneurysmal processes, leading to a dilated pupil that appears "blown." (Tso and Jampol, 1982).

Strabismus related to diabetes typically goes away completely in a few weeks or months. Diabetes that has been present for a long time may affect the iris. In people with blue eyes who have light pigmentation (a condition known as histopathologic lacy vacuolization) or in people with advanced diabetic eye disease who have rubeosis iridis (also known as ruby red eye in Latin), the iris stroma may atrophic (Tsui et al., 2022).

Neovascular glaucoma (NVG) is a serious eye condition that can lead to vision loss and severe pain. It is most commonly seen in cases of severely ischemic Proliferative retinopathy, but can also occur with other retinal vascular conditions. NVG occurs when abnormal blood vessel growth occurs in the front part of the eye known as the anterior chamber angle. This can block the drainage of fluid, leading to increased pressure inside the eye. With prompt and aggressive treatment, it is possible to reverse the process if some of the drainage angle remains open (Tsukikawa and Stacey, 2020).

6.3.2. Posterior Eye Involvement

Diabetes preferentially affects the capillary network responsible for the retinal vascular circulation. It is interesting to note that the deeper choroid and choriocapillaris are usually unaffected, possibly because these vessels differ from the inner retina's capillaries in that they are fenestrated. Until demonstrated differently, diabetes-related significant and permanent vision loss is always caused by posterior-segment ocular involvement. Retinal disorders may cause vision loss that is irreversible in a matter of weeks or months. Unless there is evidence to the contrary, patients you see who may have diabetes should always be evaluated for the possibility of impending, permanent visual loss as a result of retinal issues. It is crucial to remember that even in cases where diabetic retinopathy is properly managed, some patients may experience permanent blindness (Walsh, 1982).

Diabetic retinopathy can be classified as either moderate (double the visual angle, such as going from 20/20 to 20/40) or severe (worse than 20/200) visual loss. The primary objective of treating diabetic retinopathy is to reduce the risk of vision loss, whether it be moderate vision loss due to macular edema or severe vision loss from proliferative diabetic retinopathy (PDR).

When diabetes is present, PDR is typically the cause of highly dangerous retinopathy, which frequently manifests in its most advanced stages. The retina may not be noticeable to the patient or the primary care physician due to its anatomical posterior ocular location (Wells et al., 2016).

Sophisticated methods of examination, such as indirect ophthalmoscopy and slit-lamp biomicroscopy, are necessary to accurately assess the condition. It can easily be mistaken for common causes of vision loss like refractive error or cataract, especially by inexperienced examiners. The duration and severity of the systemic disease do not necessarily indicate whether the eye disease is permanent or treatable, so each case must be evaluated on its own merits (Williams et al., 1999).

Retinal diseases that are permanently blinding can and do occur in patients who claim they "don't even have diabetes.." This phenomenon could be explained by previously unidentified genetic factors controlling retinal vascular perfusion and neovascularization formation. Individuals with mild, late-treated Type II diabetes have gone blind; shortly after, they experience chronic renal failure (CRF), necessitating immediate hemodialysis (Figure 6.5) (Engerman et.al., 1965).

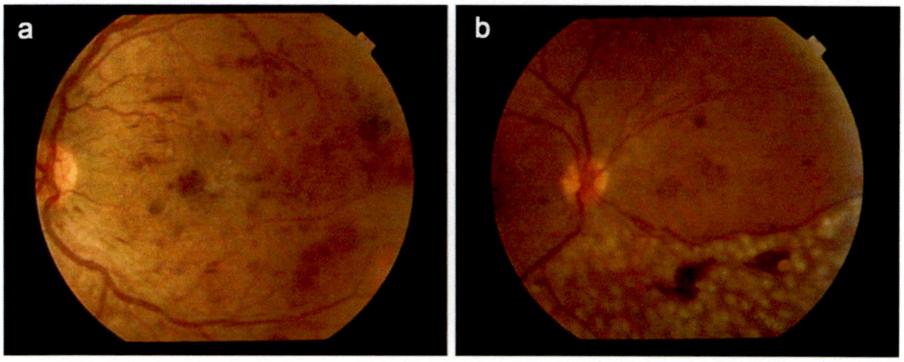

Figure 6.5. *(a) This color fundus photo of the left eye depicts a 24-year-old man with fairly good visual acuity (20/30). A casual observer might say that he had diabetic retinopathy, with "some dot-blot heme." In fact, he has very severe proliferative retinopathy, with NVD and diffuse macular edema. The conspicuous absence of lipid, bleeding and fibrosis make correct recognition difficult at first glance. (b) Photo of the same eye later that day after PRP was applied. He opted to be initially treated with simultaneous injection of intravitreal steroids.*

Source: D.R. Lazzaro and E. Shrier, Diabetes and Hypertension_ Evaluation and Management, DOI 10.1007/978-1-60327-357-2.

As long as the examination is conducted by a licensed eye care professional, annual screening exams are very beneficial. Patients need to be closely monitored by a qualified physician for the rest of their lives due to the significance of vision and the benefits of early treatment (at least twice a year when diabetic retinopathy is diagnosed). Those with true IDDM should be seen as soon as possible after diagnosis; symptoms can first appear five years after diagnosis (Wong and Mitchell, 2004).

There are three levels of nonproliferative diabetic retinopathy (NPDR): mild, or "background," moderate, and severe, or "pre-proliferative." It always comes before PDR, though it varies in how it shows up and how important it is for vision. A lot of the time, observation and reassurance are sufficient. However, its scope is occasionally overestimated. Anatomical and visual prognoses are fairly good if patients achieve good control over their blood pressure and blood sugar levels. Retinal disease paradoxically has the potential to get worse even after blood pressure, serum lipid, and glycemic index optimization (Wykoff et al., 2022).

Retinal vascular abnormalities that closely resemble those that occur in the renal glomeruli are the cause of diabetic retinopathy. Pathophysiology and pathogenesis are most likely the same. The recognized explanation includes endothelial dysfunction, pericyte loss, and thickening of the basement membrane brought on by hyperglycemia. Vascular endothelial growth factor (VEGF) is upregulated in response to hypoxia, oxidative stress, inflammation, and protein damage. Early on in nonproliferative or "background" diabetic retinopathy, there are significant alterations in native blood vessels that manifest as tiny intraretinal "dot-blot" hemorrhages and microaneurysmal saccular changes in capillaries (Engerman et al., 1965). Cotton-wool spots, which are indicative of infarct and nerve-fiber layer ischemia, are also observed; however, since they are frequently the consequence of collagen vascular diseases and hypertension, they are not pathognomonic changes of diabetes (Figures 6.6–6.8).

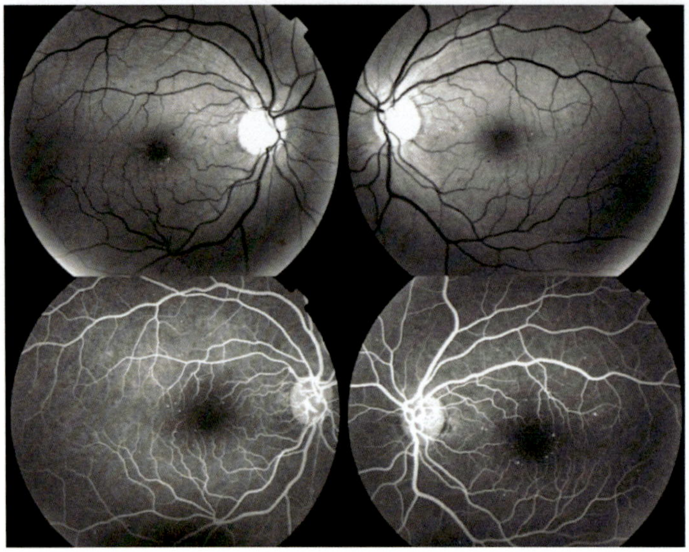

Figure 6.6. *Red-free (top) and mid-phase fluorescein angiographic images (bottom) depict microaneurysms—seen as hyper fluorescent spots. A small amount of lipid is seen inferior to the foveola top right image, indicating CSDME. This would be monitored closely, and patient would be advised of the great importance of HTN, BS and lipid control.*

Source: *D.R. Lazzaro and E. Shrier, Diabetes and Hypertension_ Evaluation and Management, DOI 10.1007/978-1-60327-357-2.*

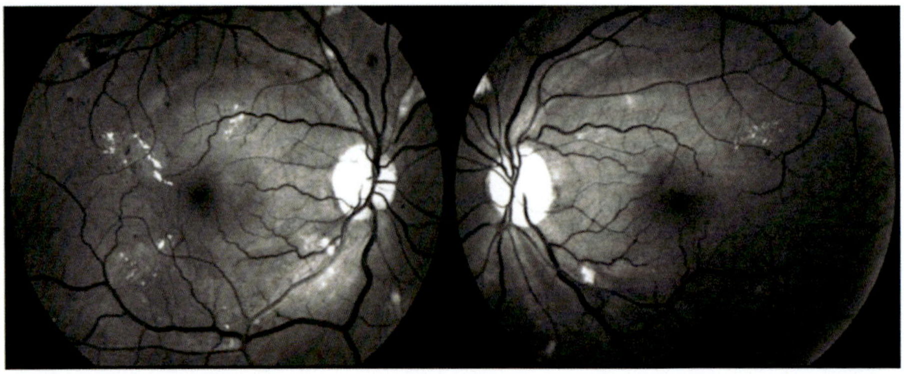

Figure 6.7. *Right (a) and left (b) eye red-free photos depicting moderate NPDR and bilateral CSDME. Lipid is threatening the foveal center (a), and a peri-foveal microaneurysm is causing foveal edema (b). Both eyes display cotton-wool spots indicative of moderate nonproliferative diabetic retinopathy. Patient was treated with focal laser (a) and intravitreal therapy (b), as the microvascular abnormality was judged too close to the fovea to treat safely with laser. Both eyes must be monitored very closely for progression to PDR. PRP laser may be necessary within months, or if patient is judged unreliable to follow-up.*

Source: *D.R. Lazzaro and E. Shrier, Diabetes and Hypertension_ Evaluation and Management, DOI 10.1007/978-1-60327-357-2.*

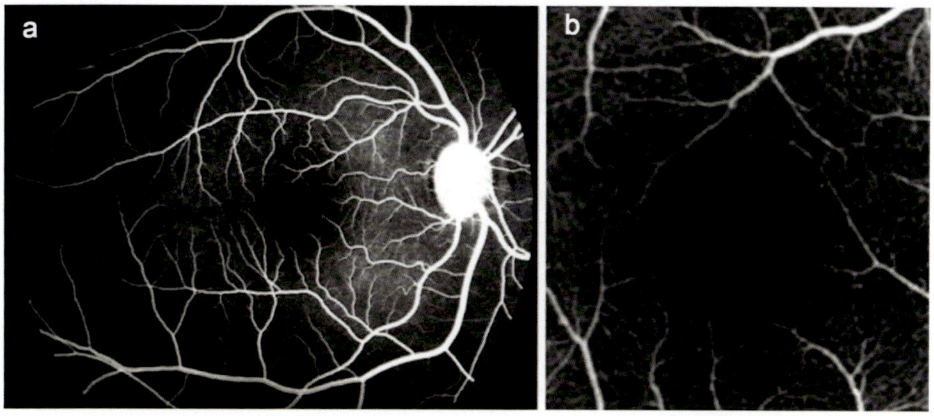

Figure 6.8. *(a) This is a normal fundus fluorescein mid-phase circulation image of the right eye . The retinal vessels show fluorescence about 1 min after fluorescein intravenous dye injection. (b) Note the healthy (magnified) appearance of the capillary network surrounding the anatomical foveola. The extent of the central black area represents the so-called foveolar avascular zone.*

Source: D.R. Lazzaro and E. Shrier, Diabetes and Hypertension_ Evaluation and Management, DOI 10.1007/978-1-60327-357-2.

Intraretinal microvascular abnormalities (IRMA), venous beading, and widespread capillary nonperfusion are examples of compensatory vascular anomalies caused by VEGF that are observed just before the proliferative type of retinopathy.

Changes in the retina often develop slowly over time and can go undetected for years, as they rarely result in noticeable vision problems. As areas of reduced blood flow in the retina increase, more VEGF and inflammatory substances are released into the vitreous, affecting the already compromised retinal capillaries. This can lead to leakage into the retina, overwhelming the ability of blood vessels and retinal pigment epithelial cells to absorb the excess fluid.

When fluid is reabsorbed, lipids separate from the suspension. The grading system for clinically significant diabetic macular edema (CSDME) includes thickening and deposition of lipids. In some cases, vision may remain normal and the condition can go unnoticed. Visual acuity is not a factor in the classification system. However, retinal thickening and lipid buildup in the macula can lead to moderate visual changes. If left untreated, severe or late-stage CSDME can result in significant vision loss and legal blindness (Wells et al., 2016).

When VEGF is overexpressed, it leads to the development of abnormal blood vessels that try to mimic the structure of the retinal capillary network. These new vessels are always considered pathological and typically result in bleeding and distortion of the retina, causing severe vision loss. They tend to grow in areas such as behind the vitreous body on the optic disc and retina, appearing as fragile capillaries known as "neovascularization of the disc" (NVD) and "neovascularization elsewhere" (NVE). The bleeding is a result of these vessels being weak and incompetent. Spontaneous bleeding may occur, especially in cases of uncontrolled hypertension, or due to vitreous traction. Tractional retinal detachment (TRD) may develop as the fibrovascular tissue of the neovascularization involutes and is constantly pulled by the vitreous body. Eventually, the vitreous may separate from the optic nerve and retina, leading to bleeding, TRD, and retinal breaks (Figure 6.9) (Kim et. al., 1999).

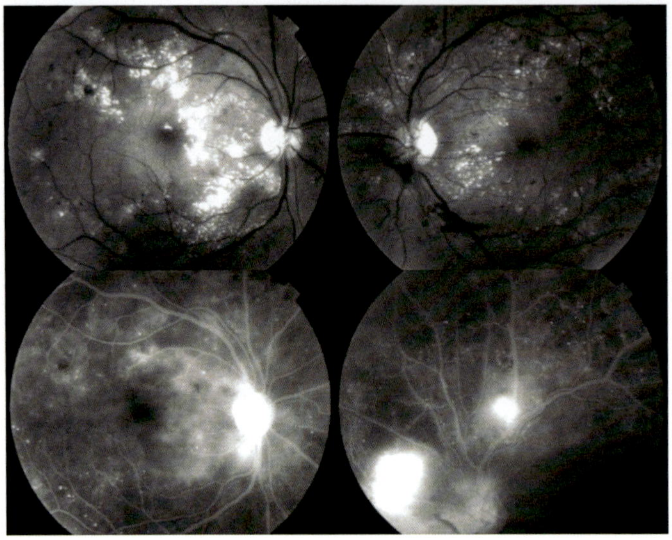

Figure 6.9. *Red-free photos (top) and late-phase fluorescein angiographic photos (bottom) of the right and left eyes. Diffuse CSDME with circinate lipid exuation is evident.*

Source: D.R. Lazzaro and E. Shrier, Diabetes and Hypertension_ Evaluation and Management, DOI 10.1007/978-1-60327-357-2.

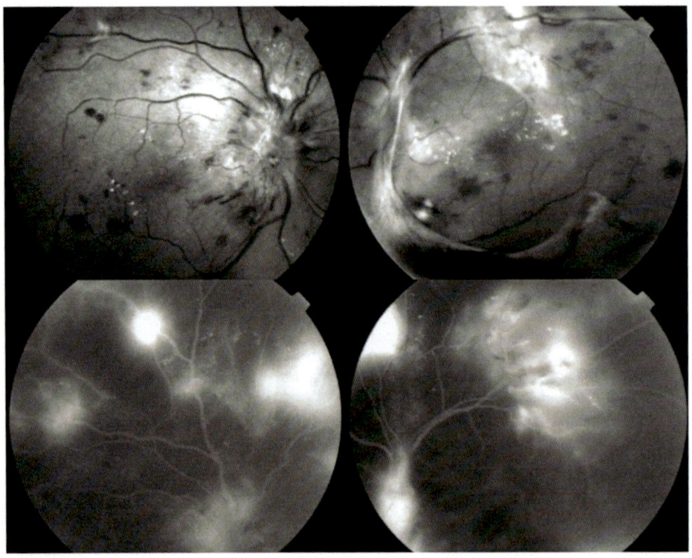

Figure 6.10. *Red-free photos (top) and late-circulation fluorescein angiographic images (bottom). Large areas of hypo fluorescence are seen consistent with nonperfusion/ischemia. Neovascularization, which is hyper fluorescent, tends to occur at borders of these areas (so-called watershed zones). Fibrosis is evident in the upper right photo, in a commonly seen con figuration. This is very severe PDR of both eyes (o.u.).*

Source: D.R. Lazzaro and E. Shrier, Diabetes and Hypertension_ Evaluation and Management, DOI 10.1007/978-1-60327-357-2.

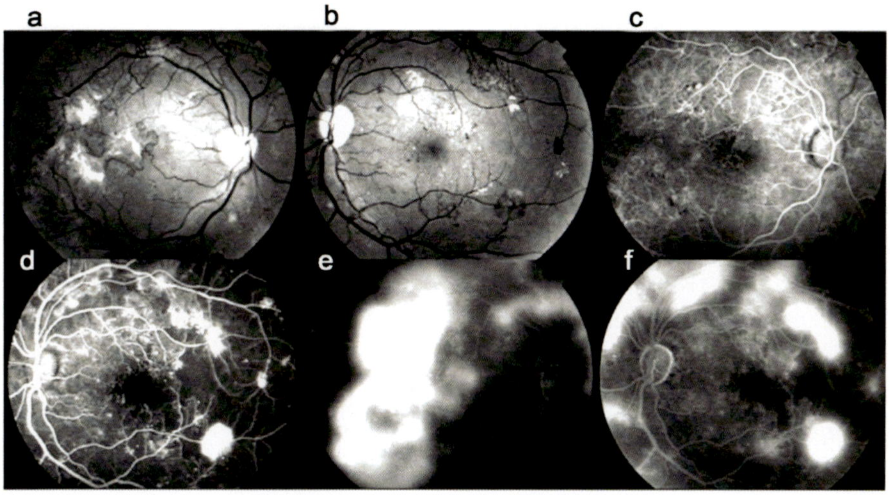

Figure 6.11. *(a – f) This 45-year-old long-standing IDDM patient has very severe, flat NVE (a , b) which has invaded the macula in the right eye (a). He recently had PRP at another facility in the o.d. (a , c) and attributes his 20/25 vision to that event. Extensive hyper fluorescent areas represent NVE (d – f). There is a conspicuous absence of NVD and VH, though, and his uncorrected vision is excellent (20/25 R and 20/20 L). He is at high risk of sudden, near simultaneous blindness. His macular disease will be treated with intravitreal therapy (Avastin) R , focal and grid laser L , and aggressive scatter PRP laser (o.u.).*

Source: D.R. Lazzaro and E. Shrier, Diabetes and Hypertension_ Evaluation and Management, DOI 10.1007/978-1-60327-357-2.

Diabetics may experience vitreous separation at a later stage due to changes in their protein composition making it stickier than normal. During vitreous surgery, abnormal splitting and lamination of the vitreous body may be observed. Failure of the vitreous to separate from the macula can lead to potential complications such as macular edema and distortion of the foveal pit, known as vitreo-macular traction syndrome (VMTS). Surgical release through pars-plana vitrectomy (PPV) is considered the best treatment for VMTS.

When diabetes is present, three-port PPV is frequently carried out. The significant cases of VMTS mentioned above, or when macular distortion is caused by contractile fibrovascular tissue, non-clearing and significant vitreous hemorrhage, TRD involving the macula, and complex retinal detachments with open retinal breaks, are among the indications for PPV in diabetics. The use and indications of PPV have somewhat expanded since it was first introduced in the 1970s and 1990s when it was thought to be safer and faster (Figures 6.10 and 6.11) (Kim et. al., 1999).

Instruments come in different sizes, ranging from 20 to 23 to 25-gauge. Only the smallest gauge requires sutures. The removal of the vitreous body's posterior hyaloid membrane and most of its substance eliminates the "scaffold" involved in the development of TRD, VMTS, and recurrent vitreous hemorrhage. However, this procedure is not without risks, such as re-bleeding (10%-20%), rare infections, macular hole, glaucoma, and optic neuropathy, all of which can lead to permanent vision loss. People who have not been treated with laser PRP may have worse outcomes. In the past, PPV for PDR carried a high risk of severe and permanent blindness, with a 10% chance of

NLP vision. Nowadays, intravitreal anti-VEGF agents are widely used for PDR before surgery in situations where there is extensive neovascularization. Thought must be given to this because rapid neovascular vessel involution and contraction can result in progressive TRD, retinal breaks, and complex retinal detachment.

Focal laser treatment is the recommended course of treatment for CSDME based on the findings of the Early Treatment of Diabetic Retinopathy Study (ETDRS). Over many years, it can cut the risk of developing moderate vision loss by roughly 50%. Applying tiny thermal laser spots under direct observation to leaky microaneurysms that are detectable at the slit-lamp and further localized on intravenous fluorescein angiography (IVFA) is known as focal laser therapy. When determining cases of coexisting macular ischemia and regions of peripheral retinal nonperfusion, IVFA is a great reSource: Diffuse macular edema patients used to have a grid-like laser pattern applied to them, but this procedure is becoming less common. When microaneurysms are not foveally involving, judicious focal laser remains the "gold standard" treatment for CSDME and is very helpful in discrete cases.

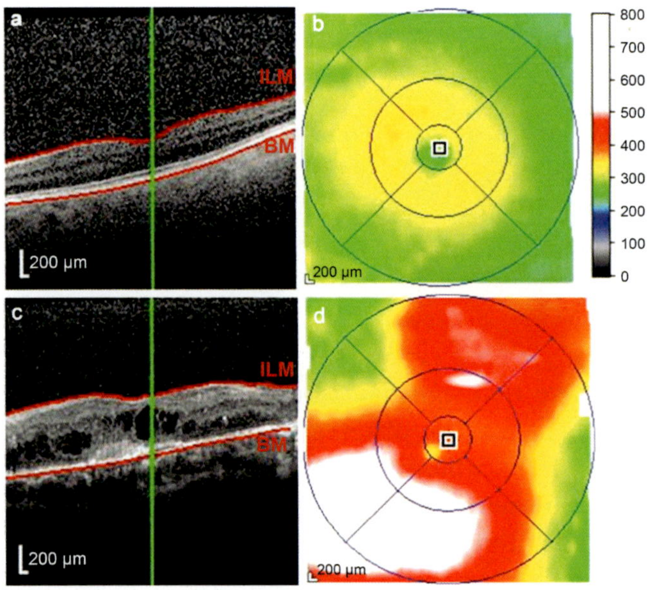

Figure 6.12. *Upper images depict SD-OCT (Heidelberg) (left) in a normal macula and its associated topographic thickness map in microns (right). Lower images depict SD-OCT (left) in chronic CSDME and associated topographic thickness map in microns (right). ILM internal limiting membrane, BM Bruch's membrane.*

Source: D.R. Lazzaro and E. Shrier, Diabetes and Hypertension_ Evaluation and Management, DOI 10.1007/978-1-60327-357-2.

When microaneurysms are situated within the foveal avascular zone and there is diffuse macular edema, focal laser treatment is less effective. Anti-VEGF intravitreal therapy (bevacizumab (Avastin) or ranibizumab (Lucentis)) is prescribed in conjunction with any kind of diabetic macular edema that is resistant to repeated focal laser treatment. Based on the ETDRS results, which indicate significant macular thickening with or without lipid presence endangering the foveal center, laser treatment is recommended. Intravitreal anti-VEGF therapy is very successful since VEGF is a strong candidate for vascular leakage from aberrant diabetic capillaries. Due to its brief duration of action (1-2 months), anti-VEGF monotherapy is less beneficial than focal laser treatment and only provides a temporary benefit.

Intravitreal steroid injection is one alternative treatment, but it comes with a high risk of ocular hypertension and the potential for cataract and glaucoma. Retinal effects are quite transient, and tachyphylaxis is frequently observed. Concocted intravitreal steroids i.e., In cases of chronic edema, sustained-release dexamethasone (Ozurdex) is the preferred treatment, particularly in cases where lipid has precipitated and deposited close to the foveal center. Focal laser, as opposed to intravitreal steroids, produces a long-lasting benefit. (Kim et. al., 1999).

When treating severe diffuse CSDME, PPV, with or without internal limited-membrane peeling, is the last resort. The best course of action after the therapeutic response to the previously mentioned modalities is to use IVFA and serial ocular coherence tomography (OCT). Although spectral domain high resolution OCT is a great advancement, IVFA is still required to evaluate the retinal circulation because it allows for noncontact measurement of the therapeutic response in the macula (Figures 6.12 and 6.13).

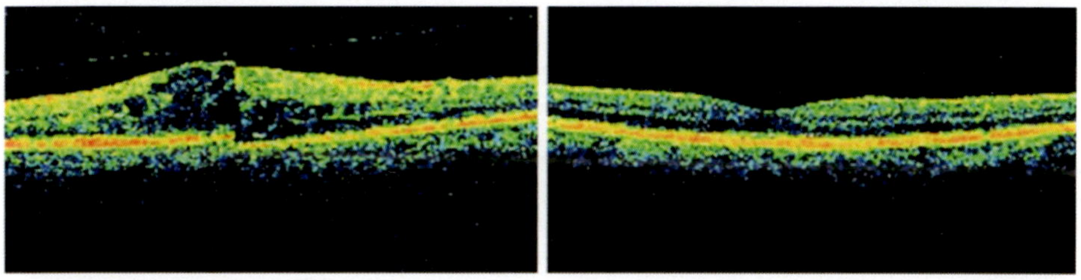

Figure 6.13. *SD-OCT image (Optovue ™) which depict macular edema of the right eye (a) and a nice foveal contour several months after focal laser of the left (b).*

Source: D.R. Lazzaro and E. Shrier, Diabetes and Hypertension_ Evaluation and Management, DOI 10.1007/978-1-60327-357-2.

Based on the findings of the diabetic retinopathy study (DRS), PDR is treated. Over a period of years, pan-retinal photocoagulation (PRP) helps lower the risk of severe vision loss. To decide whether to use a laser, factors such as the degree, location (on the disc or elsewhere), and presence of neovascularization are taken into account (Tsui et al., 2022). Additionally, the presence or absence of vitreous hemorrhage is taken into account. Based on the DRS results, this practical algorithm states that extensive necroscualrization of the disc should be treated with platelet-rich plasma (PRP), whereas more extensive necroscualrization of the disc or its association with vitreous hemorrhage are prerequisites for treatment of NVE. Patients are typically offered earlier treatment if they are deemed to be non-compliant or at high risk of progression. PRP involves applying large 300–500 mM laser spots to the peripheral retina while it is directly visible. In essence, the dying, ischemic peripheral retina—which is linked to pathologic VEGF release—is "killed off" by doing this. Lower levels of VEGF inhibit the development of macular edema and neovascularization. Moreover, the neurosensory retina "tacks down" to the underlying retinal pigment epithelium (RPE) following PRP laser treatment, theoretically reducing the likelihood of its detachment.

Because PRP laser treatment is extremely safe, effective, and long-lasting, it continues to be the "gold standard" for PDR. When indicated, PRP is typically administered in aliquots of 650–2,500 spots, depending on tolerance. Increased laser dosage may put the patient (as well as the attending physician) at risk for severe pain and bleeding. In an office setting, topical anesthesia (1% Tetracaine) is adequate to enable laser treatment. It is possible to perform peri-bulbar infiltration with a 1% lidocaine injection; however, one must take into account the possibility of severe periorbital swelling and injection-related permanent vision loss. Under monitored anesthesia, patients who are mentally challenged, emotionally unstable, or disturbed may receive treatment in an operating room or ambulatory surgery center.

It is important to note that PDR frequently results in severe and irreversible vision loss. Given the somewhat unpredictable nature of the disease, it is imperative to inform the patient of the significance of prompt and regular follow-up. In weeks to months, a fully functional adult who is employed, active, and drives can develop bilateral blindness. When uncontrolled diabetes and hypertension coexist, macular ischemia—which results from the normal foveolar avascular zone expanding—can happen. This condition causes irreversible, severe vision loss. Its occurrence in time is unpredictable (Yau et al., 2012).

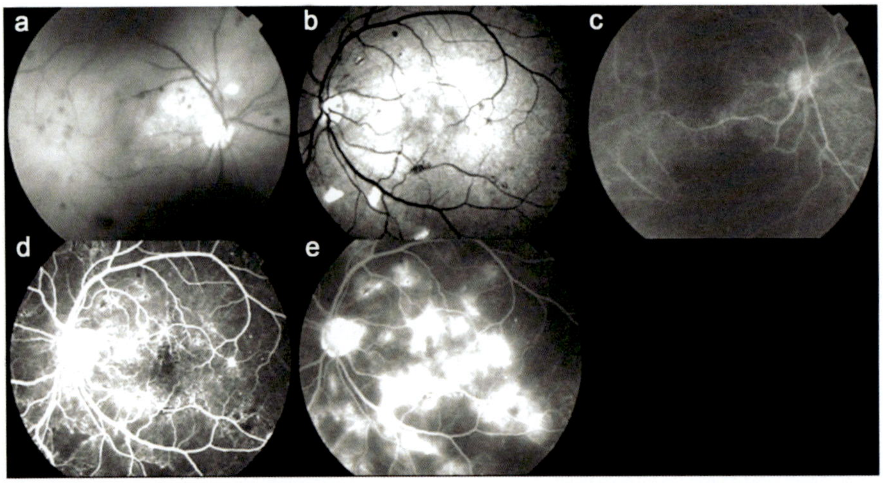

Figure 6.14. *This patient had "perfect" vision until occurrence of " floaters" R several days before presentation. He had severe PDR which was occult and unrecognized until she experienced a "sentinel bleed" in the form of VH R (a , c). Aggressive PRP will be applied in an exigent fashion, as further bleeding will necessitate urgent PPV. L will be treated with aggressive PRP (b , d , e). Surgery in this setting is quite treacherous as the risk of intra- and postoperative bleeding is high in the un- or inadequately lasered eye.*

Source: D.R. Lazzaro and E. Shrier, Diabetes and Hypertension_ Evaluation and Management, DOI 10.1007/978-1-60327-357-2.

A properly applied PRP laser is always very helpful in the setting of significant diabetic vitreous hemorrhage in PDR because it directly lowers the load of VEGF delivered to the functioning retina. If deemed necessary, it increases the likelihood of a surgical cure. Proximate treatment with vitrectomy is typically indicated in diabetic patients with minimal prior laser experience, or when significant laser cannot be safely applied due to vitreous hemorrhage (Arch Ophthalmol. 1985). Proximate surgery is indicated if the B-scan ultrasound exam is unable to confirm the status of the retina. Usually, a retinal specialist can apply some laser in a significant way. If a small amount of laser treatment was done in the past and vitreous floaters or blurry vision isn't the result of a detached retina, then observation is advised. The patient is checked on once a month. Untreated retinal regions receive fill-in PRP treatments until the bleeding stops and the neovascularization starts to recede. To maximize the gravitational inferior settling of the hemorrhage, the patient is advised to sleep with the head of the bed elevated at 30° (on two pillows) until that time (Figure 6.14).

Even with a sufficient number of laser treatments (4,000–6,000 PRP total laser spots), there is still a risk of rebleeding into the vitreous due to traction on persistent neovascular tissue. Vitreous opacities may persist to some extent indefinitely. Patients who receive significant laser treatment early on typically have a good outcome and can maintain vision necessary for important activities such as driving and reading. Severe bilateral vision loss can result in an 85% loss of body function. Strict control of diabetes, hypertension, and abnormal lipids is important for optimal outcomes. Aggressive screening and treatment can often reverse vision loss through a combination of laser treatments, injections, and surgery. Definitive treatment with pars plana vitrectomy, membrane peeling, and endolaser with gas or silicone oil treatment can significantly improve the condition and provide long-term good vision (Zheng et al., 2012).

Positively, "When they receive timely and appropriate treatment, people with proliferative retinopathy have less than a 5% chance of going blind within 5 years.." Treatments for diabetic retinopathy do not cure the condition, despite their high success rates.

6.4. DIABETES AFFECT OUR EYES

A blurred vision is one of the first symptoms of diabetes. Fluid leakage into the eye's lens, which causes the lens to swell and change shape, could be the cause of your fuzzy vision. The eyes have a hard time focusing because of these changes. Consequently, objects begin to appear hazy. Once insulin treatment has started, you may also have blurred vision as a result of fluid shifts. The illness in this instance will go away in a few weeks. Patients experience improved vision after their blood sugar levels stabilize.

A disorder where high blood sugar damages the blood vessels in the retina, the light-sensitive tissue in the back of the eye. When the condition reaches a progressive stage, the blood vessels in the retina begin to hemorrhage and cause distorted vision. It is the most common reason why diabetics lose their vision, and it is the main reason why adults become blind or have vision problems.

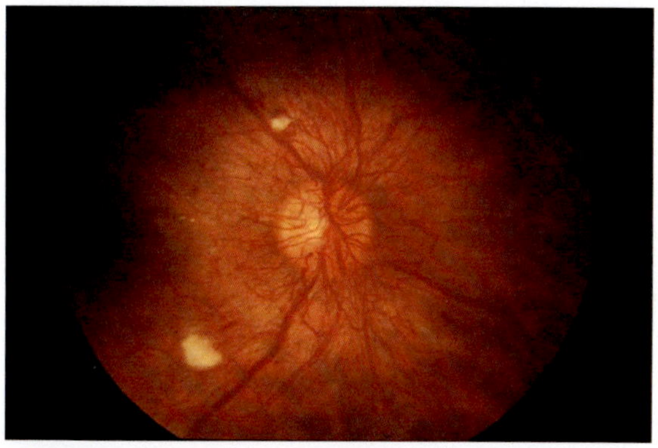

Figure. 6.15. *Affecting eyes with diabetes.*

Source: By http://www.nei.nih.gov/photo/eyedis/index.asp, Public Domain, https://commons.wikimedia.org/w/index.php?curid=862519.

6.4.1. Diabetic Macular Edema (DME)

A high percentage of vision loss associated with diabetic retinopathy is caused by a build-up of fluid in the macula, an area of the retina. This condition is known as diabetic macular edema (DME). Sharp central vision is produced by the macula, a region of the retina. In addition to blurred vision, this condition can also cause color changes and wavy vision (Zheng et al., 2018).

6.4.1.1. Proliferative Retinopathy

A condition called proliferative retinopathy, in which blood vessels leak into the center of the eye, may be the cause of blurry vision. Additionally, the patient might have problems seeing at night, seeing spots or floaters.

6.4.2. Glaucoma

A condition in which the optic nerve is damaged by intraocular pressure. A patient's risk of developing glaucoma is doubled in comparison to those without diabetes.

Other symptoms of glaucoma includes:

- Halo's around lights;
- Reddening of the eyes;
- Tunnel vision or loss of peripheral vision;
- Pain in the eye;
- Nausea or vomiting.

6.4.3. Cataracts

Cataracts result in the lens of your eyes becoming cloudy. Other symptoms of this condition include:

- Faded colours;
- Double vision, generally in one eye;
- Blurry our clouded vision;
- Halos around lights;
- Sensitivity to light;
- Prescriptions for glasses that need often replacing while vision is not improving.

Many eye conditions are more likely to develop in people with diabetes. Every year, you should have an examination of your eyes done, and part of that examination should involve dilation. Always disclose to the eye doctor the symptoms you are having as well as any medications you are taking. A prescription for new glasses or eye drops can often resolve blurred vision, which is often a minor issue. It may, nevertheless, indicate a dangerous underlying eye condition.

A Closer Look

Retinopathy

Retinopathy is a medical condition that affects the retina, the light-sensitive layer of tissue at the back of the eye responsible for vision. It encompasses a range of disorders characterized by damage to the retinal blood vessels, leading to impaired vision or blindness if left untreated. The most common types of retinopathy include diabetic retinopathy and hypertensive retinopathy, each associated with specific underlying systemic conditions.

Diabetic retinopathy is a complication of diabetes and one of the leading causes of blindness in adults. It occurs when chronically high blood sugar levels damage the retinal blood vessels, causing them to leak fluid or bleed. This can lead to swelling, abnormal blood vessel growth, and eventually, retinal detachment. Diabetic retinopathy progresses through stages, from mild non-proliferative to severe proliferative retinopathy. Early detection through regular eye exams is crucial for preventing vision loss, and treatments may include laser therapy, injections, or surgery.

Hypertensive retinopathy results from long-term high blood pressure, which causes the walls of the retinal blood vessels to thicken, narrow, or leak. This can reduce the blood flow to the retina and lead to visual disturbances. Symptoms often include blurred vision and headaches, but in severe cases, it can cause sudden vision loss. Managing hypertension through lifestyle changes and medication is essential in preventing and controlling hypertensive retinopathy.

Other forms of retinopathy include retinopathy of prematurity, affecting premature infants with underdeveloped retinal blood vessels, and radiation retinopathy, caused by exposure to radiation. Each type of retinopathy has distinct causes but generally involves damage to the retinal blood vessels and requires prompt medical attention to preserve vision.

In conclusion, retinopathy is a serious condition that underscores the importance of regular eye examinations, especially for individuals with diabetes or hypertension. Early diagnosis and timely treatment are vital to prevent progression and maintain healthy vision.

Summary

- Diabetes mellitus (DM) is a condition of defective metabolism of glucose leading to chronic hyperglycaemia due to defects in insulin production or function.
- Hypertension is persistent elevated blood pressure which puts a person at an increased risk of developing target organ damage in the vessels of the retina, brain, heart, kidneys and blood vessels.
- The arteriosclerotic changes of hypertensive retinopathy are caused by chronically elevated blood pressure.
- Hypertensive retinopathy goes through vasoconstrictive, sclerotic, and exudative phases based upon the extent of hypertension control.
- Malignant hypertension can also cause choroidopathy. Fibrinoid necrosis of choroidal arterioles leads to segmental infarction of choriocapillaris.
- Fluorescein angiography (FA) during acute malignant hypertension will demonstrate retinal capillary nonperfusion, microaneurysm formation, and a dendritic pattern of choroidal filling in the early phase.
- Diabetic retinopathy is one of the most predominant complications of diabetes and can develop in individuals who are living with either type 1 or type 2 diabetes, and it generally affects both eyes.
- Diabetes mellitus as a disease was identified as far back as 250-300 BC and was characterized by the sweet properties of urine.
- Fluorescein angiography (FA) may be used to determine the degree of ischemia or the presence of retinal vascular abnormalities.
- Diabetes affects the capillary network of the retinal vascular circulation preferentially. Interestingly, the deeper choroid and choriocapillaris are not typically affected, perhaps since these vessels are fenestrated and dissimilar to the capillaries of the inner retina.
- DME is an effect of diabetic retinopathy which refers to a build-up of fluid in the macula which is an area located in the retina, leading to swelling and is contributing a high percentage of vision loss which is linked with diabetic retinopathy.
- Blurry vision may be an indication of Proliferative retinopathy where blood vessels are leaking into the centre of the eye.

References

1. Ahn, S. J., Woo, S. J., & Park, K. H. (2014). Retinal and choroidal changes with severe hypertension and their association with visual outcome. *Investigative Ophthalmology & Visual Science, 55*(10), 7775–7785.
2. Aiello, L. P., Avery, R. L., Arrigg, P. G., et al. (1994). Vascular endothelial growth factor in ocular fluid of patients with diabetic retinopathy and other retinal disorders. *New England Journal of Medicine, 331*(22), 1480–1487.

3. American Academy of Ophthalmology (AAO). (2006). In *Basic and Clinical Sciences Course (Lifelong Education for the Ophthalmologist)*. San Francisco, CA: American Academy of Ophthalmology.
4. American College of Cardiology/American Heart Association Task Force on Clinical Practice Guidelines. (2017). *2017 ACC/AHA/AAPA/ABC/ACPM/AGS/APhA/ASH/ASPC/NMA/PCNA Guideline for the Prevention, Detection, Evaluation, and Management of High Blood Pressure in Adults: A Report of the American College of Cardiology/American Heart Association Task Force on Clinical Practice Guidelines*. American College of Cardiology.
5. Baker, C. W., Glassman, A. R., Beaulieu, W. T., Antoszyk, A. N., Browning, D. J., Chalam, K. V., Grover, S., Jampol, L. M., Jhaveri, C. D., Melia, M., Stockdale, C. R., Martin, D. F., & Sun, J. K. (2019). Effect of initial management with aflibercept vs laser photocoagulation vs observation on vision loss among patients with diabetic macular edema involving the center of the macula and good visual acuity: A randomized clinical trial. *JAMA, 321*(19), 1880–1894.
6. Baker, M. L., Hand, P. J., Liew, G., Wong, T. Y., Rochtchina, E., Mitchell, P., Lindley, R. I., Hankey, G. J., & Wang, J. J. (2010). Retinal microvascular signs may provide clues to the underlying vasculopathy in patients with deep intracerebral hemorrhage. *Stroke, 41*(4), 618–623.
7. Baker, M. L., Hand, P. J., Wang, J. J., & Wong, T. Y. (2008). Retinal signs and stroke: Revisiting the link between the eye and brain. *Stroke, 39*(4), 1371–1379.
8. Bourke, K., Patel, M. R., Prisant, L. M., & Marcus, D. M. (2004). Hypertensive choroidopathy. *Journal of Clinical Hypertension, 6*(8), 471–472.
9. Brown, D. M., Emanuelli, A., Bandello, F., Barranco, J. J. E., Figueira, J., Souied, E., Wolf, S., Gupta, V., Ngah, N. F., Liew, G., Tuli, R., Tadayoni, R., Dhoot, D., Wang, L., Bouillaud, E., Wang, Y., Kovacic, L., Guerard, N., & Garweg, J. G. (2022). KESTREL and KITE: 52-week results from two phase III pivotal trials of brolucizumab for diabetic macular edema. *American Journal of Ophthalmology, 238*, 157–172. https://doi.org/10.1016/j.ajo.2022.01.004.
10. Brown, D. M., Nguyen, Q. D., Marcus, D. M., Boyer, D. S., Patel, S., Feiner, L., Schlottmann, P. G., Rundle, A. C., Zhang, J., Rubio, R. G., Adamis, A. P., Ehrlich, J. S., & Hopkins, J. J. (2013). Long-term outcomes of ranibizumab therapy for diabetic macular edema: The 36-month results from two phase III trials: RISE and RIDE. *Ophthalmology, 120*(10), 2013–2022. https://doi.org/10.1016/j.ophtha.2013.02.034.
11. Cheung, N., Mitchell, P., & Wong, T. Y. (2010). The Lancet. *The Lancet, 376*(9735), 124–136. https://doi.org/10.1016/S0140-6736(10)60955-7.
12. Davis, M. D., Fisher, M. R., Gangnon, R. E., Barton, F., Aiello, L. M., Chew, E. Y., Ferris, F. L., & Knatterud, G. L. (1998). Risk factors for high-risk proliferative diabetic retinopathy and severe visual loss: Early Treatment Diabetic Retinopathy Study Report #18. *Investigative Ophthalmology & Visual Science, 39*(2), 233–252.
13. De Silva, D. A., Manzano, J. J., Liu, E. Y., Woon, F. P., Wong, W. X., Chang, H. M., Chen, C., Lindley, R. I., Wang, J. J., Mitchell, P., Wong, T. Y., Wong, M. C., & On behalf of the Multi-Centre Retinal Stroke Study Group. (2011). Retinal microvascular changes and subsequent vascular events after ischemic stroke. *Neurology, 77*(9), 896–903.
14. Diabetes Control and Complications Trial Research Group. (1993). The effect of intensive treatment of diabetes on the development and progression of long-term complications in insulin-dependent diabetes mellitus. *New England Journal of Medicine, 329*(14), 977–986.

15. Diabetes Control and Complications Trial Research Group. (1997). Clustering of long-term complications in families with diabetes in the diabetes control and complications trial. *Diabetes, 46*(11), 1829–1839.

16. Diabetic Retinopathy Clinical Research Network (DRCR.net), Beck, R. W., Edwards, A. R., Aiello, L. P., Bressler, N. M., Ferris, F., Glassman, A. R., Hartnett, E., Ip, M. S., Kim, J. E., & Kollman, C. (2009). Three-year follow-up of a randomized trial comparing focal/grid photocoagulation and intravitreal triamcinolone for diabetic macular edema. *Archives of Ophthalmology, 127*(3), 245–251.

17. Diabetic Retinopathy Clinical Research Network Writing Committee. (2007). Comparison of the modified Early Treatment Diabetic Retinopathy Study and mild macular grid laser photocoagulation strategies for diabetic macular edema. *Archives of Ophthalmology, 125*(4), 469–480.

18. Diabetic Retinopathy Clinical Research Network, Elman, M. J., Aiello, L. P., Beck, R. W., Bressler, N. M., Bressler, S. B., Edwards, A. R., Ferris, F. L., Friedman, S, M., Glassman, A. R., Miller, K. M., Scott, I. U., Stockdale, C. R., & Sun, J. K. (2010). Randomized trial evaluating ranibizumab plus prompt or deferred laser or triamcinolone plus prompt laser for diabetic macular edema. *Ophthalmology, 117*(6), 1064–1077.e35. https://doi.org/10.1016/j.ophtha.2010.03.056.

19. Diabetic Retinopathy Clinical Research Network. (2008). A randomized trial comparing intravitreal triamcinolone acetonide and focal/grid photocoagulation for diabetic macular edema. *Ophthalmology, 115*(9), 1447–1449.e1–10. https://doi.org/10.1016/j.ophtha.2008.04.018.

20. Diabetic Retinopathy Study Research Group. (1976). Preliminary report on effects of photocoagulation therapy. *American Journal of Ophthalmology, 81*(3), 383–396.

21. Diabetic Retinopathy Study Research Group. (1978). Photocoagulation treatment of proliferative diabetic retinopathy: The second report of the diabetic retinopathy study findings. *Ophthalmology, 85*(1), 82–106. https://doi.org/10.1016/S0161-6420(78)34016-0.

22. Diabetic Retinopathy Vitrectomy Study Research Group. (1985). Early vitrectomy for severe vitreous hemorrhage in diabetic retinopathy: Ten-year results of a randomized clinical trial, Diabetic Retinopathy Vitrectomy Study Report No. 2. *Archives of Ophthalmology, 103*(11), 1644–1652. https://doi.org/10.1001/archopht.1985.01050080062007.

23. DiMeglio, L. A., Evans-Molina, C., & Oram, R. A. (2018). Type 1 diabetes. *Lancet, 391*(10138), 2449–2462. https://doi.org/10.1016/S0140-6736(18)31320-5.

24. Do, D. V., Nguyen, Q. D., Boyer, D., Schmidt-Erfurth, U., Brown, D. M., Vitti, R., Berliner, A. J., Gao, B., Zeitz, O., Ruckert, R., Schmelter, T., Sandbrink, R., & Heier, J. S. (2012). One-year outcomes of the DA VINCI Study of VEGF Trap-Eye in eyes with diabetic macular edema. *Ophthalmology, 119*(8), 1658–1665. https://doi.org/10.1016/j.ophtha.2012.02.010.

25. Early Treatment Diabetic Retinopathy Study Research Group. (1985). Photocoagulation for diabetic macular edema: ETDRS study report number 1. *Archives of Ophthalmology, 103*(12), 1796–1806. https://doi.org/10.1001/archopht.1985.01050020076011.

26. Early Treatment Diabetic Retinopathy Study Research Group. (1987). Treatment techniques and clinical guidelines for photocoagulation of diabetic macular edema. *Ophthalmology, 94*(7), 761–774. https://doi.org/10.1016/S0161-6420(87)34015-2.

27. Early Treatment Diabetic Retinopathy Study Research Group. (1991). Early photocoagulation

for diabetic retinopathy. *Ophthalmology, 98*(5 Suppl), 766–785. https://doi.org/10.1016/S0161-6420(91)31992-4.

28. Early Treatment Diabetic Retinopathy Study Research Group. (1991). Classification of diabetic retinopathy from fluorescein angiograms. *Ophthalmology, 98*(5 Suppl), 807–822. https://doi.org/10.1016/S0161-6420(91)31993-6.
29. Early Treatment Diabetic Retinopathy Study Research Group. (1991). Fundus photographic risk factors for progression of diabetic retinopathy. *Ophthalmology, 98*(5 Suppl), 823–833. https://doi.org/10.1016/S0161-6420(91)31994-8.
30. Early Treatment Diabetic Retinopathy Study Research Group. (1991). Early photocoagulation for diabetic retinopathy. *Ophthalmology, 98*(5), 766–785. https://doi.org/10.1016/S0161-6420(91)31992-4.
31. Early Treatment Diabetic Retinopathy Study Research Group. (1995). Focal photocoagulation treatment of diabetic macular edema: Relationship of treatment effect to fluorescein angiographic and other retinal characteristics at baseline. *Archives of Ophthalmology, 113*(9), 1144–1155. https://doi.org/10.1001/archopht.1995.01100090082005.
32. Elliott, W., & Varon, J. (2020). Moderate to severe hypertensive retinopathy and hypertensive encephalopathy in adults. In *UpToDate*. Retrieved from: https://www.uptodate.com (accessed on 5 September 2024).
33. Engerman, R., & Bloodworth, J. J. (1965). Experimental diabetic retinopathy in dogs. *Archives of Ophthalmology, 73*(2), 205–210. https://doi.org/10.1001/archopht.1965.00970020147009.
34. Flynn, H. W. Jr., Chew, E. Y., Simons, B. D., Barton, F. B., Remaley, N. A., & Ferris, F. L. (1992). Pars plana vitrectomy in the Early Treatment Diabetic Retinopathy Study. *Ophthalmology, 99*(9), 1351–1357. https://doi.org/10.1016/S0161-6420(92)31721-6.
35. Garner, A., & Ashton, N. (1979). Pathogenesis of hypertensive retinopathy: A review. *Journal of the Royal Society of Medicine, 72*(6), 362–365. https://doi.org/10.1177/014107688007200606.
36. Gunn, R. M. (1892). Ophthalmoscopic evidence of (1) arterial changes associated with chronic renal diseases and (2) of increased arterial tension. *Transactions of the Ophthalmological Society of the United Kingdom, 12*, 124–125.
37. Harjasouliha, A., Raiji, V., & Gonzalez, J. (2017). Review of hypertensive retinopathy. *Disease Monographs, 63*(3), 63–69. https://doi.org/10.1016/j.disamonth.2017.01.002.
38. Hayreh, S. S., Joos, K. M., Podhajsky, P. A., et al. (1994). Systemic diseases associated with nonarteritic anterior ischemic optic neuropathy. *American Journal of Ophthalmology, 118*(6), 766–780. https://doi.org/10.1016/S0002-9394(14)70188-8.
39. Hayreh, S. S., Podhajsky, P. A., & Zimmerman, M. B. (2009). Retinal artery occlusion associated systemic and ophthalmic abnormalities. *Ophthalmology, 116*(10), 1928–1936. https://doi.org/10.1016/j.ophtha.2009.03.018.
40. Hayreh, S. S., Servais, G. E., & Virdi, P. S. (1986). Fundus lesions in malignant hypertension V. Hypertensive optic neuropathy. *Ophthalmology, 93*(1), 74–87. https://doi.org/10.1016/S0161-6420(86)33967-5.
41. Henderson, A. D., Bruce, B. B., Biousse, V., & Newman, N. J. (2011). Hypertension-related eye abnormalities and the risk of stroke. *Reviews in Neurological Diseases, 8*(1–2), 1–9.
42. Jacsobson, D. M., Vierkant, R. A., & Belongia, E. A. (1997). Nonarthritic anterior ischemic

optic neuropathy: A case-control study of potential risk factors. *Archives of Ophthalmology, 115*(11), 1403–1407. https://doi.org/10.1001/archopht.115.11.1403.

43. Jhaveri, C. D., Glassman, A. R., Ferris, F. L., Liu, D., Maguire, M. G., Allen, J. B., Baker, C. W., Browning, D., Cunningham, M. A., Friedman, S. M., Jampol, L. M., Marcus, D. M., Martin, D. F., Preston, C. M., Stockdale, C. R., & Sun, J. K. (2022). Aflibercept monotherapy or bevacizumab first for diabetic macular edema. *New England Journal of Medicine, 387*(8), 692–703. https://doi.org/10.1056/NEJMoa2204225.
44. Katakam, R., Brukamp, K., & Townsend, R. R. (2008). What is the proper workup of a patient with hypertension? *Cleveland Clinic Journal of Medicine, 75*(9), 663–672. https://doi.org/10.3949/ccjm.75a.02.
45. Keith, N. M., Wagener, H. P., & Barker, N. W. (1974). Some different types of essential hypertension: Their course and prognosis. *American Journal of Medical Sciences, 268*(6), 336–345. https://doi.org/10.1097/00000441-197412000-00002.
46. Kim, E. Y., Lew, H. M., & Song, J. H. (2012). Effect of intravitreal bevacizumab (Avastin®) therapy in malignant hypertensive retinopathy: A report of two cases. *Journal of Ocular Pharmacology and Therapeutics, 28*(3), 318–322. https://doi.org/10.1089/jop.2011.0107.
47. Kim, I., Ryan, A., Rohan, R., Amano, S., Aguilar, S., Miller, J., & Adamis, A. P. (1999). Constitutive expression of VEGF, VEGFR-1, and VEGFR-2 in normal eyes. *Investigative Ophthalmology & Visual Science, 40*(9), 2115–2121. https://doi.org/10.1167/iovs.99-0157.
48. Kishi, S., Tso, M. O., & Hayreh, S. S. (1985). Fundus lesions in malignant hypertension. I. A pathologic study of experimental hypertensive choroidopathy. *Archives of Ophthalmology, 103*(8), 1189–1197. https://doi.org/10.1001/archopht.1985.01050060078007.
49. Klein, R., Klein, B. E., Moss, S. E., & Cruickshanks, K. J. (1998). The Wisconsin Epidemiologic Study of Diabetic Retinopathy: XVII. The 14-year incidence and progression of diabetic retinopathy and associated risk factors in type 1 diabetes. *Ophthalmology, 105*(10), 1801–1815. https://doi.org/10.1016/S0161-6420(98)92012-1.
50. Klein, R., Lee, K. E., Knudtson, M. D., Gangnon, R. E., & Klein, B. E. (2009). Changes in visual impairment prevalence by period of diagnosis of diabetes: The Wisconsin Epidemiologic Study of Diabetic Retinopathy. *Ophthalmology, 116*(10), 1937–1942. https://doi.org/10.1016/j.ophtha.2009.03.012.
51. Konstantinidis, L., & Guex-Crosier, Y. (2016). Hypertension and the eye. *Current Opinion in Ophthalmology, 27*(6), 514–521. https://doi.org/10.1097/ICU.0000000000000307.
52. Lang, G. K. (2007). *Ophthalmology: A Pocket Textbook Atlas*. Thieme.
53. Lewis, R. A., Norton, E. W., & Gass, J. D. (1976). Acquired arterial macro aneurysms of the retina. *British Journal of Ophthalmology, 60*(1), 21–30. https://doi.org/10.1136/bjo.60.1.21.
54. Liang, J. C., & Goldberg, M. F. (1980). Treatment of diabetic retinopathy. *Diabetes, 29*(10), 841–851. https://doi.org/10.2337/diab.29.10.841.
55. Lindley, R. I., Wang, J. J., Wong, M. C., Mitchell, P., Liew, G., Hand, P., Wardlaw, J., De Silva, D. A., Baker, M., Rochtchina, E., Chen, C., Hankey, G. J., Chang, H. M., Fung, V. S., Gomes, L., Wong, T. Y., & Multicenter Retina and Stroke Study (MCRS) Collaborative Group. (2009). Retinal microvasculature in acute lacunar stroke: A cross-sectional study. *Lancet Neurology, 8*(7), 628–634. https://doi.org/10.1016/S1474-4422(09)70143-0.

56. Marcucci, R., Soff, F., Grifoni, E., Sodi, A., & Prisco, D. (2011). Retinal vein occlusions: A review for the internist. *Internal and Emergency Medicine, 6*(4), 307–314. https://doi.org/10.1007/s11739-011-0545-1.

57. Matthews, D. R., Stratton, I. M., Aldington, S. J., Holman, R. R., & Kohner, E. M. (2004). Risks of progression of retinopathy and vision loss related to tight blood pressure control in type 2 diabetes mellitus: UKPDS 69. *Archives of Ophthalmology, 122*(11), 1631–1640. https://doi.org/10.1001/archopht.122.11.1631.

58. Melamud, A., & Kaiser, P. K. (2006). Hypertensive retinopathy. In D. Huang, P. K. Kaiser, C. Y. Lowder, & E. I. Traboulsi (Eds.), *Retinal Imaging* (pp. 283–288). Mosby. ISBN 9780323023467.

59. Modi, P., & Arsiwalla, T. (2020). Hypertensive retinopathy. In *StatPearls*. StatPearls Publishing. Retrieved from: https://www.statpearls.com (accessed on 5 September 2024).

60. National Center for Health Statistics. (2008). *Health, United States, 2008*. Retrieved from: https://www.cdc.gov/nchs/data/hus/hus08.pdf (accessed on 5 September 2024).

61. National Diabetes Statistics Report 2020. (2020). *DiabetesResearch.org*. Retrieved from: https://www.diabetesresearch.org/file/national-diabetes-statistics-report-2020.pdf (accessed on 5 September 2024).

62. National Society to Prevent Blindness. (1980). *Vision Problems in the US: A Statistical Analysis*. National Society to Prevent Blindness.

63. Nguyen, Q. D., Shah, S. M., Heier, J. S., Do, D. V., Lim, J., Boyer, D., Abraham, P., & Campochiaro, P. A.; READ-2 Study Group. (2009). Primary end point (six months) results of the Ranibizumab for Edema of the macula in diabetes (READ-2) study. *Ophthalmology, 116*(11), 2175–2181. https://doi.org/10.1016/j.ophtha.2009.06.027.

64. Nwankwo, T., Yoon, S. S., Burt, V., & Gu, Q. (2013). Hypertension among adults in the United States: National Health and Nutrition Examination Survey, 2011–2012. *NCHS Data Brief, 133*, 1–8. Retrieved from: https://www.cdc.gov/nchs/data/databriefs/db133.pdf (accessed on 5 September 2024).

65. Panton, R. W., Goldberg, M. F., & Farber, M. (1990). Retinal arterial macro aneurysms: Risk factors and natural history. *British Journal of Ophthalmology, 74*(10), 595–600. https://doi.org/10.1136/bjo.74.10.595.

66. Pontremoli, R., Sofia, A., Tirotta, A., et al. (1996). The deletion polymorphism of the angiotensin I-converting enzyme gene is associated with target organ damage in essential hypertension. *Journal of the American Society of Nephrology, 7*(12), 2550–2558. https://doi.org/10.1681/ASN.V7122550.

67. Puklin, J. E., Tamborlane, W. V., Felig, P., Genel, M., & Sherwin, R. S. (1982). Influence of long-term insulin infusion pump treatment of type I diabetes on diabetic retinopathy. *Ophthalmology, 89*(7), 735–747. https://doi.org/10.1016/S0161-6420(82)35156-4.

68. Sapra, A., & Bhandari, P. (2020). Diabetes mellitus. In *StatPearls*. StatPearls Publishing. Retrieved from: https://www.statpearls.com (accessed on 5 September 2024).

69. Scott, I. U., Danis, R. P., Bressler, S. B., Bressler, N. M., Browning, D. J., & Qin, H.; Diabetic Retinopathy Clinical Research Network. (2009). Effect of focal/grid photocoagulation on visual acuity and retinal thickening in eyes with non-center-involved diabetic macular edema. *Retina, 29*(5), 613–617. https://doi.org/10.1097/IAE.0b013e3181a184d8.

70. Shantsila, A., & Lip, G. (2017). Malignant hypertension revisited—Does this still exist? *American Journal of Hypertension, 30*(6), 543–549. https://doi.org/10.1093/ajh/hpx008.

71. Sharp, P. S., Chaturvedi, N., Wormald, R., McKeigue, P. M., Marmot, M. G., & McHardy Young, S. (1995). Hypertensive retinopathy in Afro-Caribbeans and Europeans: Prevalence and risk factor relationships. *Hypertension, 25*(6), 1322–1325. https://doi.org/10.1161/01.HYP.25.6.1322.

72. Sinclair, S. H., Alaniz, R., & Presti, P. (1999). Laser treatment of diabetic macular edema: Comparison of ETDRS-level treatment with threshold-level treatment by using high-contrast discriminant central visual field testing. *Seminars in Ophthalmology, 14*(4), 214–222. https://doi.org/10.1076/soph.14.4.214.2296.

73. Sladek, R., Rocheleau, G., Rung, J., et al. (2007). A genome-wide association study identifies novel risk loci for type 2 diabetes. *Nature, 445*(7130), 881–885. https://doi.org/10.1038/nature05616.

74. Special Eurobarometer. (2007). *Health in the European Union*. Retrieved from: https://ec.europa.eu/commfrontoffice/publicopinion/archives/ebs/ebs_296_en.pdf (accessed on 5 September 2024).

75. Stratton, I. M., Adler, A. I., Neil, H. A., Matthews, D. R., Manley, S. E., Cull, C. A., Hadden, D., Turner, R. C., & Holman, R. R. (2000). Association of glycaemia with macrovascular and microvascular complications of type 2 diabetes (UKPDS 35): Prospective observational study. *BMJ, 321*(7258), 405–412. https://doi.org/10.1136/bmj.321.7258.405.

76. Stratton, I. M., Kohner, E. M., Aldington, S. J., Turner, R. C., Holman, R. R., Manley, S. E., & Matthews, D. R. (2001). UKPDS 50: Risk factors for incidence and progression of retinopathy in type II diabetes over 6 years from diagnosis. *Diabetologia, 44*(2), 156–163. https://doi.org/10.1007/s001250051596.

77. Stryjewski, T. P., Papakostas, T. D., & Vavvas, D. (2016). Proliferative hypertensive retinopathy. *JAMA Ophthalmology*. https://doi.org/10.1001/jamaophthalmol.2015.5583.

78. The Diabetic Retinopathy Clinical Research Network. (2015). Aflibercept, Bevacizumab, or Ranibizumab for diabetic macular edema. *New England Journal of Medicine*. https://doi.org/10.1056/NEJMoa1414264.

79. Tso, M. O., & Jampol, L. M. (1982). Pathophysiology of hypertensive retinopathy. *Ophthalmology, 89*(10), 1132–1145. https://doi.org/10.1016/S0161-6420(82)35187-7.

80. Tsui, J. C., Yu, Y., & VanderBeek, B. L. (2022). Association of treatment type and loss to follow-up with tractional retinal detachment in proliferative diabetic retinopathy [published online ahead of print, 2022 Dec 1]. *JAMA Ophthalmology*. https://doi.org/10.1001/jamaophthalmol.2022.4942.

81. Tsukikawa, M., & Stacey, A. W. (2020). A review of hypertensive retinopathy and chorioretinopathy. *Clinical Optometry, 12*, 67–73. https://doi.org/10.2147/OPTO.S183492.

82. Walsh, J. B. (1982). Hypertensive retinopathy: Description, classification, and prognosis. *Ophthalmology, 89*(10), 1127–1131. https://doi.org/10.1016/S0161-6420(82)35186-5.

83. Wells, J. A., Glassman, A. R., Ayala, A. R., Jampol, L. M., Bressler, N. M., Bressler, S. B., Brucker, A. J., Ferris, F. L., Hampton, G. R., Jhaveri, C., Melia, M., & Beck, R. W.; Diabetic Retinopathy Clinical Research Network. (2016). Aflibercept, Bevacizumab, or Ranibizumab for diabetic

macular edema: Two-year results from a comparative effectiveness randomized clinical trial. *Ophthalmology, 123*(6), 1351–1359. https://doi.org/10.1016/j.ophtha.2016.02.022.

84. Williams, K. V., Erbey, J. R., Becker, D., & Orchard, T. J. (1999). Improved glycemic control reduces the impact of weight gain on cardiovascular risk factors in type 1 diabetes: The Epidemiology of Diabetes Complications Study. *Diabetes Care, 22*(7), 1084–1091. https://doi.org/10.2337/diacare.22.7.1084.

85. Wong, T. Y., & Mitchell, P. (2004). Hypertensive retinopathy. *New England Journal of Medicine, 351*(22), 2310–2317. https://doi.org/10.1056/NEJMra032865.

86. World Health Organization. (2018). The top 10 causes of death. Retrieved from: https://www.who.int/news-room/fact-sheets/detail/the-top-10-causes-of-death (accessed on 5 September 2024).

87. Wykoff, C. C., Abreu, F., Adamis, A. P., Basu, K., Eichenbaum, D. A., Haskova, Z., Lin, H., Loewenstein, A., Mohan, S., Pearce, I. A., Sakamoto, T., Schlottmann, P. G., Silverman, D., Sun, J. K., Wells, J. A., Willis, J. R., & Tadayoni, R.; YOSEMITE and RHINE Investigators. (2022). Efficacy, durability, and safety of intravitreal faricimab with extended dosing up to every 16 weeks in patients with diabetic macular oedema (YOSEMITE and RHINE): Two randomized, double-masked, phase 3 trials. *Lancet, 399*(10326), 741–755. https://doi.org/10.1016/S0140-6736(22)00018-6.

88. Yau, J. W., Rogers, S. L., Kawasaki, R., et al. (2012). Global prevalence and major risk factors of diabetic retinopathy. *Diabetes Care, 35*(3), 556–564. https://doi.org/10.2337/dc11-1909.

89. Zheng, Y., He, M., & Congdon, N. (2012). The worldwide epidemic of diabetic retinopathy. *Indian Journal of Ophthalmology, 60*(5), 428–431. https://doi.org/10.4103/0301-4738.100542.

90. Zheng, Y., Ley, S. H., & Hu, F. B. (2018). Global aetiology and epidemiology of type 2 diabetes mellitus and its complications. *Nature Reviews Endocrinology, 14*(2), 88–98. https://doi.org/10.1038/nrendo.2017.151.

Chapter 7

ENDOCRINE HYPERTENSION IN CHILDREN

Contents

INTRODUCTION

Abnormal hormone synthesis or response is one possible cause of hypertension. The fraction of pediatric hypertension cases caused by these issues likely makes up, at most, a small portion of cases overall, but it is higher in cases of severe hypertension, cases involving very young patients, and cases that cluster in families. The adrenal gland and its hormones are involved in most cases of endocrine hypertension. The medulla, which secretes catecholamines, and the cortex, which synthesizes cortisol and aldosterone, are the two endocrine tissues that make up the adrenal gland. Although it can affect extramedullary sites as well, the adrenal medulla is the primary site of involvement for phenochromocytoma. Hypertension can be brought on by a wide range of disorders that impact the adrenal cortex. These include primary aldosteronism brought on by adenomas or hyperplasia of the zona glomerulosa, hypertensive forms of congenital adrenal hyperplasia, and Cushing syndrome (excessive glucocorticoid exposure) brought on by iatrogenic etiologies, pituitary or adrenal adenomas, or other tumors secreting excessive ACTH. Thyrotoxicosis brought on by Graves' disease or the thyrotoxic stage of Hashimoto's thyroiditis can also result in hypertension. Because the associated hypertension necessitates and typically responds favorably to specific treatment of the underlying hormonal abnormality, it is critical to accurately diagnose these disorders (Akamizu et al., 2012).

Orientation and Directional Terms

Term	Definition	Illustration
Aldosterone	Aldosterone is a steroid hormone produced by the adrenal cortex that helps regulate blood pressure, fluid and electrolyte balance, and acid-base balance. It does this by controlling the balance of salts and water in the kidneys, keeping sodium in and releasing potassium from the body.	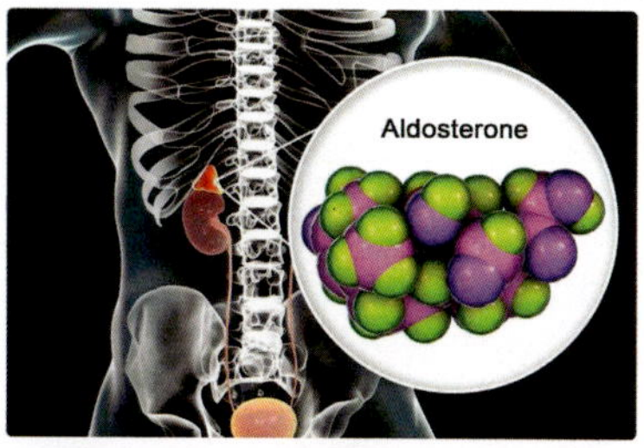
Childhood obesity	Childhood obesity is having a body mass index (BMI) at or above the 95th percentile for age and sex assigned at birth in children aged 2 years and older.	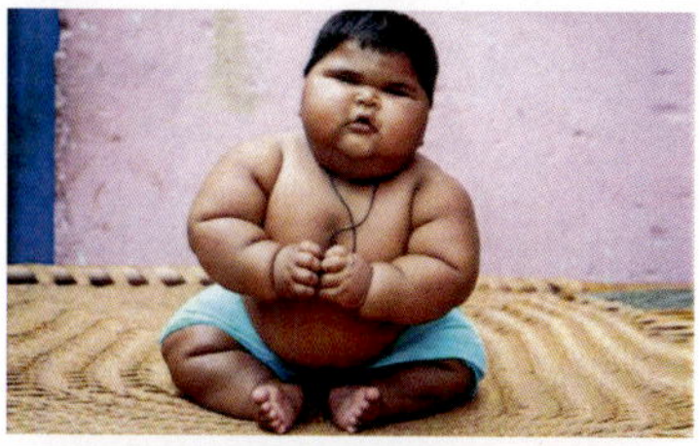
Cortisol	Cortisol is a steroid hormone that helps the body manage stress. It is produced in the adrenal glands, which sit on top of each kidney, and released into the bloodstream when a person is stressed.	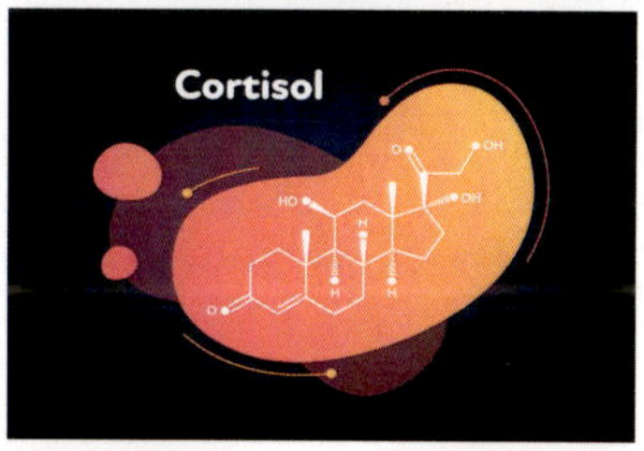
Glomerulonephritis	Glomerulonephritis is a kidney disease that involves inflammation and damage to the glomeruli, the tiny filter units in the kidneys. It can develop quickly or over time and is often caused by the immune system attacking healthy tissue.	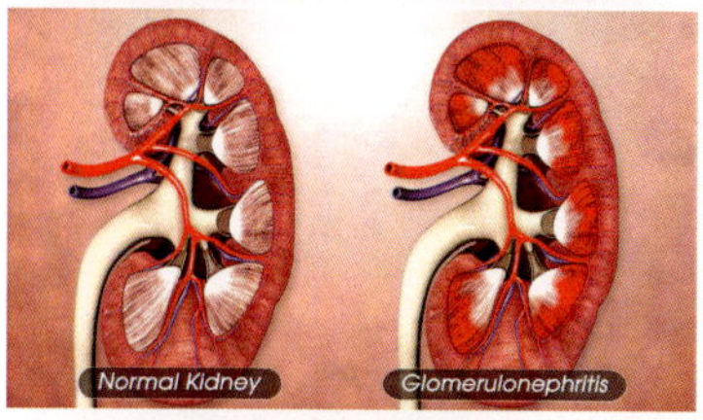
Secondary hypertension	Secondary hypertension is high blood pressure caused by another condition or disease. Conditions that may cause secondary hypertension include kidney disease, adrenal disease, thyroid problems and obstructive sleep apnea.	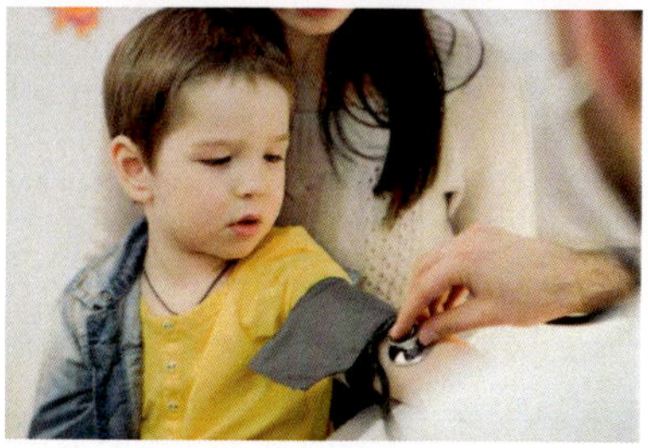

7.1. HYPERTENSION IN CHILDREN

The term "hypertension" refers to a persistent increase in either the diastolic or systolic blood pressure at rest, or both. Up until the age of 13, different blood pressure readings are deemed abnormal in children. Primary hypertension, or hypertension without a known cause, is most common in adults. It is comparatively rare for children to have secondary hypertension, or hypertension with a known cause. Although these may appear later, children typically do not experience any symptoms or complications related to hypertension during their childhood. Sphygmomanometry is used for diagnosis. To find the reasons behind secondary hypertension, tests may be conducted. Drugs, medication, and managing curable causes are all part of the treatment.

Over the past few decades, it has become evident that childhood is frequently the starting point for adult hypertension, which can be influenced by both intrauterine and neonatal conditions. Additionally, patients who had hypertension as children experience the aftereffects of their condition earlier in adulthood. For this reason, it is critical to recognize and manage childhood hypertension.

In the United States, children with hypertension typically have a prevalence of 2.2% to 3.9%, with high normal readings between 4% and 3.4%. Due to regional variations in definitions, methodology, and reference data, the prevalence worldwide is estimated to be around 4%, though this is less certain. Furthermore, the prevalence seems to be rising, most likely as a result of children becoming overweight and obese at a higher rate than in the past 30 years; among teenagers, obesity is now twice as common as it was 30 years ago. Adolescents who are obese are more likely than their peers to have high blood pressure.

7.1.1. Definition of Hypertension in Children

Since there are no outcomes data available for children with hypertension, hypertension in children under 13 is categorized normatively, meaning that it is compared to blood pressure readings in a sizable child population. Tables 7.1 and 7.2 show that normative blood pressure values in children under 13 years of age vary depending on their age, sex, and height (Barrett et al., 2019).

Table 7.1. *Blood Pressure (BP) Percentile Levels for Boys by Age and Height (Measured and Percentile)*

		Systolic BP (mm Hg)							Diastolic BP (mm Hg)						
Age (year)	BP Percentile*	Measured Height (in bold) or Height Percentile							Measured Height (in bold) or Height Percentile						
		5th	10th	25th	50th	75th	90th	95th	5th	10th	25th	50th	75th	90th	95th
1	**Measured height (cm)**	**77.2**	**78.3**	**80.2**	**82.4**	**84.6**	**86.7**	**87.9**	**77.2**	**78.3**	**80.2**	**82.4**	**84.6**	**86.7**	**87.9**
	50th	85	85	86	86	87	88	88	40	40	40	41	41	42	42
	90th	98	99	99	100	100	101	101	52	52	53	53	54	54	54
	95th	102	102	103	103	104	105	105	54	54	55	55	56	57	57
	95th + 12 mm Hg	114	114	115	115	116	117	117	66	66	67	67	68	69	69
2	**Measured height (cm)**	**86.1**	**87.4**	**89.6**	**92.1**	**94.7**	**97.1**	**98.5**	**86.1**	**87.4**	**89.6**	**92.1**	**94.7**	**97.1**	**98.5**
	50th	87	87	88	89	89	90	91	43	43	44	44	45	46	46
	90th	100	100	101	102	103	103	104	55	55	56	56	57	58	58
	95th	104	105	105	106	107	107	108	57	58	58	59	60	61	61
	95th + 12 mm Hg	116	117	117	118	119	119	120	69	70	70	71	72	73	73
3	**Measured height (cm)**	**92.5**	**93.9**	**96.3**	**99**	**101.8**	**104.3**	**105.8**	**92.5**	**93.9**	**96.3**	**99**	**101.8**	**104.3**	**105.8**
	50th	88	89	89	90	91	92	92	45	46	46	47	48	49	49
	90th	101	102	102	103	104	105	105	58	58	59	59	60	61	61
	95th	106	106	107	107	108	109	109	60	61	61	62	63	64	64
	95th + 12 mm Hg	118	118	119	119	120	121	121	72	73	73	74	75	76	76
4	**Measured height (cm)**	**98.5**	**100.2**	**102.9**	**105.9**	**108.9**	**111.5**	**113.2**	**98.5**	**100.2**	**102.9**	**105.9**	**108.9**	**111.5**	**113.2**
	50th	90	90	91	92	93	94	94	48	49	49	50	51	52	52
	90th	102	103	104	105	105	106	107	60	61	62	62	63	64	64
	95th	107	107	108	108	109	110	110	63	64	65	66	67	67	68
	95th + 12 mm Hg	119	119	120	120	121	122	122	75	76	77	78	79	79	80

5	**Measured height (cm)**	**104.4**	**106.2**	**109.1**	**112.4**	**115.**	**118.6**	**120.3**	**104.4**	**106.2**	**109.1**	**112.4**	**115.7**	**118.6**	**120.3**
	50th	91	92	93	94	95	96	96	96	51	52	53	54	55	55
	90th	103	104	105	106	107	108	108	63	64	65	65	66	67	67
	95th	107	108	109	109	110	111	112	66	67	68	69	70	70	71
	95th + 12 mm Hg	119	120	121	121	122	123	124	78	79	80	81	82	82	83
6	**Measured height (cm)**	**110.3**	**112.2**	**115.3**	**118.9**	**122.4**	**125.6**	**127.5**	**110.3**	**112.2**	**115.3**	**118.9**	**122.4**	**125.6**	**127.5**
	50th	93	93	94	95	96	97	98	54	54	55	56	57	57	58
	90th	105	105	106	107	109	110	110	66	66	67	68	68	69	69
	95th	108	109	110	111	112	113	114	69	70	70	71	72	72	73
	95th + 12 mm Hg	120	121	122	123	124	125	126	81	82	82	83	84	84	85
7	**Measured height (cm)**	**116.1**	**118**	**121.4**	**125.1**	**128.9**	**123.4**	**134.5**	**116.1**	**118**	**121.4**	**125.1**	**128.9**	**132.4**	**134.5**
	50th	94	94	95	97	98	98	99	56	56	57	58	58	59	59
	90th	106	107	108	109	110	111	111	68	68	69	70	70	71	71
	95th	110	110	111	112	114	115	116	71	71	72	73	73	74	74
	95th + 12 mm Hg	122	122	123	124	126	127	128	83	83	84	85	85	86	86
8	**Measured height (cm)**	**121.4**	**123.5**	**127**	**131**	**135.1**	**138.8**	**141**	**121.4**	**123.5**	**127**	**131**	**135.1**	**138.8**	**141**
	50th	95	96	97	98	99	99	100	57	57	58	59	59	60	60
	90th	107	108	109	110	111	112	112	69	70	70	71	72	72	73
	95th	111	112	112	114	115	116	117	72	73	73	74	75	75	75
	95th + 12 mm Hg	123	124	124	126	127	128	129	84	85	85	86	87	87	87
9	**Measured height (cm)**	**126**	**128.3**	**132.1**	**136.3**	**140.7**	**144.7**	**147.1**	**126**	**128.3**	**132.1**	**136.3**	**140.7**	**144.7**	**147.1**
	50th	96	97	98	99	100	101	101	57	58	59	60	61	62	62
	90th	107	108	109	110	112	113	114	70	71	72	73	74	74	74
	95th	112	112	113	115	116	118	119	74	74	75	76	76	77	77
	95th + 12 mm Hg	124	124	125	127	128	130	131	86	86	87	88	88	89	89

10	**Measured height (cm)**	**130.2**	**132.7**	**136.7**	**141.3**	**145.9**	**150.1**	**152.7**	**130.2**	**132.7**	**136.7**	**141.3**	**145.9**	**150.1**	**152.7**
	50th	97	98	99	100	101	102	103	59	60	61	62	63	63	64
	90th	108	109	111	112	113	115	116	72	73	74	74	75	75	76
	95th	112	113	114	116	118	120	121	76	76	77	77	78	78	78
	95th + 12 mm Hg	124	125	126	128	130	132	133	88	88	89	89	90	90	90
11	**Measured height (cm)**	**134.7**	**137.3**	**141.5**	**146.4**	**151.3**	**155.8**	**158.6**	**134.7**	**137.3**	**141.5**	**146.4**	**151.3**	**155.8**	**158.6**
	50th	99	99	101	102	103	104	106	61	61	62	63	63	63	63
	90th	110	111	112	114	116	117	118	74	74	75	75	75	76	76
	95th	114	114	116	118	120	123	124	77	78	78	78	78	78	78
	95th + 12 mm Hg	126	126	128	130	132	135	136	89	90	90	90	90	90	90
12	**Measured height (cm)**	**140.3** 101	**143** 101	**147.5** 102	**152.7** 104	**157.9** 106	**162.6** 108	**165.5** 109	**140.3** 61	**143** 62	**147.5** 62	**152.7** 62	**157.9** 62	**162.6** 63	**165.5** 63
	50th	101	101	102	104	106	108	109	61	62	62	62	62	63	63
	90th	113	114	115	117	119	121	122	75	75	75	75	75	76	76
	95th	116	117	118	121	124	126	128	78	78	78	78	78	79	79
	95th + 12 mm Hg	128	129	130	133	136	138	140	90	90	90	90	90	91	91
13	**Measured height (cm)**	**147**	**150**	**154.9**	**160.3**	**165.7**	**170.5**	**173.4**	**147**	**150**	**154.9**	**160.3**	**165.7**	**170.5**	**173.4**
	50th	103	104	105	108	110	111	112	61	60	61	62	63	64	65
	90th	115	116	118	121	124	126	126	74	74	74	75	76	77	77
	95th	119	120	122	125	128	130	131	78	78	78	78	80	81	81
	95th + 12 mm Hg	131	132	134	137	140	142	143	90	90	90	90	92	93	93
14	**Measured height (cm)**	**153.8**	**156.9**	**162**	**167.5**	**172.7**	**177.4**	**180.1**	**153.8**	**156.9**	**162**	**167.5**	**172.7**	**177.4**	**180.1**
	50th	105	106	109	111	112	113	113	60	60	62	64	65	66	67
	90th	119	120	123	126	127	128	129	74	74	75	77	78	79	80
	95th	123	125	127	130	132	133	134	77	78	79	81	82	83	84
	95th + 12 mm Hg	135	137	139	142	144	145	146	89	90	91	93	94	95	96

15	**Measured height (cm)**	**159**	**162**	**166.9**	**172.2**	**177.2**	**181.6**	**184.2**	**159**	**162**	**166.9**	**172.2**	**177.2**	**181.6**	**184.2**
	50th	108	110	112	113	114	114	114	61	62	64	65	66	67	68
	90th	123	124	126	128	129	130	130	75	76	78	79	80	81	81
	95th	127	129	131	132	134	135	135	78	79	81	83	84	85	85
	95th + 12 mm Hg	139	141	143	144	146	147	147	90	91	93	95	96	97	97
16	**Measured height (cm)**	**162.1**	**165**	**169.6**	**174.6**	**179.5**	**183.8**	**186.4**	**162.1**	**165**	**169.6**	**174.6**	**179.5**	**183.8**	**186.4**
	50th	111	112	114	115	115	116	116	63	64	66	67	68	69	69
	90th	126	127	128	129	131	131	132	77	78	79	80	81	82	82
	95th	130	131	133	134	135	136	137	80	81	83	84	85	86	86
	95th + 12 mm Hg	142	143	145	146	147	148	149	92	93	95	96	97	98	98
17	**Measured height (cm)**	**163.8**	**166.5**	**170.9**	**175.8**	**180.7**	**184.9**	**187.5**	**163.8**	**166.5**	**170.9**	**175.8**	**180.7**	**184.9**	**187.5**
	50th	114	115	116	117	117	118	118	65	66	67	68	69	70	70
	90th	128	129	130	131	132	133	134	78	79	80	81	82	82	83
	95th	132	133	134	135	137	138	138	81	82	84	85	86	86	87
	95th + 12 mm Hg	144	145	146	147	149	150	150	93	94	96	97	98	98	99

Source: *Bruce A. Kaiser. Hypertension in Children. MSD MANUALS. https://www.msdmanuals.com/en-in/professional/pediatrics/hypertension-in-children/hypertension-in-children.*

Table 7.2. *Blood Pressure (BP) Percentile Levels for Girls by Age and Height (Measured and Percentile)*

		Systolic BP (mm Hg)							Diastolic BP (mm Hg)						
Age (year)	BP Percentile*	Measured Height (in bold) or Height Percentile							Measured Height (in bold) or Height Percentile						
		5th	10th	25th	50th	75th	90th	95th	5th	10th	25th	50th	**75th**	**90th**	**95th**
1	**Measured height (cm)**	**75.4**	**76.6**	**78.6**	**80.8**	**83**	**84.9**	**86.1**	**75.4**	**76.6**	**78.6**	**80.8**	**83**	**84.9**	**86.1**
	50th	84	85	86	86	87	88	88	41	42	42	43	44	45	46
	90th	98	99	99	100	101	102	102	54	55	56	56	57	58	58
	95th	101	102	102	103	104	105	105	59	59	60	60	61	62	62
	95th + 12 mm Hg	113	114	114	115	116	117	117	71	71	72	72	73	74	74
2	**Measured height (cm)**	**84.9**	**86.3**	**88.6**	**91.1**	**93.7**	**96**	**97.4**	**84.9**	**86.3**	**88.6**	**91.1**	**93.7**	**96**	**97.4**
	50th	87	87	88	89	90	91	91	45	46	47	48	49	50	51
	90th	101	101	102	103	104	105	106	58	58	59	60	61	62	62
	95th	104	105	106	106	107	108	109	62	63	63	64	65	66	66
	95th + 12 mm Hg	116	117	118	118	119	120	121	74	75	75	76	77	78	78
3	**Measured height (cm)**	**91**	**92.4**	**94.9**	**97.6**	**100.5**	**103.1**	**104.6**	**91**	**92.4**	**94.9**	**97.6**	**100.5**	**103.1**	**104.6**
	50th	88	89	89	90	91	92	93	48	48	49	50	51	53	53
	90th	102	103	104	104	105	106	107	60	61	61	62	63	64	65
	95th	106	106	107	108	109	110	110	64	65	65	66	67	68	69
	95th + 12 mm Hg	118	118	119	120	121	122	122	76	77	77	78	79	80	81
4	**Measured height (cm)**	**97.2**	**98.8**	**101.4**	**104.5**	**107.6**	**110.5**	**112.2**	**97.2**	**98.8**	**101.4**	**104.5**	**107.6**	**110.5**	**112.2**
	50th	89	90	91	92	93	94	94	50	51	51	53	54	55	55
	90th	103	104	105	106	107	108	108	62	63	64	65	66	67	67
	95th	107	108	109	109	110	111	112	66	67	68	69	70	70	71
	95th + 12 mm Hg	119	120	121	121	122	123	124	78	79	80	81	82	82	83
5	**Measured height (cm)**	**103.6**	**105.3**	**108.2**	**111.5**	**114.9**	**118.1**	**120**	**103.6**	**105.3**	**108.2**	**111.5**	**114.9**	**118.1**	**120**
	50th	90	91	92	93	94	95	96	52	52	53	55	56	57	57
	90th	104	105	106	107	108	109	110	64	65	66	67	68	69	70
	95th	108	109	109	110	111	112	113	68	69	70	71	72	73	73
	95th + 12 mm Hg	120	121	121	122	123	124	125	80	81	82	83	84	85	85

6	**Measured height (cm)**	**110**	**111.8**	**114.9**	**118.4**	**122.1**	**125.6**	**127.7**	**110**	**111.8**	**114.9**	**118.4**	**122.1**	**125.6**	**127.7**
	50th	92	92	93	94	96	97	97	54	54	55	56	57	58	59
	90th	105	106	107	108	109	110	111	67	67	68	69	70	71	71
	95th	109	109	110	111	112	113	114	70	71	72	72	73	74	74
	95th + 12 mm Hg	121	121	122	123	124	125	126	82	83	84	84	85	86	86
7	**Measured height (cm)**	**115.9**	**117.8**	**121.1**	**124.9**	**128.8**	**132.5**	**134.7**	**115.9**	**117.8**	**121.1**	**124.9**	**128.8**	**132.5**	**134.7**
	50th	92	93	94	95	97	98	99	55	55	56	57	58	59	60
	90th	106	106	107	109	110	111	112	68	68	69	70	71	72	72
	95th	109	110	111	112	113	114	115	72	72	73	73	74	74	75
	95th + 12 mm Hg	121	122	123	124	125	126	127	84	84	85	85	86	86	87
8	**Measured height (cm)**	**121**	**123**	**126.5**	**130.6**	**134.7**	**138.5**	**140.9**	**121**	**123**	**126.5**	**130.6**	**134.7**	**138.5**	**140.9**
	50th	93	94	95	97	98	99	100	56	56	57	59	60	61	61
	90th	107	107	108	110	111	112	113	69	70	71	72	72	73	73
	95th	110	111	112	113	115	116	117	72	73	74	74	75	75	75
	95th + 12 mm Hg	122	123	124	125	127	128	129	84	85	86	86	87	87	87
9	**Measured height (cm)**	**125.3**	**127.6**	**131.3**	**135.6**	**140.1**	**144.1**	**146.6**	**125.3**	**127.6**	**131.3**	**135.6**	**140.1**	**144.1**	**146.6**
	50th	95	95	97	98	99	100	101	57	58	59	60	60	61	61
	90th	108	108	109	111	112	113	114	71	71	72	73	73	73	73
	95th	112	112	113	114	116	117	118	74	74	75	75	75	75	75
	95th + 12 mm Hg	124	124	125	126	128	129	130	86	86	87	87	87	87	87
10	**Measured height (cm)**	**129.7**	**132.2**	**136.3**	**141**	**145.8**	**150.2**	**152.8**	**129.7**	**132.2**	**136.3**	**141**	**145.8**	**150.2**	**152.8**
	50th	96	97	98	99	101	102	103	58	59	59	60	61	61	62
	90th	109	110	111	112	113	115	116	72	73	73	73	73	73	73
	95th	113	114	114	116	117	119	120	75	75	76	76	76	76	76
	95th + 12 mm Hg	125	126	126	128	129	131	132	87	87	88	88	88	88	88
11	**Measured height (cm)**	**135.6**	**138.3**	**142.8**	**147.8**	**152.8**	**157.3**	**160**	**135.6**	**138.3**	**142.8**	**147.8**	**152.8**	**157.3**	**160**
	50th	98	99	101	102	104	105	106	60	60	60	61	62	63	64
	90th	111	112	113	114	116	118	120	74	74	74	74	74	75	75
	95th	115	116	117	118	120	123	124	76	77	77	77	77	77	77
	95th + 12 mm Hg	127	128	129	130	132	135	136	88	89	89	89	89	89	89

12	**Measured height (cm)**	**142.8**	**145.5**	**149.9**	**154.8**	**159.6**	**163.8**	**166.4**	**142.8**	**145.5**	**149.9**	**154.8**	**159.6**	**163.8**	**166.4**
	50th	102	102	104	105	107	108	108	61	61	61	62	64	65	65
	90th	114	115	116	118	120	122	122	75	75	75	75	76	76	76
	95th	118	119	120	122	124	125	126	78	78	78	78	79	79	79
	95th + 12 mm Hg	130	131	132	134	136	137	138	90	90	90	90	91	91	91
13	**Measured height (cm)**	**148.1**	**150.6**	**154.7**	**159.2**	**163.7**	**167.8**	**170.2**	**148.1**	**150.6**	**154.7**	**159.2**	**163.7**	**167.8**	**170.2**
	50th	104	105	106	107	108	108	109	62	62	63	64	65	65	66
	90th	116	117	119	121	122	123	123	75	75	75	76	76	76	76
	95th	121	122	123	124	126	126	127	79	79	79	79	80	80	81
	95th + 12 mm Hg	133	134	135	136	138	138	139	91	91	91	91	92	92	93
14	**Measured height (cm)**	**150.6**	**153**	**156.9**	**161.3**	**165.7**	**169.7**	**172.1**	**150.6**	**153**	**156.9**	**161.3**	**165.7**	**169.7**	**172.1**
	50th	105	106	107	108	109	109	109	63	63	64	65	66	66	66
	90th	118	118	120	122	123	123	123	76	76	76	76	77	77	77
	95th	123	123	124	125	126	127	127	80	80	80	80	81	81	82
	95th + 12 mm Hg	135	135	136	137	138	139	139	92	92	92	92	93	93	94
15	**Measured height (cm)**	**151.7**	**154**	**157.9**	**162.3**	**166.7**	**170.6**	**173**	**151.7**	**154**	**157.9**	**162.3**	**166.7**	**170.6**	**173**
	50th	105	106	107	108	109	109	109	64	64	64	65	66	67	67
	90th	118	119	121	122	123	123	124	76	76	76	77	77	78	78
	95th	124	124	125	126	127	127	128	80	80	80	81	82	82	82
	95th + 12 mm Hg	136	136	137	138	139	139	140	92	92	92	93	94	94	94
16	**Measured height (cm)**	**152.1**	**154.5**	**158.4**	**162.8**	**167.1**	**171.1**	**173.4**	**152.1**	**154.5**	**158.4**	**162.8**	**167.1**	**171.1**	**173.4**
	50th	106	107	108	109	109	110	110	64	64	65	66	66	67	67
	90th	119	120	122	123	124	124	124	76	76	76	77	78	78	78
	95th	124	125	125	127	127	128	128	80	80	80	81	82	82	82
	95th + 12 mm Hg	136	137	137	139	139	140	140	92	92	92	93	94	94	94
17	**Measured height (cm)**	**152.4**	**154.7**	**158.7**	**163.0**	**167.4**	**171.3**	**173.7**	**152.4**	**154.7**	**158.7**	**163.0**	**167.4**	**171.3**	**173.7**
	50th	107	108	109	110	110	110	111	64	64	65	66	66	66	67
	90th	120	121	123	124	124	125	125	76	76	77	77	78	78	78
	95th	125	125	126	127	128	128	128	80	80	80	81	82	82	82
	95th + 12 mm Hg	137	137	138	139	140	140	140	92	92	92	93	94	94	94

Source: Bruce A. Kaiser. Hypertension in Children. MSD MANUALS. https://www.msdmanuals.com/en-in/professional/pediatrics/hypertension-in-children/hypertension-in-children.

Children under 13 years old have their blood pressure categorized according to their actual readings (refer to Table 7.3).

Table 7.3. *Classification of Blood Pressure (BP) in Children*

Classification	**Age 1 to < 13 Years, BP**	**Age ≥ 13 Years, BP**
Normal	< 90th percentile*	< 120/< 80
Elevated	≥ 90th percentile (or ≥ 120/80, whichever is lower) to < 95th percentile	120–129/< 80
Stage 1 hypertension	≥ 95th percentile to < 95th percentile + 12 mm Hg OR 130/80 to 139/89, whichever is lower	130/80 to 139/89
Stage 2 hypertension	≥ 95th percentile + 12 mm Hg OR ≥ 140/90, whichever is lower	≥ 140/90
** Percentiles refer to systolic BP.*		

Source: Bruce A. Kaiser. Hypertension in Children. MSD MANUALS. https://www.msdmanuals.com/en-in/professional/pediatrics/hypertension-in-children/hypertension-in-children.

7.1.2. Etiology of Hypertension in Children

Hypertension may be

- Primary (no known cause, a diagnosis of exclusion);
- Secondary (caused by another disorder, e.g., kidney disease).

Primary hypertension is the predominant etiology after the age of six, and this is especially true for adolescents. It is more common for secondary hypertension to occur before the age of six, especially in children under the age of three (Brenta et al., 2007).

7.1.2.1. Primary Hypertension

Primary hypertension is an exclusion diagnosis because, by definition, the cause is unknown. That is known to occur more frequently in kids who:

- Are overweight or obese (the most important risk factor for primary hypertension);
- Have a family history of hypertension;
- Are male;

- Are Mexican-American or non-Hispanic black (in the US);
- Have a sedentary lifestyle;
- Have unhealthy dietary habits (e.g., high salt and calorie intake);
- Had various intrauterine factors (e.g., resulting in low birth weight, prematurity, or small for gestational age);
- Have social risk factors (e.g., child abuse, family and/or interpersonal violence, food and/or housing insecurity—the number, duration, and severity of these factors have a cumulative effect).

7.1.2.2. Secondary Hypertension

Secondary hypertension has a known cause, and if the cause is treated, the hypertension might be reversible. Children's secondary hypertension is most frequently caused by the following includes:

- Renal parenchymal disease (e.g., glomerulonephritis, pyelonephritis, reflux nephropathy) or renal structural abnormalities (e.g., obstructive uropathy, polycystic kidney disease, dysplastic kidneys);
- Renovascular disease (e.g., renal artery stenosis, renal vein thrombosis);
- Cardiovascular disease (e.g., coarctation of the aorta, arteriovenous fistula);
- Endocrine disease (e.g., hyperthyroidism, mineralocorticoid excess, corticosteroid excess, catecholamine excess).

Other causes of secondary hypertension include

- Sleep-disordered breathing;
- Neurologic causes (e.g., increased intracranial pressure);
- Drugs (e.g., glucocorticoids, anabolic steroids, stimulants, oral contraceptives, nicotine, caffeine, certain illicit drugs);
- Psychologic stress or pain;
- Miscellaneous causes (e.g., neuroblastoma, tuberous sclerosis complex, Wilms tumor).

Orthopedic-related hypertension is associated with lower extremity traction or casting, typically following a femur fracture. It is believed that pressure on the femoral nerve is the cause of this kind of hypertension.

7.1.3. Pathophysiology of Hypertension in Children

The balance between cardiac output, which is influenced by myocardial contractility, heart rate, and vascular volume, and vascular resistance, which is influenced by vascular structure and function, determines blood pressure in adults as well. Sodium transport, the sympathetic nervous system, the renin-angiotensin-aldosterone system, and other mechanisms are involved. In contrast to older adults, cardiac output and volume status are more likely to be the primary causes of hypertension in children and younger adults. However, as people age, vascular structural changes such as thicker and more rigid vessel walls—which raise vascular resistance—become more significant (Castinetti et al., 2021).

7.1.3.1. Complications of Pediatric Hypertension

Complications of pediatric hypertension can be

- Acute
- Chronic

Children's acute hypertension complications are comparatively rare and typically arise from hypertensive emergencies involving end-organ damage or dysfunction. The central nervous system (encephalopathy, including seizures, lethargy, and/or coma), the heart (heart failure), the eyes (papilledema, retinal hemorrhages), and the kidneys (renal insufficiency) are among the organs affected.

In children, chronic consequences of hypertension are uncommon and usually don't show up until late adolescence or early adulthood. Children hardly ever experience the consequences of adult chronic hypertension, such as heart failure, ischemic stroke, hypertensive end-stage renal disease, and coronary artery disease. Findings in children, however, appear to indicate a potential early indicator of these complications. Echocardiography-diagnosed left ventricular (LV) hypertrophy is the most well-researched and reliable predictor. An LV mass greater than 51 g/m^2 is deemed excessive when adjusted for height, age, and sex. This research provides compelling evidence for starting antihypertensive medication in children.

Another finding by sensitive ultrasonographic techniques in certain hypertensive children is intima media thickness, which is thought to be a risk factor for cardiovascular disease in adulthood. Hypertension has been linked to a steeper decline in kidney function and an increase in urinary albumin excretion, a marker of kidney damage, in children with chronic kidney disease. Lastly, a small number of reports provide preliminary evidence that suggests hypertension contributes to deficits in neurocognitive function.

7.1.4. Symptoms and Signs of Hypertension in Children

With the rare exception of hypertensive emergencies, children's hypertension is typically asymptomatic. Other than the elevated blood pressure, the physical examination may be normal; however, there may be specific indications of hypertension and/or its causes, which should be specifically sought.

- **Eyes:** Proptosis (hyperthyroidism), hypertensive retinopathy (arteriolar spasm, hemorrhages, exudates, and rarely papilledema)
- **Head and Face:** Moon facies (corticosteroid excess, such as Cushing syndrome), tonsillar hypertrophy (sleep apnea)
- **Neck:** Thyroid enlargement and/or tenderness (hyperthyroidism)
- **Heart:** Murmur (coarctation of the aorta), friction rub (collagen vascular disease), apical heave (left ventricular hypertrophy)
- **Abdomen:** Mass (tumor, cystic kidney disease, hydronephrosis), bruit (renovascular disease)
- **Extremities:** Edema (kidney disease), joint swelling (collagen vascular disease), lower extremity traction or cast (orthopedic-related hypertension)
- **Genitalia:** Ambiguous/virilization (adrenal hyperplasia), advanced puberty (intracranial tumor)
- **Skin:** Pallor/flushing (catecholamine excess), acne/hirsutism/striae (Cushing syndrome, corticosteroid therapy), café-au-lait spots/neurofibromas (neurofibromatosis), ash-leaf spots/adenoma sebaceum (tuberous sclerosis complex), rash (systemic lupus erythematosus, immunoglobulin A–associated vasculitis)
- **Neurologic:** Muscle weakness

(hyperaldosteronism, Liddle syndrome)

- **General:** Obesity (primary/essential hypertension), growth retardation (chronic kidney disease)
- **Vital signs:** Tachycardia (hyperthyroidism, catecholamine excess), blood pressure difference between the extremities (coarctation of the aorta, mid-aortic syndromes (O'Neill JA et al., 1995))

7.1.5. Diagnosis of Hypertension in Children

- Sphygmomanometry (auscultation);
- Oscillometric devices;
- Sometimes testing for etiology.

Normative blood pressure (BP) values are used to define hypertension because BP values vary according to age, sex, and height. To rule out temporary causes of blood pressure elevation, such as recent consumption of caffeinated beverages or white coat hypertension (i.e., blood pressure elevation brought on by anxiety related to a doctor visit), hypertension should normally not be diagnosed until high blood pressure values are noted on three different visits (Feelders et al., 2019).

The right technique must be used when measuring blood pressure. Before taking a measurement, children should spend three to five minutes quietly sitting in a chair with their feet on the ground and their backs supported. Using the appropriate size cuff is crucial, so a variety of sizes—including a thigh cuff—should be offered. The inflatable bladder's length should be between 80% and 100% of the upper arm's circumference, and the cuff width should be at least 40% of that measurement. An excessively narrow cuff produces falsely high blood pressure readings, while an excessively wide cuff produces falsely low blood pressure readings. Generally speaking, every visit should involve taking at least two measurements, especially if the first one is high.

7.1.5.1. Blood Pressure Screening

Because oscillometric devices are user-friendly, less prone to observer bias, and more tolerant of younger children and infants, they are currently used for the majority of blood pressure screening procedures. Auscultation is a necessary method of confirmation for any measurement ≥ the 90th percentile since oscillometric device readings are typically higher than auscultation readings.

The 2017 guidelines for high blood pressure in children and adolescents published by the American Academy of Pediatrics (AAP) state that routine blood pressure monitoring should start at age three. Annual measurement is conducted if blood pressure falls below the 90th percentile or below the BP value that necessitates further assessment in accordance with AAP guidelines. Every visit should be the time for a child with risk factors for hypertension, such as kidney disease, heart disease, or a significant neonatal history, to be evaluated (Fleseriu et al., 2021).

To streamline the screening process, the AAP guidelines have included blood pressure values for every age group that, while not indicative of hypertension, suggest additional assessment (refer to Table 7.4). Screening professionals do not need to ascertain each child's precise BP percentile because these values represent the 90th percentile blood pressure for the smallest height cohort at each age range of 1 to 12 years. Repeat measurements and the determination of the true blood pressure percentile are usually the first steps in further evaluation, which is followed by a visit with a doctor (if the screening was conducted by other staff).

Table 7.4. *Screening Blood Pressure Values in Children That Need Additional Evaluation**

Age (years)	Boys		Girls	
	Systolic	**Diastolic**	**Systolic**	**Diastolic**
1	98	52	98	57
2	100	55	101	58
3	101	58	102	60
4 102 60			103	62
5	103	63	104	64
6	105	66	105	67
7	106	68	106	68
8	107	69	107	69
9	107	70	108	71
10	108	72	109	72
11	110	74	111	74
12	113	75	114	75
≥ 13	120	80	120	80

* Note, these values are not intended to diagnose or classify hypertension and should be used only for screening to identify children whose blood pressure requires a more thorough evaluation.

Source: Bruce A. Kaiser. Hypertension in Children. MSD MANUALS. https://www.msdmanuals.com/en-in/professional/pediatrics/hypertension-in-children/hypertension-in-children.

Further, 50% to 70% of children whose blood pressure falls between the 90th and 95th percentiles should have another auscultation examination within six months. If the blood pressure doesn't go down after six months, it is advisable to make lifestyle adjustments (diet, exercise, and weight loss if necessary) and measure the blood pressure in both the upper and lower extremities. If the patient's blood pressure doesn't go down over the course of the next six months, 24-hour ambulatory blood pressure monitoring may be performed or a specialist referral may be made. The yearly monitoring plan may be restarted, though, if blood pressure falls back below the 90th percentile during this period.

Children should be diagnosed with stage 1 hypertension if their measurements are consistently ≥ 95th percentile but < 95th percentile + 12 mm Hg. A measurement of ≥ 140/90, or ≥ 95th percentile + 12 mm Hg, whichever is lower, indicates stage 2 hypertension.

Within one to two weeks, children with stage 1 hypertension should have another examination. If blood pressure stays at stage 1, measurements of blood pressure in the upper and lower extremities, a urinalysis, and advice on lifestyle modifications should be given. Rechecking blood pressure in two to three months is recommended, and children who are still at stage 1 should be referred to a specialist for evaluation that includes determining the cause. Children who exhibit symptoms of stage 1 or stage 2 hypertension should be referred right away to a pediatrician or emergency department for potential hospitalization.

7.1.5.2. Evaluation of Cause

Any disorders that are suspected based on the history and physical examination should undergo specific testing (e.g., thyroid function tests if hyperthyroidism is suspected).

The majority of clinicians also perform an initial laboratory evaluation, which includes measuring serum blood urea nitrogen (BUN), creatinine, and electrolytes; performing a fasting lipid profile; performing a urinalysis; and, particularly in cases of childhood hypertension, abnormal urine samples in the past, or renal function issues, performing a renal ultrasonography. Nonetheless, a more focused strategy can be implemented according to risk factors, symptoms, and age (Funder, 2001).

An extensive evaluation for secondary hypertension is not necessary for children and adolescents younger than six years old with a positive family history of hypertension, asymptomatic stage 1 hypertension, obesity or overweight, and no suggestive history or physical examination findings. Initial testing for these kids can be as simple as a urine dipstick test performed in-office and the measurement of BUN, creatinine, electrolytes, and calcium. Children should be reevaluated in six months if these results are normal and there is no difference in the measurements of blood pressure in the upper and lower extremities. Dietary and lifestyle modifications (such as increased activity and weight loss if necessary) should also be initiated. After six months, additional testing should be carried out to look for additional hypertension-causing factors if the blood pressure is still elevated and the weight has either increased or stayed the same. Within a month or two, children who have three readings of asymptomatic stage 1 hypertension without a family history and who are not overweight should have this evaluation completed. Children and teenagers with symptomatic stage 1 or stage 2 hypertension should be evaluated right away.

Further evaluation includes the following tests:

- Fasting complete metabolic panel (including glucose, liver enzymes, and lipid panel), and glycosylated hemoglobin (HbA1c—for prediabetes);
- Echocardiography (for left ventricular hypertrophy);
- Urinary albumin:creatinine ratio and urinalysis;
- Renal ultrasonography.

In the event that test results are normal, diet and lifestyle modifications are maintained for an additional six months, and nutritionist consultation may be advised. However, medication therapy ought to be taken into consideration if there is proof of a coexisting condition, blood pressure is still high, and weight has not dropped.

All children ≤ 3 years old, children < 6 years old who are not overweight, and those with stage 1 hypertension with symptoms or stage 2 hypertension should have a more thorough initial evaluation, bearing in mind that the higher the blood pressure and the younger the child, the more likely it is that a secondary hypertension cause will be identified. Finally, this assessment should be completed before allowing children between the ages of 3 and 6 who are overweight and have a family history of hypertension to only undergo lifestyle modifications. These children should have the following tests:

- Comprehensive metabolic panel;
- Complete blood count;
- Urinalysis;
- Urinary albumin:creatinine ratio;
- Plasma renin activity and aldosterone levels;
- Thyroid function tests;
- Evaluation of catecholamine activity (e.g., by measuring plasma free metanephrines);
- Renal ultrasonography with Doppler flow;
- Echocardiography.

Since kidney disease accounts for the majority of the common causes of secondary hypertension in children, the other option for these kids would be an early referral to a pediatric nephrologist. In addition to other renal imaging tests, such as a technetium-99m-labeled dimercaptosuccinic acid (DMSA) renal scan (to assess for renal scarring) and/or digital subtraction angiography (to assess for renal vascular disease), a pediatric nephrologist would perform this assessment (Geller et al., 2000).

7.1.6. Treatment of Hypertension in Children

- Weight reduction;
- Dietary modification (salt and calorie reduction);
- Exercise;
- Sometimes drug treatment.

Depending on the stage of the condition, treatment for children's hypertension may involve medication, diet, exercise, and weight loss. To start a more effective and timelier course of treatment, children with stage 2 hypertension or stage 1 hypertension who also exhibit symptoms, evidence of end-organ damage, diabetes, or renal disease should be referred to a specialist.

A blood pressure of less than 90th percentile or, in the case of older children, less than 130/80 is the usual treatment objective; some centers have a lower threshold of less than 120/80. The target mean 24-hour blood pressure for kids with kidney disease is less than the 50th percentile.

All children with elevated blood pressure begin lifestyle modifications that can help lower blood pressure, such as exercise and dietary adjustments. The two most important factors in helping children lose weight are a balanced diet and regular exercise. Lower blood pressure has been linked to a diet like the DASH (Dietary Approaches to Stop Hypertension) diet, which is higher in fruits, vegetables, legumes, and low-fat dairy products and lower in salt. In addition, calorie restriction based on age, sex, and activity level should be part of dietary modifications. For children over 13, the recommended daily intake of salt is less than 2300 mg, while for younger children, it should be between 2 and 3 mEq/kg. Children between the ages of 6 and 17 ought to engage in moderate-to-intense physical exercise for 30 to 60 minutes every day, or three to five days a week, at the very least. Little ones ought to be physically active all day long.

When a trial of lifestyle modifications fails to control blood pressure, drug treatment is started sooner for some children and later for others (Gershengorn and Neumann, 2012).

7.1.6.1. Drug Treatment of Hypertension in Children

Immediate drug treatment is typically started (along with lifestyle changes) for children with

- Symptomatic hypertension at any stage or level;
- Stage 1 hypertension with any evidence of end-organ dysfunction or damage;
- Stage 2 hypertension even with an obvious, modifiable risk factor (e.g., obesity), which should be addressed while BP is being controlled;
- Any stage of hypertension if they have chronic kidney disease, diabetes, or cardiac disease.

Lifestyle modifications are started for children with high normal or borderline hypertension, or stage 1 hypertension without symptoms or end-organ dysfunction; if these do not adequately lower blood pressure within approximately six months, medication treatment will be required.

Typically, medication therapy should start with one medication at the lowest possible dosage and be increased every one to four weeks until blood pressure is under control, the medication is getting close to its maximum dosage, or side effects start to appear that interfere with the medication's use. A second medication can then be added and titrated similarly to the first medication if the BP target has not been reached. Oral medication classes that are used to treat hypertension include:

- Adrenergic modifiers (beta- and alpha-antagonist, alpha-2-agonist, beta-blocker);
- Angiotensin-converting enzyme (ACE) inhibitors;
- Angiotensin II receptor blockers (ARBs);
- Calcium channel blockers (CCBs);
- Thiazide diuretics;
- Vasodilators.

When treating persistent hypertension in children, the first line of treatment should usually involve the use of an ACE inhibitor or a calcium channel blocker (CCB). While ACE inhibitor use in children has been shown to yield greater data, ARBs are just as effective and do not induce coughing. Both drug classes appear to be equally effective when taken as a single daily dose. Patients with diabetes or chronic kidney disease should take ACE inhibitors because they may help protect the kidneys. Menstruating girls who are at risk of becoming pregnant should use CCBs because ACE inhibitors and ARBs have major side effects on the developing fetus. Additionally, CCBs have no discernible impact on blood chemistries. Although thiazide diuretics have been used as first treatments, they are rarely effective in adolescents due to their high salt intake (Hattangady et al., 2012).

If a single medication is used for initial therapy and the desired blood pressure is not reached, another medication should be added. Thiazide diuretics have shown to be effective second drugs if the first medication is an ACE inhibitor or ARB; however, a CCB could be added in its place. An ACE inhibitor or an ARB typically functions as a second medication if the first medication is a CCB; however, if there is a risk of pregnancy, these agents should be avoided and other medications, such as thiazide diuretics, can be tried in their place. Chlorthalidone is the best thiazide diuretic to use since it can be administered once daily. Vasodilators and alpha- and beta-blockers are third-line medications, which should only be used after consulting a specialist, unless there are exceptional circumstances.

7.1.7. Prevention

- Weight reduction;
- Exercise;
- Reducing salt intake;
- Reduction of cardiovascular risk factors.

Obesity in children is becoming a serious issue. Kids are consuming excessive amounts of time in front of screens. Children 8 to 10 years old spend an average of 6 hours a day, children 11 to 14 spend an average of 9 hours a day, and children 15 to 18 spend an average of 7½ hours a day, according to the Centers for Disease Control and Prevention (CDC). Only the time spent enjoying entertainment in front of a screen is included in these totals. They exclude the time spent on computers for homework at home or for educational purposes while in school. This amount of screen time is associated with overweight and obesity because it takes the place of exercise.

At least three to five days a week, children aged six to seventeen should engage in 30 to 60 minutes of moderate-to-intense physical activity. Little ones ought to be physically active all day long.

The CDC estimates that children in the US between the ages of 6 and 18 consume roughly 3,300 mg of sodium daily (Yang et al., 2012), and this is before the table is salted. The U.S. USDA and the U.S. 2020–2025 Dietary Guidelines for Americans from the Department of Health and Human Services advise children to consume less than 2,300 mg daily, and even less for those under the age of 13.

It is critical to check for smoking in children and, if required, assist in the implementation of a program to help them stop. Moreover, since alcohol, drugs, and caffeine (including energy drinks) can all contribute to hypertension, it is critical to screen for these substances.

7.2. PHEOCHROMOCYTOMA IN CHILDREN

The adrenal gland and its hormones are involved in the great majority of cases of endocrine hypertension. The medulla and cortex are the two endocrine tissues that make up the adrenal gland. Although it can affect extramedullary sites as well, the adrenal medulla is the primary site of involvement for phenochromocytoma.

7.2.1. Pathophysiology

Adrenal medullary hormones in their normal actions. Neuroendocrine (chromaffin) and glial (sustentacular) cells predominate in the medulla, with a small amount of vascular and connective tissue cells. The catecholamines dopamine, norepinephrine, and epinephrine are the main hormones produced by the adrenal medulla (Figure 7.1). In addition, the brain, sympathetic nerve endings, and chromaffin tissue outside the adrenal medulla are sites of catecholamine synthesis (Korzyńska et al., 2018).

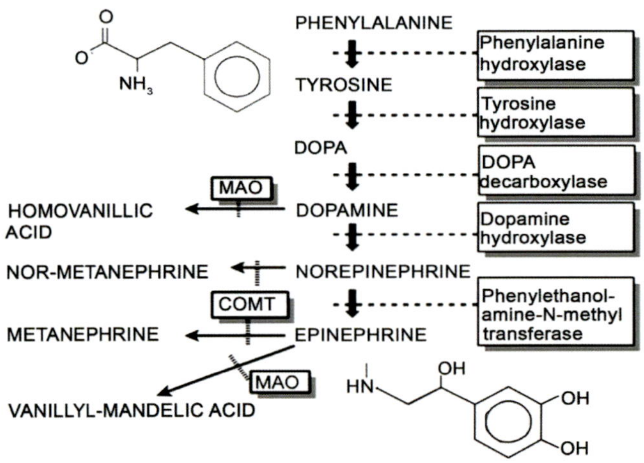

Figure 7.1. *Biosynthesis (right side of figure) and metabolism (left side of figure) of the catecholamines norepinephrine and epinephrine. COMT, catechol Omethyltransferase; MAOm monoamine oxidase. Planar structures of phenylalanine and epinephrine are shown at the top and bottom of the figure, respectively.*

Source: *Joseph T. Flynn, Julie R. Ingelfinger, and Tammy M. Brady. Pediatric Hypertension, Fifth Edition. Springer. https://doi.org/10.1007/978-3-031-06231-5.*

The adrenergic receptors that are coupled to G proteins mediate the effects of catecholamines. Only epinephrine increases cardiac output, while both norepinephrine and adrenaline raise mean arterial blood pressure. Norepinephrine raises systolic and diastolic blood pressure with only a minor decrease in pulse rate through raising peripheral vascular resistance. Epinephrine raises heart rate and lowers diastolic pressure through lowering peripheral vascular resistance. The effects of norepinephrine on blood sugar and metabolism are significantly milder than those of adrenaline.

Pheochromocytomas are tumors that secrete catecholamines and originate from chromaffin cells in the adrenal medulla; paragangliomas are the term for similar tumors that arise outside of the adrenal glands. Approximately 90% of cases have the adrenal medulla as their site of origin; however, tumors can arise anywhere along the abdominal sympathetic chain and are most likely to be found at the bifurcation or level of the inferior mesenteric artery, the organ of Zuckerkandl, which is close to the aorta. They can also show up in the cervical region, thoracic cavity, urine bladder or ureteral walls, and periadrenal area. 10% happen in children, who typically show symptoms between the ages of six and fourteen. The diameter of tumors ranges from 1 to 10 cm, and they are more common on the right side than the left. More than 20% of the children affected have bilateral adrenal tumors; 30% to 40% have tumors in both the extraadrenal and adrenal regions, and just the extraadrenal area (Lane et al., 2020).

Germline mutations are frequently linked to phenochromocytomas (Table 7.5). They can be linked to genetic syndromes like von Hippel-Lindau disease, to the MEN-2A and MEN-2B syndromes of multiple endocrine neoplasia (MEN), and, less frequently, to neurofibromatosis (type 1) or tuberous sclerosis. The classic features of von Hippel-Landau syndrome, which affects 1 in 36,000 people, include pheochromocytomas, renal clear cell carcinomas, and hemangioblastomas of the retina and central nervous system. However, the propensity of different kindreds to develop pheochromocytomas varies; in some kindreds, pheochromocytomas are the only tumors that develop. In patients with this syndrome, germline mutations in the VHL tumor-suppressor gene on chromosome 3p25–26 have been found. In families with MEN2A and MEN2B, mutations of the RET proto-oncogene on chromosome 10q11.2 have been discovered. Individuals who carry mutations at codon 634 of the RET gene are particularly at risk of developing pheochromocytoma. Patients with MEN2 are also at risk of developing parathyroid tumors and medullary thyroid carcinoma. Patients with neurofibromatosis type 1 have mutations in the NF1 gene on chromosome 17q11.2.

Table 7.5. *Genetic Causes of Endocrine Hypertension*

Syndrome	Gene	Mutation	Protein	Functional Consequence	Germline	Somatic (in Tumors)
Pheochromocytoma and Paraganglioma						
Von Hippel-Landau syndrome	VHL	Inactivating	VHL protein is an E3 ubiquitin ligase (which targets hypoxia-inducible factors for proteolysis)	Loss of tumor suppressor gene	+	+
Multiple endocrine neoplasia 2A/B	RET	Activating	RET protein is a receptor tyrosine kinase	Activated proto-oncogene	+	+

Neurofibromatosis	NF1	Inactivating	Neurofibromin-1 (GTPase activating protein; inhibits proliferative growth by blocking RAS-mediated signaling)	Loss of tumor suppressor gene	+	
Familial paragangliomas (PGL1)	SDHD	Inactivating	Succinate dehydrogenase subunit D (membrane-anchorage)	Disordered pseudohypoxia signaling pathway	+	+
PGL2	SDH5/ SDHAF2	Inactivating	Succinate dehydrogenase flavinylation factor (promotes assembly of enzyme complex)	Disordered pseudohypoxia signaling pathway	+	+
PGL3	SDHC	Inactivating	Succinate dehydrogenase subunit C (ubiquinone-binding)	Disordered pseudohypoxia signaling pathway	+	+
PGL4	SDHB	Inactivating	Succinate dehydrogenase subunit B (catalytic)	Disordered pseudohypoxia signaling pathway	+	+
Hypertensive Forms of Congenital Adrenal Hyperplasia						
11β-hydroxylase deficiency	CYP11B1	Inactivating	Steroid 11β-hydroxylase	Inability to synthesize cortisol leads to elevated levels of deoxycor-ticosterone	+	
17α-hydroxylase deficiency	CYP17A1	Inactivating	Steroid 17α-hydroxylase	Inability to synthesize cortisol leads to elevated levels of deoxycorti-costerone	+	
Apparent Mineralocorticoid Excess						
	HSD11B2	Inactivating	11β-hydro xysteroid dehydro genase 2	Cortisol activates the mineralcorticoid receptor	+	
Primary Aldosteronism						

Glucocorticoid-suppressible hyperaldosteronism	Chimeric CYP11B1/ CYP11B2	Activating	Aldosterone synthase	CYP11B2 is expressed at high levels and regulated by ACTH	+	
Familial hyperaldosteronism	CYP11B2	Activating	Aldosterone synthase	CYP11B2 is constitutively expressed at high levels	+	
Familial hyperaldosteronism	KCNJ5	Activating	Inwardly rectifying potassium channel	Increases Na^+ conductance, depolarizes cell, opens voltage sensitive calcium channel, which increases intracellular calcium and thus CYP11B2 expression	+	+
Familial hyperaldosteronism	CLCN2	Activating	Voltage sensitive calcium channel	Opens channel, increasing intracellular calcium and thus CYP11B2 expression	+	
Familial hyperaldosteronism	CACNA1H	Activating	Voltage sensitive calcium channel	Opens channel, increasing intracellular calcium and thus CYP11B2 expression	+	
Familial hyperaldosteronism	CACNA1D	Activating	Voltage sensitive calcium channel	Opens channel, increasing intracellular calcium and thus CYP11B2 expression	+	+
Aldosterone producing adenomas	ATP1A1	Inactivating	Na^+/K^+ ATPase	Reduces pump activity, lower depolarization threshold		+
Aldosterone producing adenomas	ATP2B3	Inactivating	Calcium ATPase	Intracellular calcium accumulation		+
Adrenal Cushing's Syndrome						

McCune-Albright syndrome	GNAS	Activating	Gαs stimulatory G-protein subunit	Activates adenylyl cyclase in all cells expressing the abnormal G-protein; constitutive activation of cAMPmediated signaling pathway		+
Carney complex (including primary pigmented nodular adrenocortical disease (PPNAD)	PRKAR1A	Inactivating	Regulatory subunit of protein kinase A	Constitutive activation of cAMPmediated signaling pathway	+	+
Primary bilateral macronodular adrenal hyperplasia (PBMAH)	PRKACA	Increased copy number	Catalytic subunit of protein kinase A	Constitutive activation of cAMPmediated signaling pathway	+	+
Cortisol-secreting adenomas	PRKACA	Activating	Catalytic subunit of protein kinase A	Constitutive activation of cAMPmediated signaling pathway		+
PPNAD	PDE8B, PDE11A	Inactivating	Phosphodiesterase	Increases intracellular levels of cAMP; constitutive activation of cAMP-mediated signaling pathway	+	
Multiple endocrine neoplasia type 1 (PBMAH)	MEN1	Inactivating	Menin	Loss of tumor suppressor gene	+	+
PBMAH	ARMC5	Inactivating	Armadillo repeat-containing protein 5	Loss of tumor suppressor gene	+	+
Generalized Glucocorticoid Resistance						
	NR3C1	Inactivating	Glucocorticoid receptor	Insensitivity to cortisol leads to elevated levels of deoxycorti-costerone	+	
Activating Mutation in the Mineralocorticoid Receptor						

Pregnancy-exacerbated hypertension	NR3C2	Activating	Mineralocorticoid receptor	Changes ligand specificity of receptor to recognize progesterone	+	

Source: Joseph T. Flynn, Julie R. Ingelfinger, and Tammy M. Brady. Pediatric Hypertension, Fifth Edition. Springer. https://doi.org/10.1007/978-3-031-06231-5.

In addition to paragangliomas, phenochocytomas can also occur in families, especially at sites in the head and neck. Usually, these families have mutations in the genes that encode the subunits of the mitochondrial enzyme succinate dehydrogenase (SDH), SDHC, and, very infrequently, SDHB. When SDHB mutations are present in a tumor, about half of them become malignant. The VHL and the different SDH gene products are involved in the pseudohypoxia signaling pathway, which is a common pathogenetic pathway defined as a decrease in the cytosolic oxidized to reduced forms of the nicotinamide adenine dinucleotide ratio (NAD(+)/NADH) (Redlich et al., 2021). The 3P association (3Pas) is the rare occurrence of pheochromocytomas and/or paragangliomas along with pituitary adenomas in people with germline mutations in SDH genes.

Pheochromocytomas and paraganglionomas can occur in conjunction with gastrointestinal stromal tumors (GISTs; this association is known as the Carney-Stratakis dyad), pulmonary chondromas (the Carney-Stratakis triad), and adrenocortical tumors in addition to associations with other tumors in MEN-2 patients. These correlations have a variety of genetic causes, but SDH gene mutations are frequently one of them.

7.2.2. Clinical Manifestations

It is possible that phenotypocytomas found through patient surveillance who are known carriers of tumor-suppressor gene mutations don't cause any symptoms. Some are diagnosed on abdominal CT or MRI tests done for other purposes, especially in adults (adrenal incidentaloma). If not, patients are identified as having hypertension, which is brought on by an overabundance of norepinephrine, adrenaline, and metanephrine secretion. Every patient experiences hypertension occasionally. Pheochromocytoma is characterized by paroxysmal hypertension; however, in children, the hypertension is more often sustained than paroxysmal, unlike in adults. When hypertensive paroxysms do occur, they typically start out rarely and increase in frequency over time until persistent hypertension eventually takes the lead. The patient may not have any symptoms in between episodes of hypertension. The patient reports headache, palpitations, dizziness, and abdominal pain during attacks; pallor, vomiting, and sweating also happen. Blood pressure can have a systolic range of 180–260 mmHg and a diastolic range of 120–210 mmHg (i.e., significantly higher than stage 2 hypertension); seizures and additional HEI symptoms could appear. Patients with severe hypertension may experience precordial pain, as well as pulmonary edema, hepatic and cardiac enlargement, and other complications. Exercise and over-the-counter drugs that contain stimulants like pseudoephedrine can make symptoms worse. Patients may have a strong appetite, but due to the hypermetabolic state, they may not grow or gain weight, and they may even experience severe cachexia. When polyuria and polydipsia are severe enough, they may indicate diabetes insipidus. Hemorrhages, exudate, arterial constriction, and papilledema can all be seen during an ophthalmoscopic examination (Mulatero et al., 2013).

7.2.3. Laboratory Findings

Urine is usually normal but may contain a few casts, protein, and occasionally glucose. Gross hematuria indicates that the bladder wall contains the tumor. Every now and then, polycythemia is seen. Pheochromocytomas release adrenaline and norepinephrine. While adrenal glands are the primary source of epinephrine, adrenergic nerve endings also contribute to the production of norepinephrine in plasma. Children with pheochromocytoma primarily excrete norepinephrine in their urine, as opposed to adults with the condition, who have elevated levels of both norepinephrine and epinephrine. The average urinary catecholamine excretion is higher than 300 μg/24 hours. Additionally, there is an increase in the urine excretion of metanephrine, specifically normetanephrine. As children grow older, their daily excretion of these compounds through the urine increases. The main metabolite of adrenaline and norepinephrine, vanillylmandelic acid (3-methoxy-4-hydroxymandelic acid), is excreted in the urine, but foods and fruits containing vanilla can cause falsely elevated levels of this compound, which is why it is no longer routinely measured (Nieman et al., 2015).

Plasma also shows elevated concentrations of free catecholamines and metanephrines. Measuring plasma free metanephrines and urinary fractionated metanephrines is the current consensus recommendation for diagnosis; however, some practitioners wait to collect urine for confirmation. It is important to advise the patient not to consume any caffeinated beverages or acetaminophen as these substances may cause problems for plasma normetanephrine immunoassays. An indwelling intravenous catheter should ideally be used to collect the blood sample to minimize the acute stress that comes with venipuncture.

Although extra-adrenal tumors can be challenging to identify, the majority of tumors in the adrenal gland region are easily localized using CT or MRI. Metaiodobenzylguanidine (MIBG), also known as ^{123}I or ^{131}I, is helpful in localizing small tumors because it is absorbed by chromaffin tissue throughout the body. When it comes to imaging tumors that are hard to locate, PET-CT using ^{18}F-fluorodeoxyglucose or ^{68}Ga-DOTA(0)-Tyr (3)-octreotate—a somatostatin receptor ligand—is more preferred due to its high sensitivity. Venous catheterization is now only infrequently required for tumor localization, requiring blood samples at various levels for catecholamine measurements.

7.2.4. Differential Diagnosis

There are several causes of hypertension in children that need to be taken into account, including coarctation of the aorta, renovascular or kidney disease, primary hypertension, and other types of endocrine hypertension. A pheochromocytoma's compression of a renal artery or ureter can result in an inoperable kidney. Porphyria or familial dysautonomia may be linked to paroxysmal hypertension. In the differential diagnosis, hyperthyroidism, diabetes mellitus, diabetes insipidus, and cerebral disorders must all be taken into account. In individuals with neurofibromatosis, hypertension may result from concomitant pheochromocytoma or renal vascular involvement.

Catecholamines are commonly produced by neuroblastomas, ganglioneuroblastomas, and ganglioneuromas; however, patients with pheochromocytoma typically have higher urinary levels of most catecholamines, while dopamine and homovanillic acid levels are typically higher in neuroblastomas. Neurogenic tumors that secrete substances frequently result in hypertension, flushing, pallor, rash, polyuria, and polydipsia. These tumors may be linked to chronic diarrhea, especially ganglioneuroma, which can occasionally be severe enough to indicate celiac disease (O'Neill et al., 1995).

7.2.5. Treatment

Surgery is required to remove phenochromocytomas, but cautious preoperative, intraoperative, and postoperative care are crucial. When these tumors are altered or removed, there is a noticeable rise in catecholamine secretion, which raises heart rate and blood pressure. Thus, α- and β-adrenergic blockade is necessary before surgery. Although phenoxybenzamine has been the most commonly used medication, selective α1-blockers like doxazosin and calcium channel blockers like amlodipine have also been used; however, the latter may not be covered by insurance. Since these tumors are frequently multiple in children, the best chance of finding them all is to perform a comprehensive transabdominal exploration of all the usual sites. A sharp drop in blood pressure during the procedure or within 48 hours afterward can be prevented by selecting the right anesthesia and increasing blood volume with the right fluids both before and during. Following surgery, blood pressure and volume status monitoring must be maintained. If genetic testing hasn't been done before, it should be done.

Due to the high frequency of bilateral and recurrent pheochromocytomas, some have proposed adrenal cortex sparing surgery as a means of lowering the risk of Addison disease. This method does, however, raise the possibility of tumor recurrence (Papakokkinou et al., 2021).

Even though these tumors frequently have malignant histology, the only reliable markers of malignancy are either local invasiveness that prevents total resection or the existence of metastatic disease, or both. Malignant adrenal pheochromocytomas make up about 10% of all cases, although they are uncommon in children. The mediastinum and the infradiaphragmatic para-aortic area, which includes the organ of Zuckerkandl, are extra-adrenal sites where malignant pheochromocytomas are more common. These sites are also frequently linked to mutations in the SDHB gene, which codes for a subunit of succinate dehydrogenase. Extended monitoring is recommended because functioning tumors at other sites may manifest years after the initial surgery, especially in patients with germline mutations in risk loci. Investigating the relatives of affected patients may identify other people with potentially asymptomatic, undetected tumors.

7.3. DISEASES OF THE ADRENAL CORTEX CAUSING HYPERTENSION

The adrenal cortex or adrenal medulla may be dysfunctional in cases of adrenal disorders leading to hypertension. These conditions primarily affect the adrenal cortex and result in low-renin hypertension. These disorders include congenital adrenal hyperplasia (CAH), which is caused by deficiencies in 11β-hydroxylase and 17α-hydroxylase; apparent mineralocorticoid excess; familial hyperaldosteronism type I; primary aldosteronism; Cushing's syndrome; and familial glucocorticoid resistance. Pheochromocytoma is the classic adrenal medulla disorder that causes hypertension, though catecholamine secretion may also play a role in obesity-related hypertension.

7.3.1. Physiology

Three concentric zones make up the adrenal cortex: the outermost zone is called the zona glomerulosa, followed by the zona fasciculata, which makes up about ¾ of the cortex, and the zona reticularis, which is located next to the adrenal medulla. The most powerful mineralocorticoid, aldosterone, is produced by the zona glomerulosa. Cortisol is produced by the zona fasciculata, and adrenal androgens are synthesized by the zona fasciculata and zona reticularis (Redlich et al., 2021).

7.3.1.1. Adrenal Steroidogenesis

The initial substrate for all steroid biosynthesis is cholesterol (Figure 7.2). Pregnenolone, which is produced when the side chain of cholesterol is broken down in mitochondria, diffuses out of the cells and into the endoplasmic reticulum. The zone of the adrenal cortex determines the reactions that follow.

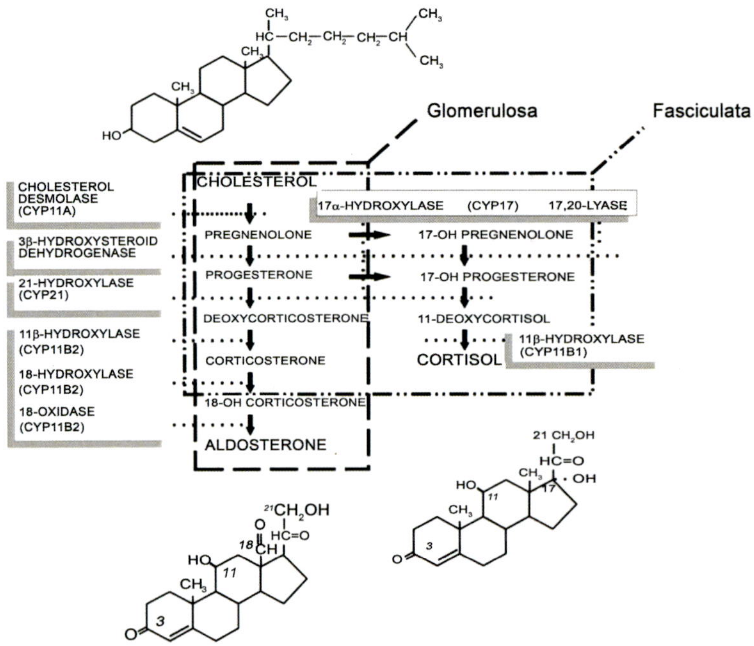

Figure 7.2. *Adrenal steroid biosynthesis. Reactions occurring in the zonae glomerulosa and fasciculata are enclosed by labeled dotted lines; several reactions take place in both zones. Additional reactions involved in androgen biosynthesis (the "backdoor pathway") are not shown. Many of the involved enzymes are cytochromes P450 (CYP). CYP11B2 mediates successive 11β-hydroxylase, 18-hydroxylase, and 18-oxidase reactions in the zona glomerulosa for the conversion of deoxycorticosterone to aldosterone. Planar structures of cholesterol, aldosterone, and cortisol are illustrated; relevant carbon positions on the latter two molecules are marked.*

Source: *Joseph T. Flynn, Julie R. Ingelfinger, and Tammy M. Brady. Pediatric Hypertension, Fifth Edition. Springer. https://doi.org/10.1007/978-3-031-06231-5.*

Pregnenolone is progressively converted to progesterone and 11-deoxycorticosterone in the zona glomerulosa. After entering mitochondria once more, deoxycorticosterone undergoes three successive oxidations: 11β-hydroxylation, 18-hydroxylation, and a further oxidation of the 18-methyl carbon to an aldehyde, all of which are carried out by aldosterone synthase (P450aldo, CYP11B2), a P450 enzyme (White, 2001).

17α-hydroxylase (P450c17, CYP17) in the endoplasmic reticulum of the zona fasciculata transforms pregnenolone into 17-hydroxypregenolone. Because the zona glomerulosa does not express this enzyme, it is unable to produce 17-hydroxylated steroids. Steroid 11β-hydroxylase (P450c11, CYP11B1) converts 17-hydroxypregnenolone to 17-hydroxyprogesterone, 11-deoxycortisol, and finally 17-hydroxypregnenolone. After entering mitochondria, this mixture is transformed into cortisol. Although it lacks 18-oxidase activity and has low 18-hydroxylase activity, this enzyme is closely related to aldosterone synthase (White, 2001). Therefore, the zona fasciculata is unable to synthesize aldosterone in normal conditions.

7.3.1.2. Regulation of Cortisol Secretion

Adrenocorticotropic hormone, also known as corticotropin, or ACTH, is primarily responsible for controlling the release of glucocorticoids. It is secreted by the anterior pituitary gland in pulses that change in amplitude throughout the day. ACTH and cortisol pulses are highest around wake-up time, lowest in the late afternoon and evening, and lowest one or two hours after sleep onset.

Through the action of a particular G proteincoupled receptor, also known as the melanocortin receptor-2 and encoded by the MCR2 gene, ACTH stimulates cyclic adenosine monophosphate (cAMP) production and adenylate cyclase. Cyclic AMP increases the expression of the steroidogenesis acute regulatory (StAR) protein, which has short-term (minutes to hours) effects on the transport of cholesterol into mitochondria. Long-term (hours to days) effects of ACTH stimulation include increased cholesterol uptake and expression of genes encoding the enzymes needed for cortisol synthesis control of the release of aldosterone. The renin-angiotensin-aldosterone system (RAAS) and potassium levels play a major role in regulating the rate of aldosterone synthesis, which is typically 100–1000 times slower than that of cortisol synthesis. ACTH only has a transient effect. The renal juxtaglomerular apparatus secretes renin in response to a decrease in intravascular volume. Angiotensinogen, also known as renin substrate, is an α2-globulin produced by the liver that is broken down by the proteolytic enzyme renin to produce the inactive decapeptide angiotensin I. Angiotensin I is quickly converted to the physiologically active octapeptide angiotensin II by the angiotensin-converting enzyme found in the lungs and other tissues. The heptapeptide angiotensin III is created by cleavage of angiotensin II. Both angiotensin II and III are strong aldosterone secretion stimulators, with angiotensin II having a greater vasopressor effect. A G protein-coupled receptor is occupied by angiotensin II and III, which activates phospholipase C. The latter protein increases intracellular calcium levels and activates calmodulin-activated (CaM) kinases and protein kinase C by hydrolyzing phosphatidylinositol bisphosphate to produce inositol triphosphate and diacylglycerol. Comparably, elevated extracellular potassium levels cause the cell membrane to depolarize and enhance the inflow of calcium via voltage-gated L-type calcium channels. The enzyme aldosterone synthase (CYP11B2), which is necessary for aldosterone synthesis, is transcriptionally activated when transcriptional regulatory factors are phosphorylated by CaM kinases (Hattangady et al., 2012).

7.3.1.3. Adrenal Steroid Hormone Actions

Formally known as NR3C2 and NR3C1, respectively, these receptors are unique to cortisol and estrogen and are part of a broader nuclear transcriptional factor superfamily. These receptors are bound by hormone molecules that permeate the cell membrane. This conformational change causes the receptors to bind DNA at particular hormone response elements. Additional transcriptional co-regulatory factors may be attracted to DNA by bound receptors.

The various genes that each hormone regulates in its various tissues dictate how each hormone is reacted to. Furthermore, distinct combinations of co-regulators exhibit expression in disparate tissues, thereby endowing each steroid hormone with an array of diverse physiological effects. Furthermore, steroids' affinity for their receptors can be altered by enzymes, which in turn can change how active the steroids are. For instance, cortisone, which is not a ligand for the glucocorticoid receptor, is converted to cortisol, an active glucocorticoid, by 11β-hydroxysteroid dehydrogenase type 1 (HSD11B1). This raises the local concentrations of glucocorticoids in many tissues, particularly the liver. On the other hand, cortisol is oxidized to cortisone by 11β-hydroxysteroid dehydrogenase type 2 (HSD11B2), especially in the kidney, which keeps high cortisol levels from occupying mineralocorticoid receptors.

7.3.1.4. Actions of Glucocorticoids

The hormones' ability to regulate glucose is referred to as glucocorticoids. But glucocorticoids, like cortisol, have a wide range of other effects as well. For example, they affect renal and circulatory function, which may help hypertension develop.

Glucocorticoids increase the left ventricular work index by exerting a positive inotropic effect on the heart (Santos and Spadari-Bratfisch, 2006). Furthermore, the effects of norepinephrine and adrenaline on the heart and blood vessels are permissive. When glucocorticoids are absent, hypotension and reduced cardiac output can occur; when glucocorticoids are overproduced, hypertension is often seen. Part of the reason for this could be the activation of the mineralocorticoid receptor, which happens when high amounts of glucocorticoids saturate renal 11β-hydroxysteroid dehydrogenase.

7.3.1.5. Actions of Mineralocorticoids

Aldosterone and, to a lesser extent, 11-deoxycorticosterone are the most significant mineralocorticoids; corticosterone and cortisol are typically not significant mineralocorticoids unless secreted in excess. By removing potassium and hydrogen ions and preserving sodium, mineralocorticoids keep the intravascular volume constant. These functions are carried out in the kidney, stomach, and sweat and salivary glands (Tomaschitz et al., 2010). In different tissues, testosterone may have different effects. The heart and vascular endothelium contain mineralocorticoid receptors, and aldosterone exacerbates myocardial fibrosis in heart failure (Funder, 2001).

The kidney's distal convoluted tubules and cortical collecting ducts are where mineralocorticoids primarily act, causing potassium secretion and sodium reabsorption. They function in a permissive manner in the medullary collecting duct, enabling vasopressin to raise the osmotic water flux (Tomaschitz et al., 2010). Thus, metabolic alkalosis, hypokalemia, and hypertension can occur in patients with excess mineralocorticoids.

It is unclear how aldosterone influences the excretion of sodium through what mechanisms. The mineralocorticoid receptor-mediated changes in gene expression are likely responsible for most of the effects of aldosterone. In fact, aldosterone causes an increase in the levels of subunits of the Na^+, K^+-ATPase, and the epithelial sodium channel (ENaC). Furthermore, aldosterone raises the expression of SGK (serum and glucocorticoid-regulated kinase), which increases the number of open sodium channels by indirectly reducing ENaC subunit turnover.

Aldosterone and cortisol have comparable in vitro affinities for the mineralocorticoid receptor; however, cortisol is a weak mineralocorticoid in vivo. The reason for this disparity is due to the conversion of cortisol to cortisone by 11βhydroxysteroid dehydrogenase type 2. While aldosterone is not a substrate for the enzyme, cortisone is not a ligand for the receptor. Cortisol can occupy renal mineralocorticoid receptors and cause sodium retention and hypertension when this enzyme is genetically deficient or is pharmacologically inhibited. The most common causes of pharmacologic inhibition are chewing tobacco with licorice flavor or overindulging in licorice (glycyrrhizic acid and glycyrrhetinic acid are the active compounds); this genetic condition is known as apparent mineralocorticoid excess syndrome.

The S810L (Ser-810 to Leu) mutation in the mineralocorticoid receptor itself causes a related syndrome by constitutively activating the receptor and changing its specificity to make progesterone a potent agonist. Pregnancy therefore makes the hypertension worse in women carrying this mutation (Geller et al., 2000).

7.4. HYPERTENSIVE FORMS OF CONGENITAL ADRENAL HYPERPLASIA

11β-hydroxylase deficiency (11OHD) and 17α-hydroxylase deficiency (17OHD) are two hypertensive forms of congenital adrenal hyperplasia (CAH). These are autosomal recessive traits that are inherited.

7.4.1. Congenital Adrenal Hyperplasia Due to 11 -hydroxylase Deficiency

Mutations in the CYP11B1 gene, which is found on chromosome 8q24, result in an 11β-hydroxylase deficiency. An estimate of its incidence ranges from 1/250,000 to 1/100,000. The 11-hydroxylation of 11-deoxycortisol to cortisol is mediated by CYP11B1. Corticotropin levels are high because 11-deoxycortisol is not converted to cortisol. As a result, precursors build up and are redirected into the biosynthesis of androgens, potentially resulting in females being born with unclear genitalia. Patients can nevertheless synthesize aldosterone normally because the disorder typically has no effect on the nearby CYP11B2 gene, which codes for aldosterone synthase. Elevated plasma levels of deoxycorticosterone and 11-deoxycortisol are observed. Plasma renin activity is suppressed due to the mineralocorticoid activity of deoxycorticosterone and its metabolites. As a result, although the capacity to produce aldosterone is unaltered, aldosterone levels are low. Although it can take years for hypertension to develop, about two thirds of patients eventually acquire it. Every now and then, hypokalemic alkalosis happens.

7.4.2. Congenital Adrenal Hyperplasia Due to 17-hydroxylase Deficiency

Mutations in the CYP17 gene are the cause of this extremely uncommon disorder. The encoded enzyme mediates two different reactions: the conversion of 17-hydroxypregnenolone to dehydroepiandrosterone via the 17,20-lyase reaction, and the 17-hydroxylation of pregnenolone and progesterone to 17-hydroxypregnenolone and 17-hydroxyprogesterone, respectively. The gonads and the adrenal cortex both express the enzyme. The majority of mutations impact both the lyase and hydroxylase functions.

Individuals lacking in 17-hydroxylase are unable to produce cortisol, but they are still able to produce corticosterone. As an active glucocorticoid, corticosterone prevents patients from developing adrenal insufficiency. The direct precursor of corticosterone, deoxycorticosterone, is overproduced. As in the case of an 11-hydroxylase deficiency, this can result in hypertension, hypokalemia, and suppression of renin and aldosterone secretion. Patients with 17-hydroxylase deficiency, however, are not able to synthesize sex hormones, unlike those with 11-hydroxylase deficiency. Males affected by this condition exhibit incomplete virilization, presenting as phenotypic females (with palpable gonads in the labia or inguinal region), or exhibit sexual ambiguity. Females affected by this condition typically exhibit delayed sexual development when they should be reaching puberty (Seidel et al., 2019).

7.4.3. Treatment

Doses of 10–15 mg/M2 /d of hydrocortisone are administered to patients. Glucocorticoids frequently treat hypertension, but if it has persisted for a long time, additional therapy may be needed. In such cases, calcium channel blockers might be helpful. Furthermore, males with this genetic condition may require supplementation of either androgen or estrogen, depending on the sex of rearing, whereas females with 17-hydroxylase deficiency require replacement of estrogen upon puberty.

7.5. PRIMARY ALDOSTERONISM IN CHILDREN

Disorders caused by excessive aldosterone secretion that are not related to the renin-angiotensin system are referred to as primary aldosteronism. Hypertension, hypokalemia, and renin-angiotensin system suppression are the hallmarks of these conditions.

7.5.1. Etiology

Aldosterone-secreting adenomas have been documented in children as young as 3 1½ years old; they are typically unilateral. They almost never develop into cancer. Children who are older are more likely to develop bilateral micronodular adrenocortical hyperplasia. It is also possible for unilateral adrenal hyperplasia to cause primary aldosteronism. Aldosterone secretion is quickly suppressed by glucocorticoid administration in glucocorticoid-remediable aldosteronism, also known as glucocorticoid-suppressible hyperaldosteronism, an autosomal dominant form of low-renin hypertension that suggests ACTH regulates aldosterone rather than the renin-angiotensin system. Uneven meiotic crossing over between the neighboring CYP11B1 (-11β-hydroxylase) and CYP11B2 (aldosterone synthase) genes is the cause of the disorder. This results in the production of a third chimeric gene that has coding sequences from CYP11B2 juxtaposed with regulatory sequences from CYP11B1. In the adrenal fasciculata, this leads to the aberrant expression of an aldosterone synthase-active CYP11B2-like enzyme.

7.5.2. Epidemiology

Although a comparatively high percentage (~3%) of glucocorticoid-remediable aldosteronism may exist in specific populations like Chile, excess aldosterone is thought to be a rare cause of hypertension in children. Between 5% and 10% of adult cases of hypertension may be related to primary aldosteronism. While bilateral hyperplasia and adenomas are typically sporadic, reports of affected kindreds have been made. Some kinds have reported having a genetic connection to chromosome 7p22, although the gene in question has not yet been found. However, mutations in multiple parts of the mechanism that potassium uses to control aldosterone secretion have been found (Korzyńska et al., 2018; Seidel and Co, 2019). Numerous kindreds have been found to carry germline mutations in the KCNJ5 gene on chromosome 11q24. These mutations change the selectivity of the potassium channel, increasing Na+ conductance and membrane depolarization, which boost the production of aldosterone and the growth of adrenal glomerulosa cells. Furthermore, a subset of sporadic aldosterone-producing adenomas has been found to have somatic mutations in the same gene (Mulatero et al., 2013). Additionally, germline mutations in the genes encoding voltage-gated chloride channel ClC-2 (CLCN2), aldosterone synthase (CYP11B2), and a subunit of the T-type voltage-gated calcium channel (CaV3.2) have been reported. Additionally, somatic mutations in ATP1A1 and ATP2B3, which encode sodium-potassium and calcium ATPases, as well as germline mutations in the CACNA1D gene, which codes for a voltage-sensitive calcium channel, have been reported. Most aldosterone-producing adenomas have mutations that activate the Wnt/β-catenin signaling pathway, either in the APC gene, which controls this pathway or in β-catenin (CTNNB1) itself.

7.5.3. Clinical Manifestations

Certain children who are impacted do not exhibit any symptoms; the diagnosis was made subsequent to the unintentional finding of mild hypertension. Some suffer from severe hypertension (240/150 mm Hg), which is accompanied by headaches, lightheadedness, and blurred vision. If there is persistent hypokalemia, it can cause polyuria, nocturia, enuresis, and polydipsia. Children with severe hypokalemia experience tetany, intermittent paralysis, growth failure, fatigue, and muscle weakness and discomfort.

7.5.4. Laboratory Findings

Hypokalemia is a common condition. Serum pH, sodium, carbon dioxide, and chloride concentrations may be higher, while magnesium and chloride levels may be lower. Serum calcium levels are normal even in children who show signs of tetany. Potassium excretion in the urine is elevated, and the urine is neutral or alkaline. Aldosterone plasma levels can range from normal to high. Urine samples taken over a 24-hour period consistently have higher levels of testosterone. Renin plasma levels are continuously low. This is a reasonably priced screening test for primary aldosteronism because the ratio of plasma aldosterone concentration to renin activity is consistently high.

There is debate regarding the best diagnostic test for primary aldosteronism. It is challenging to establish reliable reference ranges for renin and aldosterone because these levels can change depending on the time of day, posture, and sodium intake. Establishing a regular sampling schedule is preferable, such as midmorning after the patient has sat for fifteen minutes. Antihypertensive medications and other drugs that may impact aldosterone or renin secretion, such as diuretics, β-blockers, angiotensin-converting enzyme inhibitors, angiotensin receptor blockers, clonidine, and nonsteroidal anti-inflammatory agents, should be avoided for a few weeks before testing. It might be necessary to switch patients taking these medications to α-adrenergic blockers or calcium channel blockers, which have less of an impact on the biochemical measurements. Saline solution or fludrocortisone administration does not cause a decrease in aldosterone, and fluid and salt restriction has no effect on renin. 18-oxocortisol and 18-hydroxycortisol levels in the urine and plasma may rise, but not to the same degree as in glucocorticoid-suppressible hyperaldosteronism.

7.5.5. Differential Diagnosis

It is important to distinguish between primary aldosteronism and glucocorticoid-remediable aldosteronism, also known as glucocorticoid-suppressible hyperaldosteronism, which is treated with glucocorticoids only. Suspicion for the latter disorder should be raised by an autosomal dominant pattern of inheritance. Specific genetic testing or dexamethasone suppression tests are used to diagnose glucocorticoid-remediable aldosteronism. More generally, the tests previously mentioned should be used to differentiate primary aldosteronism from other types of hypertension. When evaluating patients with primary aldosteronism, computed tomography (CT) should be used. It is unable to accurately differentiate bilateral hyperplasia from the usually small aldosterone-producing adenomas, but it can rule out the presence of large tumors that would otherwise raise the possibility of adrenocortical carcinomas. Adrenal venous sampling is an invasive procedure that may not be available in all centers, but it is a reliable way to identify whether excess aldosterone secretion is coming from one gland or both. While it has been suggested as a non-invasive substitute, positron emission tomography with 11C-etomidate is currently lacking in specificity (Vassiliadi et al., 2021).

7.5.6. Treatment

To treat glucosecorticoid-remediable aldosteronism, administer 20 µg/kg/d of dexamethasone. Surgical excision is the method used to treat an aldosterone-producing adenoma. Laparotomy and adrenalectomy are the main methods used for this; successful enucleation of aldosterone-producing adenomas has also been documented. The mineralocorticoid antagonists spironolactone (1-3 mg/kg/day up to 100 mg/day) or eplerenone (25–100 mg/day in two divided doses) are used to treat hyperaldosteronism resulting from bilateral adrenal hyperplasia.

These treatments frequently normalize serum potassium and blood pressure levels. Spironolactone has been used more often, but its antiandrogenic qualities may make it inappropriate for males in their pubertal years. Although there is limited specific experience with primary aldosteronism in the pediatric age group, eplerenone is a more selective anti-mineralocorticoid that is safe for use in children. An alternative would be to use an epithelial sodium channel blocker, like amiloride, and add additional antihypertensive medications as needed

7.6. CUSHING SYNDROME IN CHILDREN

Unusually elevated blood levels of cortisol or other glucocorticoids cause Cushing syndrome. This may be the consequence of endogenous cortisol secretion, either from an adrenal tumor or from the pituitary's hypersecretion of corticotropin, also known as adrenocorticotropic hormone [ACTH] (Cushing disease) or a tumor.

Prolonged exogenous administration of glucocorticoids, particularly at high doses used to treat lymphoproliferative disorders, is the most common cause of Cushing syndrome. The most common cause of endogenous Cushing syndrome in infants and early children is a functional adrenocortical tumor. Along with symptoms of hypersecretion of other steroids, including androgens, estrogens, and aldosterone, patients with these tumors frequently show signs of hypercortisolism.

The most common cause of endogenous Cushing syndrome in children older than 7 years old is Cushing disease, which results in bilateral adrenal hyperplasia due to excessive ACTH secreted by a pituitary adenoma, despite the condition being extremely rare in infants. These adenomas are known as microadenomas because they are frequently too small to be identified by imaging methods. They are primarily composed of chromophobe cells and often exhibit positive immunostaining for proopiomelanocortin, the precursor to ACTH. A tiny percentage of these tumors occur in families with familial isolated pituitary adenoma syndrome, but the great majority are sporadic in nature. About 2% of pituitary adenomas are thought to be caused by this syndrome, which is brought on by mutations in the aryl hydrocarbon receptorinteracting protein (AIP) gene. These tumors typically secrete prolactin or growth hormone, and they very rarely secrete ACTH. In a similar vein, pituitary tumors are usually prolactinomas in patients with multiple endocrine neoplasia type 1 (MEN1), who by definition have mutations in the MEN1 (menin) gene. There have been additional gene implications.

Ectopic production of ACTH can also cause ACTH-dependent Cushing syndrome, though this is less common in children. In children, ectopic ACTH secretion has been linked to thymic carcinoid, Wilms tumor, neuroblastoma or ganglioneuroblastoma, hemangiopericytoma, and pancreatic islet cell carcinoma. In contrast to other forms of Cushing syndrome, hypertension is more common in ectopic ACTH syndrome because extremely high cortisol levels have the potential to overpower kidney 11β-hydroxysteroid dehydrogenase type 2, which enhances the mineralocorticoid (salt-retaining) effect.

Instead of a single adenomas or carcinoma, several autonomously hyperfunctioning nodules of adrenocortical tissue develop. These nodules are linked to several syndromes. They are frequently brought on by gene mutations in the cAMP-mediated signaling pathway, which is normally responsible for the regulation of cortisol secretion by ACTH. One unique variation of ACTH-independent Cushing syndrome is primary pigmented nodular adrenocortical disease (PPNAD). It can happen as a single incident or, more frequently, as a disorder that runs in the family and has additional symptoms. The small adrenal glands are characterized by numerous, tiny (less than 4 mm in diameter), pigmented (black) nodules that contain big cells with lipofuscin and cytoplasm; between the nodules, there is cortical atrophy. This adrenal disorder is a part of the Carney complex, an autosomal dominant disorder that also includes pigmented melanotic schwannomas, pituitary, thyroid, and testicular tumors, cardiac and cutaneous myxomas, and centrofacial lentigines and blue nevi.

Although there are occasional cases, the Carney complex is inherited in an autosomal dominant manner. The type 1α regulatory subunit of protein kinase A (PRKAR1A) gene on chromosome 17q22–24 and, less frequently, chromosome 2p16 have been identified as the genetic loci for the Carney complex. PPNAD is typically developed later in life in adults for patients with Carney complex and PRKAR1A mutations, while most sporadic cases and those with the disorder mapping to chromosome 2 experience PPNAD less frequently. On the other hand, PRKAR1A mutations are uncommon in children who present with PPNAD as an isolated finding, or they go on to show other Carney complex symptoms. Mutations affecting the PDE8B or PDE11A genes, which encode distinct phosphodiesterase isozymes, have been found in certain patients with isolated PPNAD. On the other hand, in cortisol-secreting adenomas, activating somatic mutations have been reported in the PRKACA catalytic subunit of protein kinase A (White, 2001).

In rare cases of McCune-Albright syndrome, there is an ACTH-independent Cushing syndrome characterized by nodular hyperplasia and adenoma formation. The syndrome typically manifests as early childhood or infancy symptoms. A somatic mutation of the GNAS gene, which codes for the G protein, $G_s\alpha$, which the ACTH receptor (MCR2) normally signals through, causes McCune-Albright syndrome. Cyclic adenosine monophosphate levels rise as a result of constitutive activation of adenylate cyclase and inhibition of guanosine triphosphatase activity. Adrenal tissue containing the mutation stimulates cortisol and cell division without the help of ACTH. Additional tissues where activating mutations may arise include the gonads, thyroid, pituitary, and bone (causing fibrous dysplasia). Clinical signs and symptoms vary depending on the tissues impacted.

The identified genes responsible for nodular adrenocortical hyperplasia primarily result in overactivity of the ACTH signaling pathway. This can be caused by either constitutively activating $G_s\alpha$ (McCune-Albright syndrome), reducing the breakdown of cyclic adenosine monophosphate and thus increasing its intracellular levels (mutations of PDE8B or PDE11A), disrupting the regulation of protein kinase A, the enzyme that is dependent on cyclic adenosine monophosphate, (PRKAR1A mutations), or by microduplications involving PRKACA. In addition, a tumor suppressor gene called Armadillo-containing repeat protein 5 (ARMC5) is mutated in about 40% of cases of primary bilateral macronodular adrenocortical hyperplasia. Lastly, MEN-1 syndrome, an autosomal dominant disorder characterized by homozygous inactivation of the menin (MEN1) tumor-suppressor gene on chromosome 11q13, may result in adrenocortical lesions such as diffuse hyperplasia, nodular hyperplasia, adenoma, and infrequently carcinoma.

7.6.1. Clinical Manifestations

Infants younger than a year old have been shown to exhibit signs of Cushing syndrome. Compared to older children, the disorder seems to be more severe and the clinical findings more pronounced in infants. The face has a round shape, prominent cheekbones, and a flushed look, or moon face. Obesity in general is prevalent in younger children. Adrenal tumor-related aberrant masculinization is common in children; consequently, hirsutism on the face and trunk, pubic hair, acne, deepening of the voice, and clitoris enlargement in girls are possible symptoms. Affected growth results in length falling below the third percentile unless significant virilization leads to normal or even faster growth. Heart failure can sometimes result from hypertension, which is a common condition. Sepsis can also be brought on by an increased vulnerability to infection.

Along with obesity, short stature is a common presenting feature in older children. The only early signs might be a slow or complete stop to growth and a gradual onset of obesity. Compared to the extremities, older children's facial and trunk obesity is typically more severe. But obesity of the upper back and neck (also known as "buffalo hump") is a general finding that shouldn't be given undue weight. It is typical to see purplish striae on the thighs, abdomen, and hips. Girls who have not reached menarche may experience amenorrhea or pubertal development may be delayed. There may be a lot of weakness, headaches, and emotional instability. Typically, there is hypertension and hyperglycemia; hyperglycemia can lead to frank diabetes. Commonly occurring osteoporosis can result in pathologic fractures.

7.6.2. Laboratory Findings

The blood levels of cortisol typically peak at 8 AM and fall to less than 50% of peak levels by midnight, with the exception of infants and young children, who may not always exhibit a consistent diurnal rhythm. Cushing syndrome patients lack this circadian rhythm, and the diagnosis is strongly suggested by midnight cortisol levels >4.4 µg/dL. Diurnal blood samples are challenging to obtain for an outpatient assessment; however, saliva samples can be collected at home at the appropriate times of the day and used to measure cortisol. Cushing syndrome is suspected when salivary cortisol levels are elevated at night.

Increased excretion of free cortisol in the urine. The most accurate way to measure this is with a 24-hour urine sample. The result is given as the ratio of cortisol excreted in micrograms to creatinine per gram. The completeness of the urine collection and body size have no bearing on this ratio (Nieman et al., 2015).

A single-dose dexamethasone suppression test is frequently beneficial; in normal individuals, but not in patients with Cushing syndrome, a dose of 25–30 μg/kg (maximum: 2 mg) given at 11 PM results in a plasma cortisol level of less than 5 μg/dL at 8 AM the following morning. To make sure the dosage is appropriate, it is wise to measure the dexamethasone level in the same blood sample.

Although a glucose tolerance test is not useful for diagnosis, it is frequently abnormal. Serum electrolyte levels are typically normal, although potassium levels may be low, particularly in patients with ectopically secreting tumors of ACTH.

Identifying whether Cushing syndrome is due to an adrenal tumor that secretes cortisol, an ectopic ACTH-secreting tumor, or a pituitary adenoma is necessary after the diagnosis has been made. ACTH concentrations may be normal in patients with ACTH-secreting pituitary adenomas, but they are typically suppressed in patients with cortisol-secreting tumors and extremely high in patients with ectopic ACTH-secreting tumors. Patients with ACTH-dependent Cushing syndrome exhibit an increased ACTH and cortisol response following an intravenous bolus of corticotropin-releasing hormone, while patients with adrenal tumors do not exhibit an increase in ACTH or cortisol. The two-step dexamethasone suppression test involves giving dexamethasone in divided doses of 30 and 120 μg/kg/24 h on separate days. The larger dose, but not the smaller dose, suppresses serum cortisol levels in children with pituitary Cushing syndrome. When using dexamethasone, patients with ACTH-independent Cushing syndrome typically do not exhibit suppressed cortisol levels. Almost all adrenal tumors larger than 1.5 cm in diameter can be detected by CT. While many are too small to be seen on MRI, pituitary adenomas that secrete ACTH can be detected; the sensitivity of detection is increased when gadolinium contrast is added. When a pituitary adenoma cannot be seen, bilateral inferior petrosal blood sampling may be necessary to measure ACTH concentrations before and after corticotropin-releasing hormone administration. However, this procedure is not commonly available in many centers, and it may also have lower specificity in pediatric patients (Vassiliadi et al., 2021).

7.6.3. Differential Diagnosis

When striae and hypertension are present in children who are obese, Cushing syndrome is often suspected. Children with Cushing syndrome are short or have a slowing growth rate; children with simple obesity are typically tall, while cortisol levels are typically normal and cortisol secretion is normally suppressed by oral administration. While salivary cortisol levels at night are normal and oral administration of low doses of dexamethasone suppresses cortisol secretion, urinary excretion of cortisol is frequently elevated in simple obesity.

Generalized glucocorticoid resistance patients have elevated cortisol and ACTH levels without clinical signs of Cushing syndrome. Patients may not show any symptoms at all or develop hypertension, hypokalemia, and precocious pseudopuberty; these side effects are brought on by increased secretion of mineralocorticoids and adrenal androgens in response to elevated levels of ACTH. There are known mutations in the glucocorticoid receptor.

7.6.4. Treatment

The preferred course of treatment for pituitary Cushing disease in children is transsphenoidal pituitary microsurgery (Nieman et al., 2015). 60% to 80% of cases are successful overall when followed up for less than ten years. Most of the time, low postoperative serum or urine cortisol concentrations indicate long-term remission. Pituitary radiation therapy and reoperation are used to treat relapses.

Cyproheptadine is a centrally acting serotonin antagonist that inhibits the release of ACTH and has been used to treat adult Cushing disease; however, remissions are typically not maintained when treatment is stopped. Children are seldom treated with this agent. Preoperatively, inhibitors of adrenal steroidogenesis (etomidate, aminoglutethimide, ketoconazole, and metyrapone) have been used to lower perioperative morbidity and mortality and restore normal circulating cortisol levels (Castinetti et al., 2021). A few cases have involved the use of glucocorticoid receptor antagonist mifepristone.

Adults with persistent disease following surgery or those for whom surgery is contraindicated may use the somatostatin analog pasireotide, which has been approved (Feelders et al., 2019).

The adrenal glands may need to be removed if a pituitary adenoma is not responsive to treatment or if an ectopic metastatic tumor secretes ACTH. This is frequently a laparoscopic procedure. Nelson syndrome is a condition that occurs in approximately 25% of adults who have undergone adrenalectomy for Cushing syndrome. It is characterized by marked hyperpigmentation and increased ACTH secretion by an unresected pituitary adenoma following adrenalectomy (Papakokkinou et al., 2021).

An alternative to adrenalectomy may be one of several medications that block adrenocortical function. Together with the previously listed agents, the FDA has approved mitotane, which is toxic to adrenocortical cells, and osilodrostat, which inhibits aldosterone synthase [CYP11B2] and 11-hydroxylase [CYP11B1]. As of 2021, levoketoconazole, a stereoisomer of ketoconazole, is in an advanced stage of development and inhibits several steroidogenic enzymes (Fleseriu et al., 2021).

Sufficient preoperative and postoperative corticosteroid replacement therapy is necessary for the management of patients undergoing adrenalectomy. Cortisol replacement (10 mg/M^2/24 h in three divided doses after the immediate postoperative period) is necessary until the hypothalamic-pituitary-adrenal axis recovers, which may take 12 months or longer. Tumors that produce corticosteroids typically cause atrophy of the normal adrenal tissue. Particularly in infants with Cushing syndrome, postoperative complications can include sepsis, pancreatitis, thrombosis, inadequate wound healing, and abrupt collapse. While there is significant growth for catching up, pubertal development, and increased bone density, adult height is frequently compromised and bone density stays abnormal.

7.7. GENERALIZED GLUCOCORTICOID RESISTANCE

Chrousos syndrome, another name for generalized glucocorticoid resistance, is an uncommon genetic disorder that results in partial insensitivity to glucocorticoids in target tissues. It is typified by a wide range of clinical manifestations and can be inherited or incidental.

7.7.1. Pathophysiology

Target-tissue insensitivity to glucocorticoids is present in patients with generalized glucocorticoid resistance. Although there are occasional cases, the condition is typically inherited in an autosomal dominant manner. The HPA axis is activated when the hypothalamus and pituitary are unable to produce the normal negative feedback of cortisol, which leads to an increase in ACTH and cortisol concentrations. The NR3C1 gene encodes the glucocorticoid receptor, and mutations in this receptor can interfere with transcriptional activation, ligand binding, DNA binding, or any combination of these, thereby impairing the receptor's ability to function and causing generalized glucocorticoid resistance. The majority of mutations are heterozygous; glucocorticoid receptors typically bind DNA as dimers; in the case of a heterozygous mutation, 3 out of every 4 dimers will contain at least 1 abnormal receptor molecule.

7.7.2. Clinical Manifestations

Adrenal hyperplasia, or increased production of adrenal steroids with mineralocorticoid activity (e.g., cortisol, deoxycorticosterone, and corticosterone) and androgens and precursors (e.g., androstenedione, DHEA, and DHEA sulfate) is brought on by excess ACTH secretion. Because of the insensitivity to glucocorticoids, high cortisol concentrations do not cause Cushing syndrome; on the other hand, most indications of adrenal insufficiency are absent, with the exception of recurrent chronic fatigue and sporadic anxiety (one extremely rare patient with a homozygous null mutation was reported to have neonatal hypoglycemia). Conversely, the androgen and mineralocorticoid receptors typically bind to their ligands with sensitivity. Symptoms of excess mineralocorticoids include hypokalemic alkalosis and hypertension. Adrenal androgen excess may result in oligospermia in males, acne, hirsutism and infertility in both sexes, irregular menstrual cycles, ambiguous genitalia in females, and gonadotropin-independent precocious puberty in children of either gender. Periodically, there are pituitary adenomas that secrete ACTH and testicular adrenal rest tumors.

7.7.3. Laboratory Findings

Elevated serum cortisol concentrations and increased 24-hour urinary free cortisol excretion in the absence of Cushing syndrome suggest the diagnosis of generalized glucocorticoid resistance. Other adrenal steroids also have higher levels. Plasma levels of ACTH can range from low to high. The HPA axis is resistant to dexamethasone suppression, and the circadian rhythm of ACTH and cortisol secretion is maintained, albeit at higher than normal concentrations. NR3C1 gene sequencing can validate the diagnosis.

7.7.4. Differential Diagnosis

It is important to distinguish between relatively mild cases of Cushing syndrome (whether due to an adrenal tumor or pituitary adenoma) and generalized glucocorticoid resistance. The latter is more likely to be linked to poor linear growth or excessive weight gain. Adrenocortical tumors can secrete androgens and mineralocorticoids like deoxycorticosterone, but they also frequently suppress ACTH levels. The tumor is typically visible on CT or MRI scans. When 11β-hydroxylase deficiency causes congenital adrenal hyperplasia, the condition can manifest as hypertension and androgen excess; however, cortisol levels are low and cortisol precursors (17-hydroxyprogesterone, 11-deoxycortisol) are elevated. Patients who are obese may also have hyperandrogenism and hypertension, but dexamethasone should easily suppress cortisol secretion (Nieman et al., 2015).

7.7.5. Treatment

Treatment aims to reduce excessive ACTH secretion, which in turn reduces the production of more adrenal steroids that have androgenic and mineralocorticoid properties. For this, high doses of a pure glucocorticoid agonist, like dexamethasone (usually ~20–40 μg/kg/day), must be administered with caution to titrate and suppress endogenous corticosteroid secretion without producing symptoms of glucocorticoid excess, like excessive weight gain or suppression of linear growth.

7.8. HYPERTHYROIDISM IN CHILDREN

When the thyroid gland produces too much thyroid hormone, the condition known as hyperthyroidism results. Thyroid hyperactivity is another name for this illness. Increased metabolism is a result of hyperthyroidism. It may result in a variety of symptoms, including rapid or irregular heartbeat, hand tremors, and weight loss.

7.8.1. Pathophysiology

7.8.1.1. Synthesis, Regulation, and Actions of Thyroid Hormones

Follic cells are where thyroid hormones are made. Thyroid peroxidase iodinates the adjacent tyrosine residues on thyroglobulin, which contains approximately 120 tyrosines. Subsequently, the adjacent phenolic rings undergo conjugation, releasing the hormones through proteolysis. There are two active hormones: triiodothyronine (T3) and thyroxine (T4). Triiodothyronine is about four times more active than thyroxine but has a much shorter half-life. Both are created from scratch, and type 1 and especially type 2 deiodinases change T4 into T3.

Thyrotropin-releasing hormone (TRH) and thyroid-stimulating hormone (TSH) control synthesis at the hypothalamic and pituitary levels, respectively. As a result, TSH levels are suppressed in patients with hyperthyroidism and elevated in those with primary hypothyroidism. TSH stimulates the synthesis of thyroid hormone by signaling through a G-protein coupled receptor on the surface of follicular cells (Gershengorn and Neumann, 2012).

Members of the nuclear hormone receptor superfamily make up the thyroid hormone receptors through which thyroid hormones operate. The two different genes THRA and THRB encode receptors that are expressed in different tissues. The retinoid X receptor (RXR) can bind DNA in monomers, homodimers, or heterodimers. Thyroid hormones raise rates of cellular metabolism and have significant permissive effects on somatic growth, skeletal maturation, and neural development (Brenta et al., 2007). The fact that they control catecholamine sensitivity in the neurological and cardiovascular systems is crucial in this context. Therefore, the signs and symptoms of hyperthyroidism (also known as thyrotoxicosis) are strikingly similar to those of excess catecholamines, as observed in pheochromocytoma.

7.8.1.2. Thyrotoxicosis

Thyrotoxicosis is caused by two autoimmune diseases. Antibodies to the thyroid stimulating hormone (TSH) receptor interact with the receptor to activate it in a manner similar to that which would result from occupation by its physiological ligand (TSH), which is the cause of Graves' disease. These are known as TSH receptor antibodies (TRAb) or thyroid-stimulating antibodies (TSI). Although hypothyroidism is more frequently linked to chronic lymphocytic (Hashimoto's) thyroiditis, it can also manifest as a thyrotoxic phase, in which thyroid cells undergo cytotoxic lymphocyte-induced autoimmune destruction, causing the thyroid cells to release triiodothyronine (T3) and thyroxine (T4). Thyrotoxicosis can be brought on by hyperfunctioning, or "hot," thyroid nodules, which are uncommon in children. Finally, amiodarone, an anti-arrhythmia medication that contains iodine, may result in hypothyroidism or, less frequently (2%) hyperthyroidism (Barrett et al., 2019).

7.8.2. Clinical Manifestations

Most patients have experienced weight loss. They have a wide pulse pressure, tachycardia, and hypertension, mostly systolic. An uncommon consequence is atrial fibrillation. Thyroid enlargement is not always present and can vary greatly. The consistency of the gland can range from firm to micronodular; a single palpable nodule should prompt a thyroid scan and raise suspicions of a hyperfunctioning nodule. Over the thyroid, there is frequently a bruit or thrill. There is hyperdynamic precordium. Patients exhibit signs of anxiety and frequently report a history of subpar academic performance and difficulty focusing in class. They have quick reflexes and are typically tremulous, with tremors most easily induced by having the patient extend their hands or tongue. They also frequently have mild to moderate clonus.

When a patient looks quickly downward, it can often induce a lid lag (the lids do not drop as they would normally). Additional ocular symptoms such as proptosis, puffy eyelids, and conjunctival injection strongly suggest Graves' disease.

A severe form of thyrotoxicosis known as "thyroid storm" can cause fever, severe tachycardia, high-output congestive heart failure, diarrhea, or dysfunction of the liver in addition to other symptoms. It could be present at the time of diagnosis or could be brought on by radioactive iodine or surgery used to treat hyperthyroidism. One way to grade severity is by applying the Burch-Wartovsky scale. There is a significant (~10%) chance of dying from it (Akamizu et al., 2012).

7.8.3. Laboratory Findings

TSH levels are typically too low to be detected. Both free and total T4 levels are high. Since T3 has a much shorter half-life than T4, it is especially helpful for tracking the short-term response to treatment. Total T3 levels are also elevated. Thyroid-stimulating antibodies, such as thyroid-stimulating immunoglobulin or thyroid-stimulating hormone receptor antibodies, are only elevated in Graves' disease and are useful for differentiating between the two conditions. Levels of antibodies to thyroid proteins, such as anti-thyroid peroxidase and anti-thyroglobulin, are typically elevated in both Graves' disease and Hashimoto's thyroiditis. Even during the thyrotoxic phase, radioactive iodine (^{123}I) uptake is reduced in Hashimoto's thyroiditis but elevated in Graves' disease. A hot nodule may be seen on a thyroid scan following the administration of ^{123}I or ^{99}mTc.

7.8.4. Treatment

To treat hypertension, tachycardia, and tremulousness, beta blockade is commonly used with 25–50 mg of atenolol daily. With particular treatment, this is continued until thyroid hormone levels have returned to normal. More intensive therapy for thyroid storm may be necessary, such as intravenous fluids, sodium iodide, corticosteroids, antipyretics, and occasionally inotropic drugs. In patients with thyroid storm, beta blockade should be cautiously induced with shorter acting agents like propranolol or esmolol due to the potential for aggravating heart failure. For thyrotoxicosis, there are three long-term therapies available. Drugs called thionamides are effective in treating Graves' disease and the thyrotoxic stage of Hashimoto's thyroiditis because they inhibit the synthesis of thyroid hormones. Methimazole, initially administered at ~0.05 mg/kg/d in two divided doses, is the primary agent used in the United States; propylthiouracil was once widely used but is no longer advised due to the risk of liver failure, especially in children. It is important to keep an eye on transaminases and complete blood counts because methimazole frequently results in rashes or other allergic reactions and can also cause agranulocytosis or liver failure. Usually, once the patient reaches euthyroid status, the medication dose can be lowered. The fact that 20%–30% of pediatric Graves' disease patients eventually experience remission and are able to stop taking their medication entirely justifies continuing medication treatment for an extended period of time, if necessary, rather than always moving forward with definitive treatment. After a few months, patients with Hashimoto's thyroiditis usually "burn out" and need to be weaned off methimazole. Levothyroxine is typically required for thyroid replacement (Yang et al., 2012).

There is some debate regarding the relative merits of two other approaches that are primarily pertinent to Graves' disease. With comparatively little overall radiation exposure, radioactive iodine (^{131}I), which is specifically absorbed by the thyroid gland, can cause thyroid cell ablation. 25 years ago, it was a rare treatment for children; today, teens and older schoolchildren are accepted to use it, even as a first line of treatment. Rather than attempting to make the patient euthyroid, the goal of total thyroid ablation can reduce the risk of developing a thyroid adenoma. However, based on data from atomic bombs and Chernobyl, the author believes that there may be a risk of subsequent thyroid tumors before the age of eight. Therefore, if methimazole is well tolerated, it is advisable to delay treatment until the patient is older rather than starting it too early in infancy. As an alternative, surgery to remove the thyroid may be performed (Zaat et al., 2021). Although there is little chance of long-term complications, a skilled surgeon is needed to prevent hypoparathyroidism or damage to the recurrent laryngeal nerve. The preferred course of treatment for a hyperfunctioning nodule is hemisphereectomy.

Lastly, researchers are looking into other medication therapies, especially those that block the thyroid-stimulating hormone receptor (Lane et al., 2020).

A Closer Look

Gordon Syndrome

Gordon syndrome is an autosomally dominant inherited syndrome characterized by hyperkalemia in all and varying degrees of hyperchloremic acidosis, HT, short stature, mental subnormality and muscle weakness in the presence of normal renal glomerular function. This was first described by Gordon in 1960s, but the pathophysiology still remains unclear. Some proposed mechanisms are a defect in WNK kinases and their targets in the renal tubule, which causes sodium retention, volume expansion and HT. This in turn leads to suppressed renin concentration which prevents the kaliuretic action of aldosterone, leading to hyperkalemia. Low levels of atrial natriuretic hormone (ANH) and/or reduced responsiveness to ANH, impaired cell membrane transport and impaired prostaglandin metabolism have all been proposed as pathogenetic mechanisms in Gordon syndrome. The biochemical features are exactly opposite to that of Bartter's syndrome which is caused by loss of function mutation of Na Cl cotransporter in the renal tubules

HT in Gordon syndrome is usually severe and is seen more frequently in males. It may not manifest in childhood in all cases, but is seen commonly in young adulthood. Hence, the diagnosis is often missed and it masquerades as essential HT unless hyperkalemia is detected. The HT is extremely sensitive to salt intake and restriction of dietary salt leads to reversal of HT and hyperkalemia. HT usually ameliorates during pregnancy but the hyperkalemia persists, and such babies tolerate hyperkalemia better and do not usually develop cardiac arrhythmias. Hypercalciurea and low bone mass are also seen as characteristic features in most families. Patients not responding to dietary salt restriction need thiazide diuretics which are usually started at 50% of the age- and weight-adjusted dosage because of the extreme sensitivity of the HT to thiazide diuretics. Growth rate may also normalize with thaizide diuretics (Zaat et al., 2021).

Summary

- Hypertension may be caused by abnormal synthesis of, or response to, various hormones. The proportion of pediatric hypertension cases resulting from such problems probably represents at most a small percentage of cases overall, but a higher fraction of cases of severe hypertension, those occurring in the very young, or cases clustering in families. Most endocrine hypertension involves the adrenal gland and its hormones. The adrenal gland is composed of two endocrine tissues: the medulla (secreting catecholamines) and the cortex (synthesizing cortisol and aldosterone).
- Hypertension is sustained elevation of resting systolic blood pressure, diastolic blood pressure, or both; the pressures considered abnormal in children vary based on age up to age 13. Hypertension with no known cause (primary) is most common as with adults.
- The vast majority of endocrine hypertension involves the adrenal gland and its hormones. The adrenal gland is composed of two endocrine tissues: the medulla and the cortex. Pheochromocytoma is mainly a disease of the adrenal medulla, although extramedullary sites may be involved.
- Adrenal disorders causing hypertension can be related to the dysfunction of either the adrenal cortex or the adrenal medulla. These disorders, including congenital adrenal hyperplasia (CAH), owing to 11β-hydroxylase deficiency and to 17α-hydroxylase deficiency; apparent mineralocorticoid excess; familial hyperaldosteronism type I; primary aldosteronism; Cushing's syndrome; and familial glucocorticoid resistance, primarily affect the adrenal cortex and cause low-renin hypertension. The classic disorder of the adrenal medulla resulting in hypertension is pheochromocytoma, although hypertension in obesity might also be associated with catecholamine secretion.
- Deficiency of 11β-hydroxylase is caused by mutations in the CYP11B1 gene located on chromosome 8q24. Its incidence has been estimated to be 1/250,000 to 1/100,000. CYP11B1 mediates 11-hydroxylation of 11-deoxycortisol to cortisol. Because 11-deoxycortisol is not converted to cortisol, levels of corticotropin are high. In consequence, precursors accumulate and are shunted into androgen biosynthesis, so that females may be born with ambiguous genitalia.
- 17-hydroxylase deficiency is a very rare disorder caused by mutations in the CYP17 gene. The encoded enzyme catalyzes two distinct reactions: 17-hydroxylation of pregnenolone and progesterone to 17-hydroxypregnenolone and 17-hydroxyprogesterone, respectively, and the 17,20-lyase reaction-mediating conversion of 17-hydroxypregnenolone to dehydroepiandrosterone. The enzyme is expressed in both the adrenal cortex and the gonads. Most mutations affect both the hydroxylase and lyase activities.
- Primary aldosteronism encompasses disorders caused by excessive aldosterone secretion independent of the renin–angiotensin system. These disorders are characterized by hypertension, hypokalemia, and suppression of the renin– angiotensin system.
- Cushing syndrome is the result of abnormally high blood levels of cortisol or other glucocorticoids. This can be iatrogenic or the result of endogenous cortisol secretion, due

either to an adrenal tumor or to hypersecretion of corticotropin (adrenocorticotropic hormone [ACTH]) by the pituitary (Cushing disease) or by a tumor.

- Generalized glucocorticoid resistance, also known as Chrousos syndrome, is a rare genetic condition that causes partial insensitivity to glucocorticoids in target tissues. It can be familial or sporadic, and is characterized by a broad clinical spectrum.
- Hyperthyroidism happens when the thyroid gland makes too much thyroid hormone. This condition also is called overactive thyroid. Hyperthyroidism speeds up the body's metabolism. That can cause many symptoms, such as weight loss, hand tremors, and rapid or irregular heartbeat.

References

1. Akamizu, T., Satoh, T., Isozaki, O., Suzuki, A., Wakino, S., Iburi, T., Tsuboi, K., Monden, T., Kouki, T., Otani, H., Teramukai, S., Uehara, R., Nakamura, Y., Nagai, M., & Mori, M. (2012). Diagnostic criteria, clinical features, and incidence of thyroid storm based on nationwide surveys. *Thyroid, 22*(7), 661–679. https://doi.org/10.1089/thy.2011.0334.
2. Barrett, B., Hawkes, C. P., Isaza, A., & Bauer, A. J. (2019). The effects of amiodarone on thyroid function in pediatric and young adult patients. *Journal of Clinical Endocrinology & Metabolism, 104*(12), 5540–5546. https://doi.org/10.1210/jc.2019-00466.
3. Brenta, G., Danzi, S., & Klein, I. (2007). Potential therapeutic applications of thyroid hormone analogs. *Nature Clinical Practice Endocrinology & Metabolism, 3*(9), 632–640. https://doi.org/10.1038/ncpendmet0587.
4. Castinetti, F., Nieman, L. K., Reincke, M., & Newell-Price, J. (2021). Approach to the patient treated with steroidogenesis inhibitors. *Journal of Clinical Endocrinology & Metabolism, 106*(8), 2114–2123. https://doi.org/10.1210/clinem/dgab129.
5. Feelders, R. A., Newell-Price, J., Pivonello, R., Nieman, L. K., Hofland, L. J., & Lacroix, A. (2019). Advances in the medical treatment of Cushing's syndrome. *Lancet Diabetes & Endocrinology, 7*(4), 300–312. https://doi.org/10.1016/S2213-8587(18)30374-7.
6. Fleseriu, M., Auchus, R. J., Pivonello, R., Salvatori, R., Zacharieva, S., & Biller, B. M. K. (2021). Levoketoconazole: A novel treatment for endogenous Cushing's syndrome. *Expert Review of Endocrinology & Metabolism, 16*(3), 159–174. https://doi.org/10.1080/17446651.2021.1884188.
7. Funder, J. (2001). Mineralocorticoids and cardiac fibrosis: The decade in review. *Clinical and Experimental Pharmacology & Physiology, 28*(12), 1002–1006. https://doi.org/10.1046/j.1440-1681.2001.03568.x.
8. Geller, D. S., Farhi, A., Pinkerton, N., Fradley, M., Moritz, M., Spitzer, A., Meinke, G., Tsai, F. T. F., Sigler, P. B., & Lifton, R. P. (2000). Activating mineralocorticoid receptor mutation in hypertension exacerbated by pregnancy. *Science, 289*(5476), 119–123. https://doi.org/10.1126/science.289.5476.119.
9. Gershengorn, M. C., & Neumann, S. (2012). Update in TSH receptor agonists and antagonists. *Journal of Clinical Endocrinology & Metabolism, 97*(12), 4287–4292. https://doi.org/10.1210/jc.2012-2797.

10. Hattangady, N. G., Olala, L. O., Bollag, W. B., & Rainey, W. E. (2012). Acute and chronic regulation of aldosterone production. *Molecular and Cellular Endocrinology, 350*(2), 151–162. https://doi.org/10.1016/j.mce.2011.10.030.

11. Korzyńska, W., Jodkowska, A., Gosławska, K., Bogunia-Kubik, K., & Mazur, G. (2018). Genetic aspects of primary hyperaldosteronism. *Advances in Clinical and Experimental Medicine, 27*(8), 1149–1158. https://doi.org/10.17219/acem/69013.

12. Lane, L. C., Cheetham, T. D., Perros, P., & Pearce, S. H. S. (2020). New therapeutic horizons for Graves' hyperthyroidism. *Endocrine Reviews, 41*(6), 873–884. https://doi.org/10.1210/endrev/bnaa021.

13. Mulatero, P., Monticone, S., Rainey, W. E., Veglio, F., & Williams, T. A. (2013). Role of KCNJ5 in familial and sporadic primary aldosteronism. *Nature Reviews Endocrinology, 9*(2), 104–112. https://doi.org/10.1038/nrendo.2012.248.

14. Nieman, L. K., Biller, B. M., Findling, J. W., Murad, M. H., Newell-Price, J., Savage, M. O., & Tabarin, A. (2015). Treatment of Cushing's syndrome: An endocrine society clinical practice guideline. *Journal of Clinical Endocrinology & Metabolism, 100*(8), 2807–2831. https://doi.org/10.1210/jc.2015-1818.

15. O'Neill, J. A., Berkowitz, H., Fellows, K. J., & Harmon, C. M. (1995). Midaortic syndrome and hypertension in childhood. *Journal of Pediatric Surgery, 30*(2), 164–171. https://doi.org/10.1016/0022-3468(95)90555-3.

16. Papakokkinou, E., Piasecka, M., Carlsen, H. K., Chantzichristos, D., Olsson, D. S., Dahlqvist, P., Petersson, M., Berinder, K., Bensing, S., Höybye, C., Engström, B. E., Burman, P., Follin, C., Petranek, D., Erfurth, E. M., Wahlberg, J., Ekman, B., Åkerman, A. K., Schwarcz, E., Johannsson, G., Falhammar, H., & Ragnarsson, O. (2021). Prevalence of Nelson's syndrome after bilateral adrenalectomy in patients with Cushing's disease: A systematic review and meta-analysis. *Pituitary, 24*(6), 797–809. https://doi.org/10.1007/s11102-021-01138-w.

17. Redlich, A., Pamporaki, C., Lessel, L., Frühwald, M. C., & Vorwerk, P. (2021). Pseudohypoxic pheochromocytomas and paragangliomas dominate in children. *Pediatric Blood & Cancer, 68*(7), e28981. https://doi.org/10.1002/pbc.28981.

18. Santos, I. N., & Spadari-Bratfisch, R. C. (2006). Stress and cardiac beta-adrenoceptors. *Stress, 9*(2), 69–84. https://doi.org/10.1080/10253890500499453.

19. Seidel, E., Schewe, J., & Scholl, U. I. (2019). Genetic causes of primary aldosteronism. *Experimental & Molecular Medicine, 51*(1), 1–12. https://doi.org/10.1038/s12276-019-0220-1.

20. Tomaschitz, A., Pilz, S., Ritz, E., Obermayer-Pietsch, B., & Pieber, T. R. (2010). Aldosterone and arterial hypertension. *Nature Reviews Endocrinology, 6*(2), 83–93. https://doi.org/10.1038/nrendo.2009.271.

21. Vassiliadi, D. A., Mourelatos, P., Kratimenos, T., & Tsagarakis, S. (2021). Inferior petrosal sinus sampling in Cushing's syndrome: Usefulness and pitfalls. *Endocrine, 73*(3), 530–539. https://doi.org/10.1007/s12020-021-02649-0.

22. White, P. C. (2001). Steroid 11 beta-hydroxylase deficiency and related disorders. *Endocrinology and Metabolism Clinics of North America, 30*(1), 61–79. https://doi.org/10.1016/s0889-8529(08)70019-0.

23. Yang, Q., Zhang, Z., Kukline, E. V., et al. (2012). Sodium intake and blood pressure among U.S. children and adolescents. *Pediatrics, 130*(4), 611–619. https://doi.org/10.1542/peds.2011-3870.

24. Zaat, A. S., Derikx, J. P. M., Zwaveling-Soonawala, N., van Trotsenburg, A. S. P., & Mooij, C. F. (2021). Thyroidectomy in pediatric patients with Graves' disease: A systematic review of postoperative morbidity. *European Thyroid Journal, 10*(1), 39–51. https://doi.org/10.1159/000510952.

Chapter 8

ENDOCRINE HYPERTENSION IN PREGNANT WOMAN

Contents

INTRODUCTION

Endocrine hypertension during pregnancy is a complex condition characterized by elevated blood pressure due to hormonal imbalances. This form of hypertension is often associated with disorders such as primary aldosteronism, pheochromocytoma, Cushing's syndrome, and hyperthyroidism. Each of these conditions contributes to hypertension through different mechanisms. Primary aldosteronism, for instance, involves excess production of aldosterone, leading to sodium retention, increased blood volume, and consequently, high blood pressure. Pheochromocytoma, a rare adrenal gland tumor, secretes excessive catecholamines, causing episodic or sustained hypertension with symptoms like palpitations, headaches, and sweating. Cushing's syndrome results from elevated cortisol levels, which can increase blood pressure through various pathways, including increased vascular sensitivity to catecholamines and enhanced renal sodium retention. Hyperthyroidism raises blood pressure by increasing cardiac output and heart rate, among other effects (Sibai, 2002).

The diagnosis of endocrine hypertension in pregnant women poses significant challenges due to overlapping symptoms with pregnancy-related physiological changes. Accurate diagnosis is critical, as untreated endocrine hypertension can lead to severe maternal and fetal complications, including preeclampsia, eclampsia, placental abruption, intrauterine growth restriction, and preterm delivery. A thorough medical history, physical examination, and appropriate laboratory tests are essential for identifying the underlying endocrine disorder. For example, measuring plasma aldosterone concentration and plasma renin activity can help diagnose primary aldosteronism, while elevated urinary metanephrines and catecholamines are indicative of pheochromocytoma. Elevated 24-hour urinary free cortisol or late-night salivary cortisol can confirm Cushing's syndrome, and thyroid function tests are used to diagnose hyperthyroidism.

Management of endocrine hypertension in pregnancy requires a multidisciplinary approach involving obstetricians, endocrinologists, and cardiologists. The treatment strategy depends on the specific endocrine disorder and the gestational age. For instance, surgical removal of pheochromocytoma is preferred before pregnancy or during the second trimester if detected early, while medical management with alpha-blockers is necessary if surgery is not feasible. For primary aldosteronism, potassium-sparing diuretics may be used, although their safety in pregnancy must be carefully considered. In the case of Cushing's syndrome, surgical or medical treatment may be required based on the severity of hypercortisolism and its impact on both the mother and the fetus. Hyperthyroidism is typically managed with antithyroid medications, with propylthiouracil preferred during the first trimester and methimazole thereafter. Close monitoring of blood pressure, fetal growth, and maternal well-being is crucial throughout pregnancy to minimize complications and ensure optimal outcomes for both mother and child.

Orientation and Directional Terms

Term	Definition	Illustration
Pregnancy	Pregnancy (or gestation) is calculated as 40 weeks and starts from the first day of your last menstrual period. Pregnancy is classified into 3 stages known as trimesters. The gender and inherited characteristics of the baby are decided at the moment of conception.	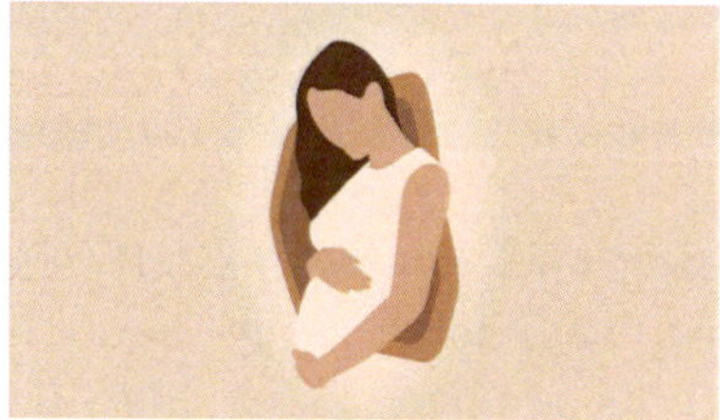
Cushing's syndrome(CS)	Cushing's syndrome (CS) is a rare problem caused when the adrenal gland(s) makes too much of a hormone called cortisol. CS is most often due to a tumor or mass found in the pituitary gland, but can also be caused by tumors in the adrenal glands themselves.	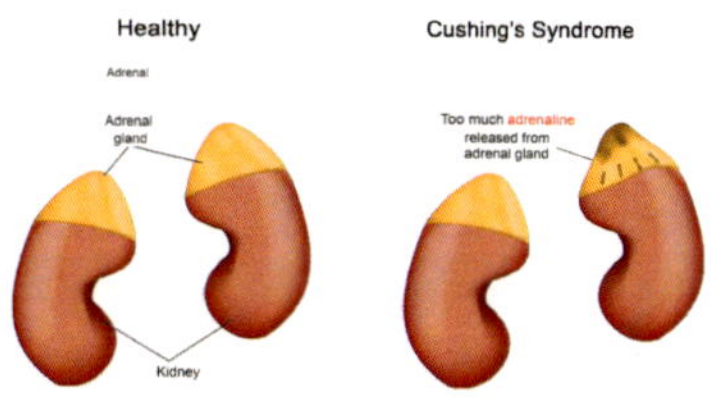
Primary aldosteronism(PA)	Primary aldosteronism is an endocrine problem in which the adrenal glands produce too much of a hormone called aldosterone. This can cause high blood pressure and other symptoms. You have two adrenal glands located just above your kidneys.	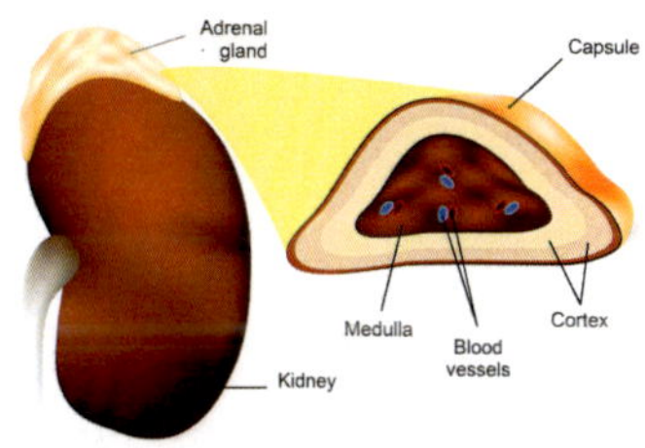
Chronic hypertension	Women who have chronic hypertension and become pregnant need to be closely monitored. Chronic hypertension puts women at a higher risk of developing pre-eclampsia or other blood pressure conditions during pregnancy. Chronic hypertension is also associated with increased risks of pregnancy complications like stillbirth, placental abruption, and fetal growth restriction.	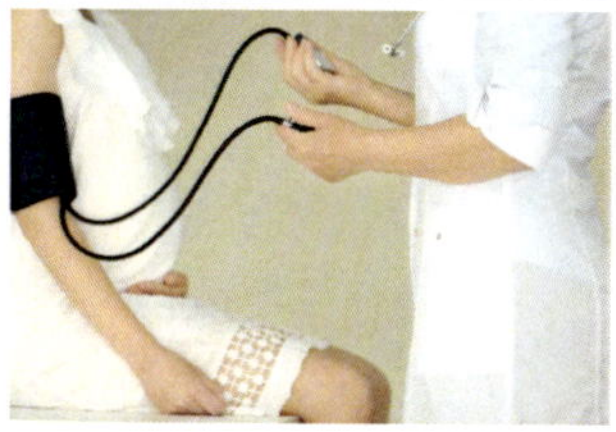
Blood pressure	Blood pressure is the amount of force your blood uses to get through your arteries. When your heart pumps, it uses force to push oxygen-rich blood out to your arteries. They bring it to your body's cells and tissues. If your blood pressure is too high, it can cause health issues.	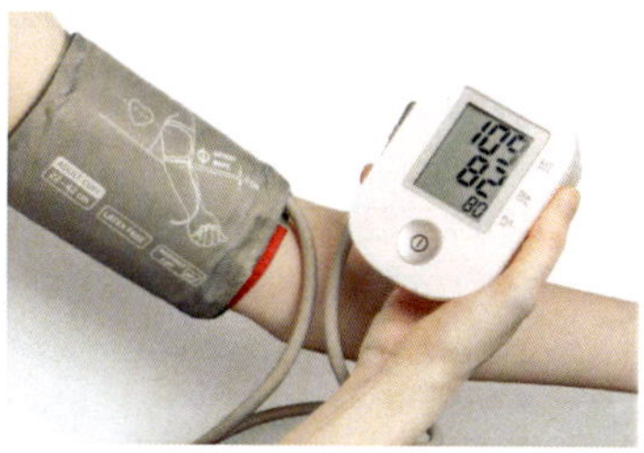

8.1. CHRONIC HYPERTENSION IN PREGNANCY

Pregnancy-related chronic hypertension is defined as hypertension that existed before 20 weeks of gestation or before conception. Up to 5% of pregnant women have chronic hypertension; rates vary depending on the population under study and the diagnostic standards applied. When high blood pressure is known to occur before conception, chronic hypertension complicating pregnancy is diagnosed. Elevated blood pressure found before 20 weeks of gestation is frequently the result of chronic hypertension when prepregnancy blood pressure is unknown. However, gestational hypertension or early preeclampsia should also be taken into consideration if blood pressure was normal during the first trimester and then increases before 20 weeks of gestation. A blood pressure measurement of 140 mm Hg or higher at the systolic or 90 mm Hg at the diastolic levels, or both, is considered hypertension. Although a distinction is not made between chronic, gestational, or preeclamptic hypertension, blood pressure is classified as mild to moderate (systolic, 140–159 mm Hg or diastolic, 90–109 mm Hg) or severe (systolic, 160 mm Hg or higher, diastolic, 110 mm Hg or higher) during pregnancy. Up to 10% of women with chronic hypertension may have underlying renal or endocrine disorders, which can cause secondary hypertension. However, the majority of these women will have essential hypertension, also known as primary hypertension (Vanek et al., 2004).

When pre-pregnancy hypertension is well-documented and women are already taking antihypertensive medication, the diagnosis of chronic hypertension can be made with ease. When hypertension is detected in the first trimester of pregnancy, the most likely diagnosis is also chronic hypertension. Pregnant women with prepregnancy undiagnosed hypertension may have problems if they experience the pregnancy-associated physiologic drop in blood pressure and then initially present in the second trimester with normal blood pressure. These women were assumed to be normotensive, and if their blood pressure rises during the third trimester, they might be mistakenly diagnosed with superimposed preeclampsia instead of gestational hypertension or, if proteinuria is present, preeclampsia. Therefore, it is possible that chronic hypertension won't be identified until much later on. In other cases, women who have a history of hypertension before becoming pregnant may show normal blood pressure during the whole pregnancy, but after giving birth, their blood pressure may return to what it was before the pregnancy.

8.1.1. Maternal and Fetal Outcomes

The distinction between women with superimposed preeclampsia and those with uncomplicated chronic hypertension has not always been made in reports of the outcomes of pregnancies complicated by chronic hypertension. Preeclampsia has been linked to preexisting hypertension as a known risk factor. 13–40% of women with chronic hypertension develop superimposed preeclampsia, depending on the diagnostic criteria, duration, and severity of the hypertension. The etiology can range from essential to secondary. The fact that some studies use a broad definition of superimposed preeclampsia is a major contributing factor to this wide variation in incidence.

Adverse maternal-fetal outcomes are more common in women with chronic hypertension who develop superimposed preeclampsia; however, it is unclear what risks are associated with uncomplicated chronic hypertension on its own. Uncomplicated chronic hypertension was still linked to a higher risk of cesarean delivery (odds ratio [OR], 2.7; 95% confidence interval

[CI], 2.4–3.0) and postpartum hemorrhage (OR, 2.2; 95% CI, 1.4–3.7) when compared to women without hypertension, according to an analysis of 1,807 deliveries in women with chronic hypertension. Additional unfavorable outcomes for mothers who have chronic hypertension include accelerated hypertension that leads to damage to target organs (such as the heart, brain, or kidneys), though this is very rare in the absence of preeclampsia. Pregnant women who have secondary hypertension or higher blood pressure before conception are more likely to experience severe hypertension during pregnancy. An elevated risk of gestational diabetes is linked to chronic hypertension (OR, 1.8; 95% CI, 1.4–2). This could be due to similar pathogenetic mechanisms (like obesity) and risk factors (like insulin resistance) for both conditions. Women with chronic hypertension have a threefold increased risk of abruptio placentae, although the majority of this increased risk is linked to superimposed preeclampsia. Hospitalization for hypertension is more common in pregnant women with chronic hypertension.

Preeclampsia superimposed on chronic hypertension predisposes most of the increased attributable risk associated with prenatal mortality. When comparing women with uncomplicated chronic hypertension to those with superimposed preeclampsia, the relative risk of perinatal death is estimated to be around 3:06. In addition, compared to controls with normotension, there is a higher risk of perinatal death in women with uncomplicated hypertension (relative risk, 2.3). Fetal growth restriction is typically associated with preeclampsia that has been superimposed and is more common in patients with chronic hypertension. Antihypertensive drug exposure in utero has also been linked to a risk of chronic hypertension in pregnancy, which has been shown to cause fetal malformations and growth restriction. The issue of whether antihypertensive medications have an impact on growth is still debatable, despite the fact that the majority of medications deemed safe for use during pregnancy have not been linked to fetal abnormalities. Clinical trials using a restricted number of agents, mainly methyldopa, have assessed the long-term outcomes of exposed offspring.

8.1.2. Preconception Counseling

Preconception counseling should cover the warning signs and symptoms of preeclampsia as well as the risks of chronic hypertension. The presence of diabetes, obesity, or renal disease; a history of preeclampsia, especially early preeclampsia; the degree and duration of hypertension before pregnancy; and the existence of secondary hypertension, such as pheochromocytoma and renovascular hypertension, are maternal characteristics that raise the risk of superimposed preeclampsia. Pregnancy should be avoided while taking known fetal harmful medications that are frequently prescribed to women with chronic hypertension. Specifically, it is not recommended to use angiotensin-converting enzyme (ACE) inhibitors, angiotensin receptor blockers, or mineralocorticoid antagonists. There is conflicting evidence regarding the safety of using statins during pregnancy, which is why they should be avoided. Statins are commonly prescribed to people with hypertension who also have elevated cholesterol.

8.1.3. Antepartum Management

8.1.3.1. Initial Evaluation of Women with Known or Suspected Chronic Hypertension

To rule out secondary (and potentially treatable) hypertension when appropriate and to look for evidence of target organ damage, unless such evaluations were previously completed, all women with preexisting hypertension should be evaluated either before pregnancy or early in the pregnancy, according to the guidelines set forth by the National High Blood Pressure Education Program and the Seventh Report of the Joint National Committee on Prevention, Detection, Evaluation, and Treatment of High Blood Pressure. Whether superimposed preeclampsia is suspected later in pregnancy, baseline values for serum creatinine, electrolytes, uric acid, liver enzymes, platelet count, and urine protein (either dipstick test or quantification of urine protein) should be recorded to use as comparators. To prevent gestational diabetes in women who are obese, have a history of the disease, or have a strong family history of type 2 diabetes mellitus, glucose tolerance testing should be done early in pregnancy. For women with severe hypertension that has persisted for a long time (more than 4 years), good clinical practice recommends assessing left ventricular function using either echocardiography or electrocardiography.

8.1.3.2. Screening for Secondary Hypertension

Chronic kidney disease is the most common cause of secondary hypertension, and routine blood tests and urinalyses make screening for this condition simple. If a urinalysis results in a proteinuria result (1+ or higher), the amount of proteinuria should be determined by measuring the protein/creatinine ratio in a spot urine sample or by collecting a 24-hour urine sample. Renal ultrasonography should be done to rule out polycystic kidney disease, the most common genetic type of kidney disease, if signs of chronic kidney disease are found (elevated serum creatinine or abnormal urinalysis), or if there is a strong family history of kidney disease. Primary aldosteronism, renovascular hypertension, pheochromocytoma, and Cushing disease are additional conditions that can cause secondary hypertension in women of childbearing age. Additional diagnostic testing should be taken into consideration if any of the suggestive clinical characteristics of secondary hypertension—resistant hypertension, hypokalemia, palpitations, age under 35, and absence of family history of hypertension—appear. Certain diagnoses, such as pheochromocytoma and renovascular hypertension, are linked to poor maternal and fetal outcomes, according to case series and case reports. However, these outcomes can be improved if the underlying disorder is treated. The task force recommends referral to a hypertension specialist if secondary hypertension is a possibility because there is variation in the suggested methods for diagnosing secondary hypertension (Sibai et al., 2009).

8.1.3.3. Monitoring Blood Pressure

Every pregnant woman has her blood pressure checked once a month as part of routine obstetric care. Good clinical practice requires more frequent monitoring for women whose blood pressure is above target, even though this approach hasn't been tested for enhancing pregnancy outcomes. Superimposed preeclampsia can happen before 24 weeks of gestation; in fact, anecdotal reports of cases before 20 weeks of gestation exist, despite the fact that most cases occur near term. Therefore, the second half of pregnancy may be especially benefiting from more monitoring. The task force recommends this strategy for pregnant women due to the substantial body of research on hypertension in non-pregnant patients that shows how home blood pressure monitoring can help patients meet their goals and track their reactions to treatment.

- **White Coat Hypertension:** It is defined as elevated BP primarily in the presence of health care providers, may account for up to 10%–15% of individuals with office hypertension. The prevalence in pregnancy is not known. Ambulatory

BP monitoring is the preferred test to diagnose white coat hypertension in an individual who is not pregnant. White coat hypertension should be suspected if BP is higher in the doctor's office compared with other settings. Failure to recognize white coat hypertension may result in overtreatment of BP and unnecessary adverse effects of treatment.

8.1.3.4. Treatment

Hypertension significantly increases the risk of stroke, coronary heart disease, congestive heart failure, kidney disease, and death. Lowering blood pressure has been proven to prevent these complications in individuals with hypertension who are not pregnant. The progression of vascular damage and cardiovascular issues related to hypertension occurs over the course of many years. Stage 1 hypertension (blood pressure of 140-159 mm Hg systolic/90-99 mm Hg diastolic) is associated with a 40% higher risk of stroke compared to individuals of the same age without hypertension, typically becoming evident after 10 years of untreated hypertension. It takes years of treatment in non-pregnant individuals to see the benefits of lowered blood pressure. However, in pregnancy, the focus is on preventing immediate complications of hypertension for the woman and ensuring a healthy pregnancy. Treatment goals also involve minimizing risks to the fetus, including potential harm from antihypertensive medications. While preventing long-term cardiovascular issues for the mother is important, it is not the primary concern during pregnancy.

- **Nonpharmacologic Treatment:** Two main approaches are used to treat hypertensive individuals who are not pregnant: (1) lowering blood pressure; and (2) reducing additional cardiovascular risk factors. Nonpharmacologic strategies that have been effective in lowering blood pressure in non-pregnant individuals include regular aerobic exercise, preserving an ideal body weight, consuming alcohol in moderation, following certain diets (like the DASH [Dietary Approaches to Stop Hypertension] diet, which emphasizes a diet rich in fruits, vegetables, low-fat dairy products, and high fiber), and cutting back on sodium. Certain methods have not been tested in a pregnancy-related setting or are not suitable for use during pregnancy. In hypertensive individuals who are not pregnant, weight loss and regular aerobic exercise have been demonstrated to be beneficial because they lower blood pressure and have a positive impact on weight and insulin sensitivity. Pregnant women without medical or obstetric complications are advised to engage in moderate-level physical activity. Pregnancy-related exercise regimens have been tested, mainly as a preventative measure against excessive weight gain. The effectiveness of this method for reducing blood pressure in expectant mothers with chronic hypertension has not been studied. Exercise may help prevent preeclampsia, according to observational studies and small clinical trials; however, the effects of exercise on women with chronic hypertension have not been specifically addressed in these studies. There hasn't been enough research done to determine whether moderate or intense aerobic exercise is harmful to women with chronic hypertension.

- **Antihypertensive Pharmacologic Treatment:** Treatment of severe hypertension: The task force discovered little information about the precise blood pressure level at which pregnant women with chronic hypertension should begin antihypertensive medication. Although the exact blood pressure level at which the risk of these adverse events increases is unknown and is likely to vary depending on comorbidities and other factors like baseline blood pressure and the rate of increase, severe elevations in blood pressure are linked to acute maternal cerebrovascular and coronary events. When the systolic blood pressure in an adult non-pregnant patient is 140 mm Hg or higher, or the diastolic blood pressure is 90 mm Hg or higher, antihypertensive therapy is advised. This recommendation is backed by extensive clinical trials that have amply demonstrated the therapeutic benefits of the intervention (Sibai et al., 1998).

The ideal blood pressure for pregnant women with preexisting (chronic) hypertension has not been the subject of many clinical trials. Preeclampsia and gestational hypertension, as well as women with chronic hypertension, have been included in the majority of studies that address this. The effectiveness of antihypertensive medication has been compared to placebo or no medication at all, and the results of these trials have been inconsistently measured (e.g., development of superimposed preeclampsia, progression of hypertension, and fetal weight and survival). A Cochrane systematic review of medication therapy for severe hypertension during pregnancy included few women with chronic hypertension out of 35 trials totaling 3,573 participants. In most studies, medication therapy was not started until the third trimester, or when diastolic blood pressure levels reached or exceeded 100–110 mm Hg. If they were included, there was no reported subgroup analysis, and women with chronic hypertension were generally excluded. As a result, there is little data on when to start antihypertensive medication in pregnant patients who have chronic hypertension. It is unlikely that further placebo-controlled trials for the treatment of severe hypertension will be started, and considering the ethical implications, it is not advised. Indirect evidence from treating pregnant patients with new acute onset severe gestational hypertension or preeclampsia serves as the basis for recommendations for treating women with chronic hypertension who have significantly elevated blood pressure. A lower diastolic blood pressure threshold of 105 mm Hg is recommended for treatment due to the limitations of the data and the increased probability of outpatient therapy with less frequent blood pressure monitoring among pregnant women with chronic hypertension.

- **Treatment of Mild to Moderate Hypertension:** It is less clear when and how to use antihypertensive medications in pregnant women with chronic hypertension who do not have significantly elevated blood pressure. For women with chronic hypertension who have mild to moderately elevated blood pressure (systolic blood pressure of 140 mm Hg or higher and less than 160 mm Hg or diastolic blood pressure of 90 mm Hg or higher and less than 110 mm Hg), the use of antihypertensive therapy during pregnancy must

> be justified by the improvement in perinatal outcomes and the benefit to the mother that results from treatment, outweighing any potential risks to the safety of the fetus and newborn. This includes the possibility that medication-induced drops in maternal systemic blood pressure could compromise uteroplacental blood flow.

Antihypertensive medication did not improve maternal or perinatal outcomes, according to data from seven placebo-controlled randomized trials involving 650 women with mild to moderate chronic hypertension. The risk of developing severe hypertension was found to be decreased by treatment, but the incidence of preeclampsia was not affected, according to a Cochrane systematic review of antihypertensive drug therapy for mild to moderate hypertension in pregnancy (including all diagnoses) that included 46 trials (4,282 women). On perinatal outcomes, such as preterm birth, small-for-gestational-age (SGA) infants, and fetal death, there were no effects observed, either positive or negative. Just five of the included studies had a specific focus on women with chronic hypertension.

In this subgroup, treatment reduced the risk of progressing to severe hypertension (RR, 0.57; 95% CI, 0.34–0.98), in line with the overall findings, but had no impact on perinatal outcomes. There were no side effects from the treatment. Therefore, the evidence that is currently available points to a possible maternal benefit of antihypertensive treatment by slowing the development of severe hypertension, but there is no evidence of a direct benefit to the fetus or a notable improvement in perinatal outcomes for women who have chronic hypertension. Two meta-regression analyses examined the effect of lowering blood pressure specifically on fetal birth weight, despite the 2007 Cochrane review's lack of evidence of fetal harm associated with blood pressure lowering. These analyses included seven trials involving women with chronic hypertension and 38 trials involving women with late-onset hypertension during pregnancy. An average drop in baby birth weight of 145 g was linked to a drop in mean arterial pressure of 10 mm Hg. In women with chronic hypertension, however, the correlation between a drop in BP and SGA was less compelling, perhaps as a result of the study's limited power. Antihypertensive medication use during the second or third trimester of pregnancy was significantly associated with an increased risk of SGA (OR, 1.53; 95% CI, 1.17–1.99), according to a 2010 case–control analysis of the Quebec Pregnancy Registry data. This association persisted even after adjusting for potential confounders.

The possibility of drug-induced teratogenicity is a significant concern when treating maternal hypertension during pregnancy. There is conflicting evidence. According to two population-based studies (Arias et al., 1979), exposure to any antihypertensive medication may be linked to an increased risk of fetal cardiac abnormalities. However, other studies did not support these findings. These population-based studies have several limitations, such as the small total number of malformations; additionally, it is impossible to determine whether these are effects of a particular medication, effects of elevated blood pressure, or, conversely, effects of low blood pressure secondary to treatment. Despite the small increase in malformations, these data highlight the need for more carefully planned prospective trials to fully understand the benefits and risks of prescribing any medication during pregnancy, especially in the first trimester. Thus, starting antihypertensive therapy for mild to moderate chronic hypertension during pregnancy is not advised unless blood pressure approaches 160 mm Hg systolic or higher, 105 mm Hg diastolic or higher, or both, in the lack of compelling evidence.

- **Blood Pressure Targets for Antihypertensive Treatment:** The optimal target blood pressure in pregnant women with chronic hypertension after antihypertensive therapy is started is rarely discussed in the literature. An analysis of 256 women's Cochrane reviews compared "tight" (systolic blood pressure less than 130 mm Hg and diastolic blood pressure less than 80 mm Hg) and "less tight" (systolic blood pressure less than 140 mm Hg and diastolic blood pressure less than 90 mm Hg) blood pressure control. The trials were two pilot randomized trials that included women with either mild to moderate chronic or birth hypertension. There were no notable negative effects found, and there wasn't enough data to determine the ideal blood pressure control required to enhance the outcomes for mothers and their fetuses or newborns (Ferrer et al., 2000).
- **Treatment of Women Receiving Antihypertensive Therapy Before Pregnancy:** There is not enough information available to inform decisions about whether to continue or stop therapy for women who take medication for well-controlled or mild hypertension before becoming pregnant. There was no increase in preeclampsia, abruptio placentae, or perinatal death when compared to untreated groups in a review of 298 women whose medication dosage was decreased or stopped. A recent case-control study also discovered no correlation between the first trimester cessation of antihypertensive medication and preeclampsia or eclampsia. It is reasonable practice to stop taking medications during the first trimester and resume them if blood pressure approaches the severe range, although individual decisions must be made. Systolic blood pressure of less than 140 mm Hg and diastolic blood pressure of less than 90 mm Hg are the lower blood pressure goals for women with end-organ damage, such as chronic renal disease or cardiac disease, to prevent the disease's progression during pregnancy and its related complications. As previously mentioned, evaluation of kidney and heart end-organ damage should occur either before or during the early stages of pregnancy, or both. Women should be closely monitored if medications are stopped. A thorough review of the medical history is helpful, as is a baseline assessment of cardiac and renal function (echocardiography or electrocardiography, serum creatinine, creatinine clearance, and urinary protein excretion). It is obvious that in this situation, the decision to receive therapy or not should be made after a thorough discussion with the expectant patient.

8.1.3.5. Types of Antihypertensive Medication

The aim of treatment is a crucial factor to take into account when selecting an antihypertensive drug for the treatment of chronic hypertension in pregnancy. This goal can be either acutely lowered severe hypertension in a hospital setting (Table 8.1) or chronically treated to keep blood pressure levels below the severe range, frequently in an outpatient setting (Table 8.2).

- **Drugs for Urgent Lowering of Blood Pressure:** A Cochrane systematic review comparing antihypertensive drugs with one another for the acute lowering of severely elevated blood pressure during pregnancy included 35 randomized controlled trials with 3,573 women. Women with known chronic hypertension or those who had previously used antihypertensive therapy were excluded from the majority of these trials, which only included women with preeclampsia or gestational hypertension in the third trimester. Among the drugs that were compared were calcium channel blockers, labetalol, and hydralazine. The systematic review's conclusions indicate that there is insufficient data to support any of these drugs' superior safety or effectiveness. Thus, the authors draw the conclusion that the selection of an antihypertensive drug should be based on the drug's potential side effects and contraindications as well as the experience and familiarity of the individual clinician with it. It is reasonable to extrapolate management recommendations based on these data, given the unlikely nature of future trials focusing specifically on acute treatment of pregnant women with chronic hypertension. In the hospital setting, oral nifedipine, intravenous hydralazine, or intravenous labetalol are suitable first-line medications for acute blood pressure reduction (Table 8.1). The use of nifedipine and intravenous magnesium sulfate together raises the possibility of hypotension and neuromuscular blockade. Although one review found that taking these medications together does not raise these risks, it is still advisable to closely monitor women who are taking both because of the plausible mechanism (both are calcium antagonists). In light of these findings, the choice and method of drug administration for women who need antihypertensive medications for severe hypertension should be based primarily on the physician's experience and familiarity with the prescribed medication, any adverse effects or contraindications, local availability, and cost.
- **Drugs for Continuous Management:** Pregnant women with chronic hypertension are treated outpatient with oral agents. Labetalol (included in one trial) and methyldopa (included in five trials) have been the subject of randomized controlled trials of medication therapy. In the largest trial involving pregnant women with chronic hypertension, 263 women were randomized to receive labetalol, methyldopa, or no treatment at all; no differences were observed in terms of safety or outcome. Table 8.2 summarizes commonly used oral agents for the management of chronic hypertension in pregnancy.

Methyldopa is a centrally acting alpha-2 adrenergic agonist that is still widely used due to its extensive history of use in pregnancy and its safety information for younger patients. Since the indirect mechanism of action takes several hours to take effect, blood pressure control is gradual. Methyldopa has been specifically studied prospectively in a mixed group of hypertensive women and in chronic hypertension in comparison to placebo. The uteroplacental, fetal, or fetal well-being hemodynamics do not appear to be negatively impacted (Zetterstrom et al., 2005).

Table 8.1. *Antihypertensive Agents Used for Urgent Blood Pressure Control in Pregnancy*

Drug	Dose	Comments
Labetalol	10–20 mg IV, then 20–80 mg every 20–30 min to a maximum dose of 300 mg or Constant infusion 1–2 mg/min IV	Considered a first-line agent Tachycardia is less common and fewer adverse effects Contraindicated in patients with asthma, heart disease, or congestive heart failure
Hydralazine	5 mg IV or IM, then 5–10 mg IV every 20–40 min or Constant infusion 0.5–10 mg/h	Higher or frequent dosage associated with maternal hypotension, headaches, and fetal distress—may be more common than other agents
Nifedipine	10–20 mg orally, repeat in 30 minutes if needed; then 10–20 mg every 2–6 hours	May observe reflex tachycardia and headaches

Abbreviations: IM, intramuscularly; IV, intravenously.

Source: https://www.preeclampsia.org/frontend/assets/img/advocacy_resource/HypertensioninPregnancy_1583246906.pdf.

Table 8.2. *Common Oral Antihypertensive Agents in Pregnancy*

Drug	Dosage	Comments
Labetalol	200–2,400 mg/d orally in two to three divided doses	Well tolerated Potential bronchoconstrictive effects Avoid in patients with asthma and congestive heart failure
Nifedipine	30–120 mg/d orally of a slow-release preparation	Do not use sublingual form
Methyldopa	0.5–3 g/d orally in two to three divided doses	Childhood safety data up to 7 years of age May not be as effective in control of severe hypertension
Thiazide diuretics	Depends on agent	Second-line agent
Angiotensin-converting enzyme inhibitors/ angiotensin receptor blockers		Associated with fetal anomalies Contraindicated in pregnancy and preconception period

Source: https://www.preeclampsia.org/frontend/assets/img/advocacy_resource/HypertensioninPregnancy_1583246906.pdf.

Infants exposed to methyldopa in utero showed comparable birth weight, neonatal complications, and development at one year when compared to those who received no therapy. A 7-year-old children's follow-up study revealed no differences in the children's neurocognitive development or IQ when compared to controls. Hepatic necrosis and dysfunction as well as hemolytic anemia are serious side effects. The Cochrane analysis of a subset of studies suggests that methyldopa may be less effective than the combined β-blocker and calcium channel blocker classes in preventing severe hypertension (OR, 0.75; 95% CI, 0.59–0.94).

Pregnant women frequently use labetalol, a nonselective β-blocker that can block vascular alpha receptors. Comparing methyldopa or placebo to perinatal outcomes in women with chronic hypertension revealed no discernible differences in perinatal outcomes. In women with chronic hypertension, labetalol is a reasonable option, according to comparisons with placebo or other antihypertensive agents for mild to moderate hypertension during pregnancy. Lethargy, exhaustion, insomnia, and bronchoconstriction are among the side effects. Women who suffer from asthma, heart disease, or congestive heart failure should not take labetalol. Pregnancy has made extensive use of beta-blockers alone because they are a useful tool for lowering blood pressure. If β-blockers are compared to a placebo or no treatment, there could be a higher rate of SGA infants (RR, 1.34; 95% CI, 1.01–1.79).

The use of calcium channel blockers in pregnant patients with chronic hypertension has not been thoroughly researched. Nifedipine was the most often prescribed calcium channel blocker in the comparison trials for mild to moderate hypertension in pregnancy, and extrapolation from these trials shows no increase in unfavorable perinatal outcomes. Moreover, it doesn't seem that nifedipine negatively impacts umbilical or uterine blood flow. Diuretics are typically regarded as second-line medications for the management of pregnancy-related hypertension. Diuretics have the potential to deplete intravascular volume, which could restrict fetal growth. This has sparked theoretical worry. However, data from a Cochrane systematic review of diuretics for the prevention of preeclampsia and a meta-analysis of nine randomized trials do not support this. Diuretics can therefore be used during pregnancy, but dosage adjustments must be made to reduce side effects and risks like hypokalemia. In women with known salt-sensitive hypertension, they might be especially helpful, especially when there is a decline in renal function (Rey and Couturier, 1994).

Angiotensin-converting enzyme inhibitors and angiotensin receptor blockers used in the second and third trimesters of pregnancy are associated with fetal abnormalities (including renal failure, oligohydramnios, pulmonary hypoplasia, calvarial abnormalities, and fetal growth restriction) as well as postdelivery effects such as oliguria and anuria. Serious concerns also have been raised regarding first-trimester exposure and congenital anomalies. Based on a review of 29,096 Tennessee Medicaid records, 209 infants were exposed to ACE inhibitors in the first trimester with an RR for congenital malformations of 2.71 (95% CI, 1.72–4.27) compared with women not taking antihypertensive drugs. Cardiac and central nervous system anomalies were most common. In the Kaiser Northern California database, first-trimester ACE inhibitor use was associated with a higher rate of cardiac malformations compared with normal controls (adjusted OR, 1.54; 95% CI, 0.9–2.62), but not significantly higher than women with chronic hypertension with or without other medications (adjusted OR, 1.14; 95% CI, 0.65–1.98).

The task force advises against using ACE

inhibitors, angiotensin-receptor blockers, and related drug classes like renin inhibitors and mineralocorticoid receptor antagonists while pregnant based on the data that is currently available. Women of reproductive age should refrain from using these medications because half of pregnancies are unplanned. Women should be advised of the risks associated with these medications and advised to use effective contraception if they are absolutely necessary or cannot be avoided (such as in the case of proteinuric renal disease). Extensive counseling regarding the risks and benefits of continuing ACE inhibitors until conception is warranted in certain, rare cases (Williams et al., 1991).

Prevention of Superimposed Preeclampsia: Numerous dietary changes, the addition of extra vitamins, and pharmaceuticals have all been assessed in extensive randomized controlled trials aimed at preventing preeclampsia. The task force was unable to find many studies that were limited to women with chronic hypertension; nevertheless, trials involving high-risk women have included hypertensive women as a subgroup. The use of antiplatelet agents, such as low-dose aspirin, has been shown through meta-analyses and systematic reviews to be associated with a slight but statistically significant reduction (17%) in preeclampsia. A reduction of up to 25% (95% confidence interval: 34%–15%) may be experienced by women who are deemed to be at high risk, including those who have chronic hypertension. There were also minor effects (roughly a 10% reduction) on fetal outcomes (preterm birth or fetal survival). According to a different meta-analysis, starting low-dose aspirin earlier in pregnancy had more advantages. The prevention of preeclampsia through calcium supplementation has also been the subject of extensive research. A Cochrane meta-analysis of 13 studies involving over 15,000 women found that a 1 g or more calcium supplement was linked to a 50% reduction in blood pressure and the onset of preeclampsia. The largest effects were seen in high-risk women (RR = 0.22; 95% CI, 0.12–0.42) and women with low baseline calcium intake (RR = 0.36; 95% CI, 0.20–0.65) (five trials, 587 women). There was a slight decrease in preterm birth (RR, 0.76; 95% CI, 0.60–0.97) among women who were recruited to four small trials (568 women; RR, 0.45; 95% CI, 0.24–0.83) who were at high risk of developing preeclampsia. Tested preventive measures, mostly for low-risk women, have not demonstrated any improvement in maternal and fetal outcomes or a decrease in the incidence of preeclampsia.

8.1.3.6. Fetal Surveillance for Women with Chronic Hypertension

Pregnant women with chronic hypertension are more likely to experience fetal growth restriction. The incidence of SGA infants ranges from 8% to 15% in patients with mild chronic hypertension, but it can reach up to 40% in women with severe chronic hypertension. Growth-restricted fetuses have a higher chance of perinatal illness. Prenatal interventions aimed at reducing perinatal risks should ideally be made possible by the identification of fetal growth restriction. Fundal height measurement and ultrasonographic fetal weight estimation are the two main screening techniques for fetal growth restriction. Measurements of fundal height are more appropriate for women who are not at high risk of fetal growth restriction. For high-risk women, the sensitivity of fundal height measurement to identify fetal growth restriction is insufficient. Ultrasonography is the recommended screening method in pregnancies at high risk of fetal growth restriction due to maternal disease, such as hypertension. According to observational data, serial ultrasonographic measurements of the fetal weight or abdominal circumference are the most reliable indicators of fetal growth restriction. It is unknown when and how frequently exams should be performed. Ultrasonography for fetal growth is timed and performed based on the clinical situation, including the degree of hypertension, previous obstetric history, and coexisting morbidities.

Whether prenatal identification of fetal growth restriction reduces perinatal mortality is still unknown. After 24 weeks of gestation, screening with ultrasonography as opposed to not screening did not improve perinatal outcomes in a systematic review involving over 27,000 lowrisk women. There is no data available to address this issue in high-risk pregnancies. Expert opinion suggests that a 20% reduction in the stillbirth rate can be achieved through early detection and appropriate management of fetal growth restriction. Increased placental resistance and fetal vascular response can be identified prenatally by Doppler velocimetry studies of the fetoplacental unit. When a fetus has growth restriction, umbilical artery Doppler velocimetry is frequently used in conjunction with prenatal testing to determine the best time to deliver the baby. Fetal compromise is indicated by both reversed and absent end-diastolic flow. The timing of the delivery is determined by the gestational age and the degree of the umbilical artery Doppler velocimetry abnormality, in the event that it is abnormal. The use of umbilical artery Doppler testing compared with either no Doppler or nonstress test (NST) alone reduced perinatal mortality by 29% (RR, 0.71; 95% CI, 0.52–0.98) without increasing rates of induction of labor (RR, 0.89; 95% CI, 0.80–0.99) or cesarean delivery (RR, 0.92; 95% CI, 0.84–0.97) in a systematic review of 10,156 high-risk pregnancies from 18 randomized studies. The quality of the studies included in this analysis was low, and they did not only focus on patients with hypertension who did not have fetal growth restriction (Ananth et al., 1997). In high-risk pregnancies, fetal antenatal surveillance using an NST, biophysical profile (BPP), or a modified BPP may be helpful in lowering perinatal morbidity and mortality. Data regarding the best time to start prenatal testing, how often to test, and which prenatal test is most useful are lacking in patients with chronic hypertension. Pregnancy-related morbidity is frequently reduced by antepartum fetal surveillance with either, based on observational studies in populations at high risk of intrauterine fetal death. Either fetal growth restriction or superimposed preeclampsia characterizes patients with chronic hypertension who are most at risk of perinatal mortality. In 2,105 high-risk women, six randomized or quasi-randomized trials comparing NSTs with no or concealed NSTs revealed no difference in perinatal mortality (RR, 2.05; 95% CI, 0.95–4.42) or potentially preventable deaths (RR, 2.46; 95% CI, 0.96–6.30). In a systematic review of five trials involving 2,974 high-risk women, BPPs were compared with NSTs or modified BPPs; the results showed no significant difference in perinatal deaths between the groups (RR, 1.33; 95% CI, 0.60–2.98).

8.1.4. Intrapartum Management

It has not been investigated when a woman with chronic hypertension should give birth to minimize maternal and fetal morbidity and mortality, whether or not there are complications for either mother or fetus. Women with hypertensive disorders of pregnancy, such as gestational hypertension and preeclampsia, with or without preexisting hypertension, were included in the trials. Although the population affected by hypertensive disorders of pregnancy is diverse, data are frequently extrapolated to include women who have chronic hypertension. According to a small clinical trial, the risk of unfavorable perinatal outcomes is comparable for women with chronic hypertension who do not have any obstetric complications. Results from a population-based cohort study indicate that

38–39 weeks of gestation is the ideal window of time for women with simple hypertension. This gestational age group reduces neonatal morbidity and optimizes fetal outcomes when delivery occurs. An increased risk of neonatal complications and death within the first year of life is linked to late preterm birth, according to a systematic review of 22 studies involving nearly 30 million infants. Patients with isolated, uncomplicated chronic hypertension should not be delivered before 38–39 weeks of gestation unless there is a known benefit to the mother or fetus and a known risk of neonatal complications.

8.2. SUPERIMPOSED PREECLAMPSIA

Women with chronic hypertension who develop preeclampsia are said to have superimposed preeclampsia. It can be difficult to distinguish benign gestational increases in blood pressure and proteinuria, which are frequently seen in women with chronic hypertension, from superimposed preeclampsia. To raise awareness and avoid disastrous outcomes for the mother and fetus, it may be preferable to over diagnose given the increased risk of unfavorable pregnancy outcomes with superimposed preeclampsia. As an alternative, a more focused and stratified strategy based on severity and adverse outcome predictors could be helpful in directing clinical care and preventing needless preterm births.

Based on these considerations, the task force proposes that superimposed preeclampsia be stratified into two groups to guide management: (1) superimposed preeclampsia; and (2) superimposed preeclampsia with severe features. Superimposed preeclampsia is likely when any of the following are present:

- A sudden increase in BP that was previously well controlled or escalation of antihypertensive medications to control BP;
- New onset of proteinuria or a sudden increase in proteinuria in a woman with known proteinuria before or early in pregnancy.

The diagnosis of superimposed preeclampsia with severe features is established when any of the following are present:

- Severe-range BP despite the escalation of antihypertensive therapy;
- Thrombocytopenia (platelet count less than 100,000/microliter);
- Elevated liver transaminases (two times the upper limit of normal concentration for a particular laboratory);
- New-onset and worsening renal insufficiency;
- Pulmonary edema;
- Persistent cerebral or visual disturbances.

It is important for clinicians to understand that the diagnosis of superimposed preeclampsia is frequently ambiguous and that the disease's clinical spectrum is wide. Moreover, end-organ involvement and unfavorable outcomes can develop in women with superimposed preeclampsia. Therefore, even in cases where the diagnosis is suspected and not conclusive, there is a need for enhanced surveillance but not for intervention (e.g., delivery). More research is required to improve the diagnosis, possibly incorporating indicators that indicate a poor prognosis (Taguchi et al., 2008).

8.2.1. Initial Evaluation of Women with Superimposed Preeclampsia

Women who have superimposed preeclampsia should be evaluated initially in a hospital setting to verify the diagnosis, assess the condition of the mother and fetus, and keep an eye out for the disease's progressive worsening. Preeclampsia symptoms (neurologic symptoms, epigastric or right upper quadrant pain, nausea and vomiting, vaginal bleeding, and fetal movement) should be discussed during the clinical workup. Serial blood pressure readings ought to be taken. Preeclampsia symptoms and related complications should be looked for during a physical examination. A 24-hour urine collection or a protein/creatinine ratio should be used to evaluate proteinuria. A complete blood count with platelets, liver transaminases, lactic dehydrogenase, and creatinine assessment should all be part of the laboratory evaluation. Since hyperuricemia is linked to poor outcomes in superimposed preeclampsia as well as early renal dysfunction, which may be present with chronic hypertension, uric acid assessment may also be beneficial if uric acid concentrations are known from early pregnancy. It is ideal to compare these lab results with baseline data from the early stages of pregnancy. The diagnosis of end-organ involvement, hemolysis, elevated liver enzymes, and low platelet count (HELLP) syndrome, or superimposed preeclampsia can be confirmed if the abnormalities are of recent onset. Before making a final diagnosis, results should be carefully interpreted if abnormalities are long-standing or of unknown duration. Fetal growth and well-being should be evaluated when superimposed preeclampsia is suspected, even though they are not included in the diagnostic criteria. If fetal status is a concern, further testing, interventions, or both, may be necessary.

8.2.2. Antihypertensive Treatment for Superimposed Preeclampsia

Lowering blood pressure after superimposed preeclampsia is diagnosed has not been particularly addressed in clinical trials evaluating antihypertensive therapy that included women with chronic hypertension. Therefore, based on the evidence about preeclampsia and chronic hypertension in pregnancy, recommendations regarding antihypertensive treatment are derived for this group. For women with hypertension (systolic blood pressure of 160 mm Hg or higher, or diastolic blood pressure of 105 mm Hg or higher), or at even lower levels if end-organ involvement is evident, pharmacologic antihypertensive therapy should be used to prevent acute maternal cerebrovascular and coronary events.

Treatment does not appear to help reduce the risk of unfavorable perinatal outcomes in women with systolic blood pressure of 140–160 mm Hg or diastolic blood pressure of 90–105 mm Hg, but it does slow the development of severe hypertension. When superimposed preeclampsia is present, antihypertensive medication should be started or doses increased in response to worsening blood pressure; this should all happen in a hospital setting, with close monitoring for worsening maternal-fetal status. Intravenous or oral medication (intravenous labetalol, intravenous hydralazine, or oral nifedipine) can be used to lower severe hypertension acutely (Table 8.2). Initially, oral agents like methyldopa, nifedipine, or labetalol are typically used in the long-term management of blood pressure to keep levels below the severe range (Table 8.2).

8.2.3. Antepartum Management of Superimposed Preeclampsia

The administration of antenatal corticosteroids and the use of magnesium sulfate for seizure prophylaxis are general considerations in the antepartum management of women with superimposed preeclampsia. The severity of the disease and the gestational age determine the timing and ongoing management of the baby.

8.2.3.1. Antenatal Corticosteroids

Women with superimposed preeclampsia diagnosed before 37 weeks of gestation are at increased risk of preterm delivery. Therefore, antenatal corticosteroids should be administered at less than 34 weeks of gestation for fetal lung maturity benefit to decrease neonatal morbidity and mortality.

8.2.3.2. Magnesium Sulfate for Seizure Prophylaxis

Maternal mortality in the 0-1% range and significant morbidity, such as renal failure, pulmonary edema, aspiration pneumonia, stroke, and cardiopulmonary arrest, are linked to eclampsia. Additionally, there is proof of long-term maternal sequelae, including cognitive decline and the persistence of white-matter lesions. It has been demonstrated that when it comes to preventing seizures in preeclamptic women, magnesium sulfate is more effective than several other treatments.

According to observational and small retrospective studies, the frequency of eclampsia in women with superimposed preeclampsia and chronic hypertension varies from 0% to 2%. For the subgroup of women with superimposed preeclampsia, there doesn't seem to be any data that particularly addresses the use of magnesium sulfate for seizure prophylaxis at this time. Thus, management must be guided by evidence from the general preeclampsia literature. The task force advises intrapartum–postpartum parenteral magnesium sulfate to be administered to women with chronic hypertension and severe features of preeclampsia to prevent eclampsia. The task force as a whole is opposed to the use of magnesium sulfate for seizure prophylaxis during labor and delivery in this subgroup since there are no data that directly address superimposed preeclampsia without any severe features. The decision to start magnesium during labor and delivery should take into account signs and symptoms that are typically thought to be premonitory to eclampsia, such as neurologic symptoms, clonus, and pain in the right upper quadrant, as well as a worsening clinical course to severe disease (Blumenthal et al., 2010).

8.2.3.3. Timing and Indications for Delivery

The timing and indications for delivery in cases of superimposed preeclampsia depend on many factors, including gestational age, disease severity, disease progression, and continuous monitoring of the health of the mother and fetus. The possible benefits to the fetus and newborn must be balanced against the risks of maternal and fetal morbidity and mortality when attempting to extend pregnancy.

- **Gestational Age of 37 Weeks or Older:** Delivery is suggested for superimposed preeclampsia diagnosed at term (37 weeks of gestation or more). Neonatal outcomes are favorable, and continuation of pregnancy incurs risk to the woman and her fetus.
- **Gestational Age of Less Than 37 Weeks:** It makes sense to manage expectantly while closely monitoring both the mother and the fetus in the absence of severe symptoms and with a reassuring fetal status. Data to support the outpatient management of superimposed preeclampsia are scarce. If an outpatient strategy is chosen, the mother must follow her home blood pressure monitoring regimen, report any symptoms, see her doctor one or two times a week, have weekly lab tests, and have fetal surveillance. Women with superimposed preeclampsia with worsening disease, severe features, or concern for fetal well-being should be monitored as inpatients.

It is unclear whether 34 or 37 weeks of gestation is the ideal time to deliver a baby in cases of superimposed preeclampsia when there is no sign of severe features or deteriorating disease. A retrospective cohort study using a perinatal database found no difference in perinatal outcomes between preeclampsia and superimposed preeclampsia; however, there was an increased rate of cesarean delivery (46.2% versus 36.3%; P<0.001), neonatal intensive care unit admission (16.3% versus 11.4%; P<0.002), and delivery at less than 34 weeks of gestation (17.3% versus 8.7%; P<0.001). These findings raise the possibility of needless iatrogenic preterm births with superimposed preeclampsia since women with superimposed preeclampsia have a higher risk of intervention-related events and morbidity than women with preeclampsia. Preeclampsia without severe features should be delivered at 37 weeks of gestation, according to extrapolation from the general preeclampsia literature, and severe preeclampsia (which should be expectedly managed) at 34 weeks of gestation. The task force recommends treating superimposed preeclampsia with severe features like severe preeclampsia and treating superimposed preeclampsia without severe features like preeclampsia without severe features. Further studies and research are required to more clearly define the risks and benefits of continuing a pregnancy in women with superimposed preeclampsia between 34 and 37 weeks of gestation. 37 weeks of gestation is recommended for delivery if the disease has stayed stable and there is no sign of progression or severe features (Martin et al., 2010).

8.2.4. Management of Superimposed Preeclampsia with Severe Features

Before 34 weeks of gestation, there are three options for managing superimposed preeclampsia with severe features: short-term prolongation to benefit the fetus from steroids, long-term prolongation (expectant management) to increase gestational age and improve neonatal outcomes, or immediate delivery following maternal stabilization. The timing and indications for delivery are based on indirect evidence from the management of preeclampsia due to the dearth of prospective studies and clinical trials in women with superimposed preeclampsia. Severe preeclampsia is managed based on several observational studies and two large randomized trials involving 133 women. Any combination of uncontrollably high blood pressure, eclampsia, pulmonary edema, disseminated intravascular coagulation, new or worsening renal dysfunction, or both, abruptio placentae, or nonreassuring fetal status should result in an immediate delivery following maternal stabilization due to the significant morbidity that can occur to both the mother and the fetus. An attempt to attain some degree of steroid benefit and immediate delivery are not always clearly distinguished in these studies. A portion of women with severe disease may be able to postpone delivery to benefit from antenatal corticosteroid use (48 hours), given the benefits of the medication for the unborn child and some evidence in favor of expectant management of HELLP syndrome and fetal growth restriction. Thrombocytopenia, elevated liver transaminases, neurologic or epigastric pain symptoms, HELLP syndrome or partial HELLP syndrome, and fetal growth restriction are potential candidates for short-term pregnancy prolongation with close inpatient monitoring and easily accessible tertiary obstetric, neonatal, and anesthesia services. Should the mother's or the fetus's condition worsen, delivery is advised. If you want to prevent seizures, you should take parenteral magnesium sulfate.

There is little information available in the literature about managing expectant mothers who have superimposed preeclampsia and were diagnosed before 34 weeks of pregnancy to obtain the benefits of steroids after 48 hours.

Therefore, the management approach relies on the extrapolation of both direct evidence from retrospective studies of expectant management of superimposed preeclampsia and indirect evidence from the management of severe preeclampsia. In two randomized trials of severe preeclampsia at less than 34 weeks of gestation, expectant management beyond the 48 hours of antenatal corticosteroid administration was linked to a significant prolongation of pregnancy, a decrease in neonatal respiratory distress syndrome, fewer days spent in the neonatal intensive care units, and a higher birth weight with reasonable maternal safety in the expectantly managed group. If blood pressure was under control, there was no indication of severe end-organ involvement, and the fetal status was encouraging without growth restriction, then women with severe preeclampsia were candidates for expectant management.

In studies on the expectant management of preeclampsia, the subgroup of women with superimposed preeclampsia diagnosed before 34 weeks of gestation is usually excluded, and if included, their outcomes are typically not reported separately. The management of pregnant patients with superimposed preeclampsia is mentioned in prospective studies of women with chronic hypertension, but this topic is not thoroughly covered. For instance, superimposed preeclampsia was present in 22% of the 861 women with chronic hypertension who were prospectively enrolled in the Vitamins in Preeclampsia Trial, and 51% of these women gave birth before 37 weeks of gestation. An expectant management approach was likely used in at least a subset of patients with superimposed preeclampsia, as evidenced by the average antenatal inpatient stay of 7.3 days. A retrospective case series on the treatment of preeclampsia in expectant mothers focused on a subgroup of 29 women who had preeclampsia on top of it. In this series, women with superimposed preeclampsia did not differ in the rates of abruptio placentae, oliguria, or HELLP syndrome, but their latency periods were similar (8.4 days versus 8.5 days) compared to women with severe preeclampsia.

The subjects of a different retrospective review were American women who had superimposed preeclampsia and were expecting to give birth before 37 weeks of gestation but were expected to be managed beyond 48 hours to obtain steroid benefits. With a wide range of 2–34 days, the mean time from diagnosis to delivery in this series of 41 women was 9.7 days, and the median gestational age at diagnosis was 31.6 weeks. A total of 17.9 days were spent on average in the neonatal intensive care unit, with two cases of abruption placentae, one case of pulmonary edema, one case of progression to HELLP syndrome, and no perinatal deaths. The rate of adverse outcomes and latency periods appear to be similar to those seen with expectant management of preterm severe preeclampsia, despite the small sample size and numerous limitations of these studies. Based on the rationale for preterm severe preeclampsia, expectant management in hospitalized women with superimposed preeclampsia before 34 weeks of gestation seems appropriate. To calculate the risks and advantages of this strategy, prospective studies are required (Duley et al., 2013).

Inpatient management with delivery at 34 weeks of gestation is advised for women with severe features of superimposed preeclampsia undergoing expectant management before 34 weeks of gestation. The morbidity linked to severe preeclampsia and the methodology employed in randomized clinical trials serve as the foundation for this. Similar to the expectant management of severe preeclampsia, parenteral magnesium sulfate is advised during the first assessment and stabilization phase, which typically lasts for 24 hours, before expected management. Delivery should occur after the mother's condition has stabilized, just like in the case of severe preeclampsia. This also applies to superimposed preeclampsia with severe features that is newly diagnosed after 34 weeks of gestation.

8.3. MANAGEMENT OF WOMEN WITH CHRONIC HYPERTENSION IN THE POSTPARTUM PERIOD

Even if they were not treated for chronic hypertension before or during pregnancy, women with this condition typically need to be treated with antihypertensive medications in the postpartum phase. Antihypertensive drugs that are safe for breastfeeding (i.e., they typically don't get secreted into breast milk) should be prescribed because the American College of Obstetricians and Gynecologists promotes breastfeeding for all mothers and their babies. As far as the task force is aware, there are no clinical trials that concentrate on the treatment of postpartum hypertension in pregnant women who had hypertension of any kind. In the first one to two weeks after giving birth, blood pressure is typically higher in the postpartum period than it was in the antepartum period. Maintaining blood pressure within a safe range, which is less than 160 mm Hg systolic and 100 mm Hg diastolic, requires adjusting medication. When a woman has chronic hypertension—especially if she has preeclampsia on top of it—she should avoid using nonsteroidal anti-inflammatory drugs during the postpartum phase. There is a wealth of evidence showing nonsteroidal anti-inflammatory drugs raise blood pressure and cause sodium retention in non-pregnant patients. While the postpartum period has not been studied for the use of these medications, other approaches are advised (Leather et al., 1968).

If there are indications of either a recent or persistent superimposed preeclampsia, such as HELLP syndrome signs and symptoms, visual disturbances, shortness of breath, and severe headache, magnesium sulfate is recommended. Older women, have comorbid conditions (such as obesity, diabetes, or kidney disease), or whose hypertension began earlier in pregnancy may be more susceptible to persistent increases in blood pressure after giving birth. Additionally, eclampsia and unfavorable cerebrovascular events linked to pregnancy have been found to be more common in the postpartum phase. Although the contribution of blood pressure control to averting these consequences has not been thoroughly investigated, antihypertensive drugs may be taken more often during the postpartum phase, and blood pressure should be lowered if cerebral symptoms are evident. The woman should be referred to a hypertension specialist to rule out secondary causes if her postpartum hypertension persists despite taking two antihypertensive medications at appropriate doses.

8.3.1. Breastfeeding

Although the task force is not aware of any clinical trials that have evaluated either maternal or fetal outcomes in this patient population, good clinical practice suggests that women with chronic hypertension should be encouraged to breastfeed. Breast milk contains many, if not most, of the antihypertensive drug types, albeit in trace amounts. Generally speaking, medications attached to plasma proteins do not pass into breast milk. Drugs soluble in lipids have the potential to reach higher concentrations than drugs soluble in water. The levels of methyldopa in breast milk are minimal, and it is thought to be safe. Breast milk contains high concentrations of atenolol and metoprolol and low concentrations of propranolol and labetalol, among other β-blockers. Many believe that both captopril and enalapril are safe for nursing because of their low concentrations in breast milk; however, other medications are more suitable for women who need higher dosages. The presence of calcium channel blockers in breast milk has only been reported in small amounts, and no negative effects have been noted. Even though diuretics typically have a low concentration in breast milk, they can still decrease milk production and make it more difficult to breastfeed. Clinical trials assessing the effects of infants exposed to antihypertensive drugs in breast milk are not known to the task force.

8.4. ENDOCRINE CAUSES OF HYPERTENSION IN PREGNANCY

Pregnancy-related hypertension accounts for less than 1% to 2% of cases; however, certain causes of endocrine-mediated hypertension carry a nearly 30% risk of maternal and fetal death if undiagnosed and untreated. Cushing syndrome (CS) from excessive cortisol, primary aldosteronism (PA) from excess aldosterone, and pheochromocytoma and paraganglioma from excess catecholamines are examples of endocrine causes of hypertension. The elevated morbidity and mortality rates of these disorders highlight the significance of prompt diagnosis and treatment, despite their rarity.

While the importance of recognizing endocrine causes of hypertension is clear, there are many challenges to diagnosis and successful management. The physiologic changes that occur during pregnancy alter normal hormone dynamics, resulting in difficultly interpreting the biochemical assays usually used for diagnosis. Additionally, many of the preferred imaging modalities are contraindicated during pregnancy, limiting localization. Finally, typical management strategies used to treat endocrine causes of hypertension must be modified or delayed during pregnancy due to risk to the mother and the fetus. In this review, we will discuss the unique challenges of diagnosing hypertension due to excess aldosterone, cortisol or catecholamines during pregnancy and aim to provide practical insight into management strategies (Alison et al., 2020).

8.4.1. Primary Aldosteronism (PA)

With PA accounting for around 10% of all cases of secondary hypertension in the non-pregnant population, it is the most common cause of hypertension. Less than 50 instances of PA in pregnancy have been documented in the literature, despite this high prevalence. This could be because the severity of PA varies and the renin-angiotensin-aldosterone system (RAAS) undergoes numerous changes during pregnancy that complicate the diagnosis of PA. Through RAAS regulation, aldosterone keeps potassium levels in check and blood pressure stable. Renin, which is produced by the kidney in situations of perceived hypoperfusion or low tubular sodium and suppressed by hyperperfusion or elevated sodium delivery to the macula densa, is the first factor that triggers the RAAS. The first of two steps in the conversion of angiotensinogen to angiotensin II is catalyzed by renin, and angiotensin II increases the release of aldosterone from the adrenal glands zona glomerulosa. Elevated potassium levels also stimulate the kidney's aldosterone system, which increases blood volume and sodium retention while also increasing potassium excretion in the urine (Arias and Zamora, 1979).

The RAAS is activated during a typical pregnancy because of an increase in renin production from the placenta and uterus as well as an increase in angiotensinogen production in the liver. By 10 weeks of gestation, renin activity has quadrupled and reaches a plateau at 22 weeks. Due to progesterone's competitive inhibition of aldosterone at the mineralocorticoid receptor (MR) in the distal convoluted tubule and cortical collecting duct, the effect of increased aldosterone is attenuated by the end of pregnancy, when serum aldosterone can reach concentrations ten times higher than those of non-pregnant individuals. Accordingly, hypokalemia or hypertension are rarely brought on by the level of aldosterone elevation seen in a typical pregnancy (Figure 8.1).

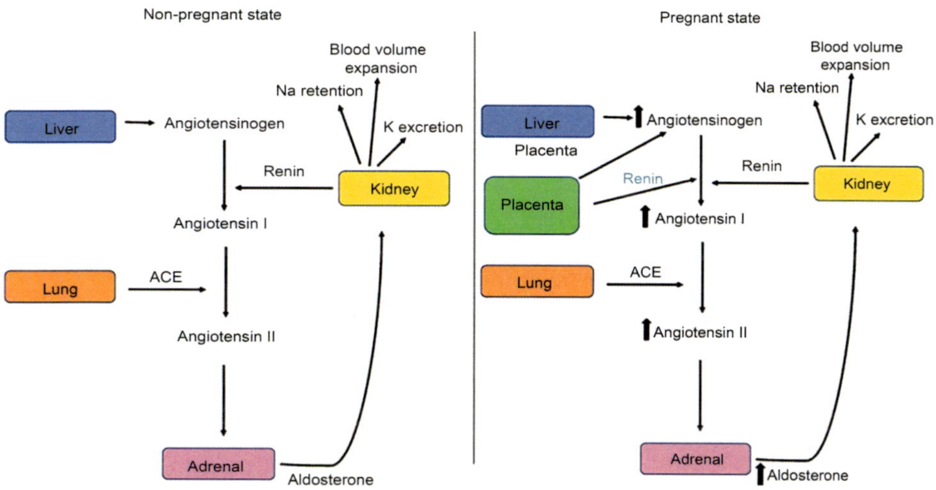

Figure 8.1. *Changes to RAAS during pregnancy. The placenta produces renin, leading to increased aldosterone, while the increased estrogen of pregnancy increases angiotensinogen production in the liver. Increased aldosterone in normal pregnancy does not lead to hypertension, although the mechanism for this is not entirely clear. RAAS, renin-angiotensin-aldosterone system; ACE, angiotensin-converting enzyme.*

Source: https://www.ncbi.nlm.nih.gov/pmc/articles/PMC7082268/.

Due to progesterone's anti-mineralocorticoid action, some patients with PA who were diagnosed before becoming pregnant showed clinical improvement. PA has a variable course during pregnancy. Severe hypertension and hyperkalemia occur in other cases. More than half of the case reports that are currently available in the literature and describe PA during pregnancy ended in a delivery before 38 weeks.

Other associated negative outcomes include intrauterine fetal demise in 9.4% of cases and intrauterine growth retardation, as well as rare instances of maternal renal failure and maternal pulmonary edema. It is unclear if PA increases the risk of pre-eclampsia, as hypertension with proteinuria is common in hyperaldosteronism. However, in one study of 35 pregnancies in patients with glucocorticoid-remediable aldosteronism (GRA), a hereditary form of PA, there was no increased risk of pre-eclampsia.

The initial stage of diagnosing PA in pregnancy involves measuring elevated aldosterone and suppressed plasma renin activity (PRA) or renin mass, just like in the non-pregnant population. Non-pregnancy reference ranges cannot be used for screening because both renin and aldosterone are elevated during pregnancy. Aldosterone and renin reference ranges during pregnancy are not established, however some have proposed that a PRA of less than 4ng/mL/h is suggestive of PA. Confirmatory testing (like salt loading), adrenal vein sampling (AVS), and/or imaging for subtype differentiation are the next steps in the diagnosis process for the non-pregnant population. Because there is a chance that confirmatory testing will exacerbate the volume expansion that has already occurred during pregnancy, it is not advised to do so. Because AVS exposes users to excessive radiation, it is not advised. These restrictions frequently cause a definitive diagnosis to be postponed until after delivery, which probably accounts for the low number of pregnancy-related PA cases that are reported.

A wide range of treatment strategies for PA during pregnancy, including no treatment, medical management and adrenalectomy. Regardless of treatment method, blood pressure control is the most critical aspect of management. The stillbirth rate in mothers with poorly controlled hypertension is 9.4%, while good fetal outcomes have been observed in cases when blood pressure is well controlled. In most cases, if good blood pressure control can be achieved, surgical evaluation and management may be postponed until after delivery (Affinati AH, Auchus, 2020).

Table 8.3. Diagnostic and Treatment Considerations for Endocrine Hypertension in Pregnancy

	Primary Aldosteronism	**Cushing syndrome**	**Pheochromocytoma**
Best diagnostic approach	Plasma aldosterone and renin measurement	Late-night salivary cortisol followed by ACTH and MRI for localization	24-h urine or plasma metanephrines followed by MRI for localization
Caveats for diagnosis in pregnancy	Confirmatory testing and AVS not recommended	DST is unreliable due to elevated cortisol, ACTH and CBG	Medications and physiologic stress may elevate catecholamines
	Elevated aldosterone may be normal	Salivary cortisol and ACTH levels may be elevated in normal pregnancy	Radionuclide imaging for localization is contra-indicated in normal pregnancy
	Renin may not be completely suppressed due to secretion by placenta and uterus	IPSS is not recommended for evaluation of CD	
Treatment	Medical management with amiloride	Surgery before 24th week gestation	Surgery before 24th week gestation
	If hypertension uncontrolled and nodule present, may consider laparoscopic adrenalectomy	Medical management with metyrapone if pre-surgical treatment is necessary or surgery is not possible	Presurgical preparation includes alpha-blockade followed by beta-blockade

Source: https://www.ncbi.nlm.nih.gov/pmc/articles/PMC7082268/.

Although spironolactone is a pregnancy risk category C medication, it is not advised as first line therapy for pregnant women with PA. Spironolactone is the preferred treatment for PA in the non-pregnant population. Results of spironolactone treatment include feminization of the male fetus and a reduction in the live birth rate in animals. Though there has been at least one case of neonatal genital ambiguity after spironolactone treatment, there have been case reports of women treated with the drug during pregnancy who gave birth to healthy male infants without deformities. Eplerenone is an additional MRA that may be used in PA, but research on animals has shown that it increases post-implantation reabsorption while decreasing fetal weight. There are no extensive human studies on the use of eplerenone during pregnancy, although there is a case report of eplerenone used in PA during pregnancy without any issues.

Rather, the recommended medication is amiloride, a potassium-sparing diuretic used in cases of MRA intolerance, because it is safe to use during pregnancy (Table 8.3). Numerous case reports exist detailing the use of amiloride to treat severe hypertension in pregnancy resulting from various etiologies, as well as hyperaldosteronism, without causing harm to the developing foetus. If there is no other viable medical treatment for hypertension, surgery might be required. Although MRI cannot differentiate between an aldosterone-producing adenoma and a non-functional (incidental) adenoma, it is the preferred imaging study in these cases to assess for an adrenal adenoma. If detected, the best course of action is to surgically remove the adenoma during the second trimester. The literature contains multiple case reports of adrenal adenoma removal that resulted in a notable improvement in hypokalemia and hypertension. Out of the six patients who had adrenalectomy, five had their hypertension under control and had an average term length of 33.07 wGA at delivery. An emergency delivery resulted in the infant's death in a patient who had resistant hypertension and documented adrenal adenoma but did not receive surgery.

8.4.2. Cushing Syndrome (CS)

Although CS in pregnancy is uncommon because high cortisol disrupts the reproductive axis, it can have a substantial negative impact on maternal and fetal health. Cushing disease (CD), a pituitary adenoma that secretes adrenocorticotropic hormone (ACTH), is the most common cause of excess cortisol in the non-pregnant population. However, CD is not commonly diagnosed during pregnancy because menstrual abnormalities result from ACTH-mediated hypersecretion of adrenal androgens. About half of all cases of CS in pregnancy are caused by adrenal adenoma, 30% by CD, and 1-3% by ectopic ACTH syndrome, which is usually connected to cancer. Furthermore, hypercortisolism caused by pregnancy accounts for 13% of cases of CS. This condition is primarily brought on by aberrantly high expression of the luteinizing hormone/chorionic gonadotropin (LH/CG) receptor on an adrenal adenoma, or less frequently, throughout the adrenal glands. This leads to an excess of cortisol when the elevated human CG of pregnancy stimulates these receptors (Pickard et al., 1990).

It is critical to identify cortisol excess because untreated CS during pregnancy has serious repercussions. Among patients without treatment, 40.5% have hypertension, while in patients with cured CS, the percentage is 2.3%. Similar increases are seen in the rates of pre-eclampsia (26.3%) and diabetes mellitus (369.9%). Rarely, serious mental health issues, infections from cuts, osteoporosis, and heart failure can occur. The risk of fetal loss is predicted by the etiology of CS, with pregnancy-induced CS and ectopic ACTH production increasing the risk of fetal loss by three to four times compared to CD. In CD, spontaneous abortion or stillbirth occurs in 17% of pregnancies, and the rate of preterm delivery is 33%.

Because the symptoms of cortisol excess and normal pregnancy overlap, clinical recognition of CS may be delayed during pregnancy. Pregnancy frequently brings on the typical CS symptoms of weight gain, striae, round faces, and glucose intolerance. Further research should be done if CS exhibits more particular symptoms that are uncommon during pregnancy. These include virilization, poor wound healing, ecchymoses, proximal myopathy, purple (not flesh-toned) striae wider than 1 cm, especially if outside the abdomen, such as the breast and axilla; and neuropsychiatric symptoms. As with PA, diagnosis of CS can be difficult due to the changes in the hypothalamic-pituitary-adrenal (HPA) axis that occur during pregnancy. Hypothalamic corticotropin releasing hormone (CRH) stimulates pituitary ACTH production, which then drives cortisol secretion from the adrenal gland. Cortisol is then transported to the peripheral tissues bound to corticosteroid-binding globulin (CBG). Pregnancy results in alterations to each of these components.

The placenta secretes CRH during pregnancy, which raises the amount of CRH in the bloodstream overall. Additionally, during pregnancy, ACTH rises and peaks at delivery. Elevated estrogen levels cause CBG to become more glycosylated, which inhibits CBG cleavage and causes concentrations to increase two to three times. The overall levels of cortisol in the serum rise as a result. These modifications have an impact on the widely used CS screening exams (Figure 8.2).

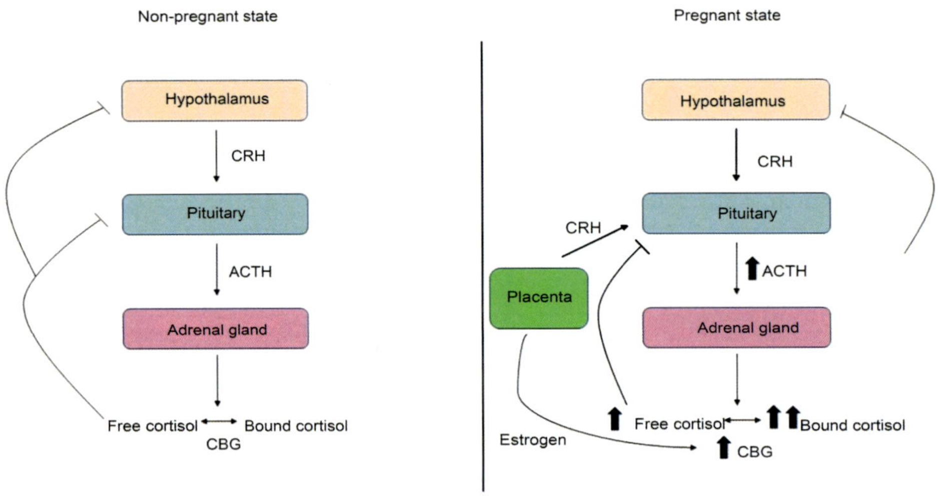

Figure 8.2. *Changes to HPA axis during pregnancy. The placenta produces CRH, increasing ACTH and cortisol levels. Elevated estrogen concentration during pregnancy increases CBG levels and increases the proportion of bound cortisol to free cortisol. CRH, corticotropin releasing hormone; ACTH, adrenocorticotropic hormone; CBG, corticosteroid-binding globulin; HPA, hypothalamic-pituitary-adrenal.*

Source: *https://www.ncbi.nlm.nih.gov/pmc/articles/PMC7082268/.*

The dexamethasone suppression test (DST), late-night salivary cortisol measurement, and 24-hour urine free cortisol (UFC) measurement are screening tests for CS in the non-pregnant population. The UFC exhibits predictable changes during pregnancy and has been used extensively in the literature. UFC usually increases 1–6 times during the second and third trimesters; therefore, CS should not be diagnosed unless the UFC is at least 2-3 times the upper limit of normal. Salivary cortisol concentrations reflect plasma free cortisol values and avoid the influence of elevated CBG on serum total cortisol measurements because saliva is an ultrafiltrate of plasma. The use of late-night salivary cortisol to diagnose CS during pregnancy has been documented in many case reports; however, there is disagreement over the diagnostic cut-off values. According to some reports, salivary cortisol levels during pregnancy do not change significantly, and normal adult levels can be used. A detailed analysis of these studies indicates that salivary cortisol levels in pregnant women vary widely, with some exhibiting elevated levels even in the absence of clinical hypercortisolism. Other authors have suggested that normal values in pregnant women are <6.9 nmol/L in the first trimester, <7.2 nmol/L in the second trimester, and <9.1 nmol/L in the third trimester. Based on these data and similar studies, these values have been shown to produce specificities ranging from 80% to 92%.

The circadian rhythm of cortisol, which peaks in the early morning and falls in the late evening, is preserved during the first and second trimesters of pregnancy but is lost or attenuated in convulsions. To rule out CS, early studies recommended measuring salivary cortisol in the AM and PM and dropping it by 50% from morning to evening. However, this strategy has not been applied in the more recent literature. Following exposure to dexamethasone, which is expected to suppress ACTH and cause low serum cortisol, the DST measures the levels of cortisol in the serum. Pregnant patients should refrain from taking the DST because the elevated CBG causes elevated serum cortisol levels regardless of free cortisol levels, which makes it challenging to interpret incomplete cortisol suppression. This dynamic test of adrenal function is further complicated by the fact that ACTH is also more difficult to suppress during pregnancy, possibly as a result of placental CRH production (Fardella et al., 2000).

After hypercortisolism has been identified, figuring out its cause is essential to administering the right care. CS can be classified as either ACTH-independent (usually of adrenal origin) or ACTH-dependent (caused by pituitary disease or ectopic ACTH expression). Because placental CRH and ACTH can result in elevated ACTH levels even in patients with adrenal CS, differentiating between these two during pregnancy may also be difficult. When there is an elevated cortisol level, ACTH levels over 35 pg/mL generally indicate an ACTH-dependent source of cortisol excess, whereas ACTH levels under 5 pg/mL are consistent with adrenal cortisol surplus. Several dynamic confirmatory tests that are commonly used for patients who are not pregnant have not been thoroughly studied during pregnancy and are therefore not advised.

The recommended imaging test for CS with elevated ACTH is sella MRI. Pregnancy causes the pituitary gland to enlarge, so this must be taken into account when analyzing pituitary MRI results. Most corticotrope adenomas that cause CD are tiny (<5 mm) and frequently do not change the pituitary's geometry. Rather, these tumors are usually detected by low enhancement after gadolinium contrast is administered as opposed to the normal gland. Sadly, pregnant women must avoid gadolinium contrast, which significantly reduces the sensitivity of sella MRI in detecting CD tumors. Although CD can be confirmed in the non-pregnant population with inferior petrosal sinus sampling (IPSS), pregnant women usually avoid this procedure because of the high radiation risk. Although IPSS techniques have been reported to reduce fetal radiation exposure, the results of these treatments have not been good for the fetus. The recommended imaging studies for adrenal CS are adrenal MRI without contrast and abdominal ultrasonography (Rossi et al., 2006).

Treatment for pituitary and adrenal CS can be achieved safely and effectively through surgical management. Whatever the method, the operation must be carried out in the second trimester, ideally before the 24th week of pregnancy. Preterm birth risk has been found to be higher in certain reports involving third trimester surgery, which may be related to the procedure itself or the extended duration of hypercortisolism. The genesis of CS determines the best surgical approach; unilateral adrenalectomy is recommended for adrenal adenoma. Bilateral adrenalectomy, which leaves patients with permanent adrenal insufficiency, is the most effective treatment for pregnancy-induced CS in the absence of a discrete adenoma. There has been prior review of specific surgical considerations for these procedures in pregnant women.

Medical treatment has been reported to have varying degrees of success in situations where surgical management is either not possible or cannot be delayed. Metyrapone is the drug most frequently used to control CS during pregnancy. Metyrapone has been administered without causing birth defects during the first trimester before surgery as well as the whole pregnancy. Metyrapone's availability and cost may restrict its use. Metyrapone has occasionally been linked to elevated blood pressure, most likely as a result of increased levels of 11-deoxycorticosterone, a steroid intermediate that functions as a mineralocorticoid agonist. Only one or two cases each of the use of other medications, such as ketoconazole, mitotane, and cabergoline, have been documented. The teratogenicity of these drugs has generally led to their avoidance. Due to its concurrent progesterone antagonistic action, mifepristone, a glucocorticoid antagonist used in CS in the non-pregnant population, should be avoided. This is the rationale behind its use as an abortificant.

Maternal and fetal outcomes improve with treatment for CS. In comparison to women whose CS was not treated, the odds ratio for fetal loss was 0.25–0.34 for those with treated CS. Patients with active CS have much higher rates of gestational diabetes, gestational hypertension, preeclampsia, and cesarean sections than patients with cured CS, whose rates are more in line with those of the general population. Although both surgical and medical options have been reported, there is no consensus regarding the optimal treatment strategy due to the condition's rarity and the variety of strategies employed in the literature.

8.4.3. Pheochromocytoma and Paraganglioma

Catecholamine excess can be caused by paraganglioma (originating from sympathetic ganglia) or pheochromocytoma (originating from the chromaffin cells in the adrenal gland). Pregnancy-related pheochromocytoma and paraganglioma incidences are estimated to be 1 in 15,000 to 45,000; however, the repercussions of an undiagnosed case can be catastrophic for the mother and the fetus. Strong vasoconstrictors, catecholamines also improve cardiac contractility. Therefore, serious cardiovascular consequences may result from failing to diagnose these tumors before delivery. If the tumor was not discovered before delivery, the rates of maternal and fetal death in the earliest pheochromocytoma studies (before the 1970s) were 48% and 54%, respectively. The associated mortality rates significantly dropped to 5% and 15% if diagnosed before term. According to more recent research, if the tumor is discovered early on, there is a 100% chance of maternal survival; however, if it is not identified, the death rate remains at 29%. The cause of death is hypertensive crisis, which results in shock, arrhythmias, cardiomyopathy, acute coronary syndrome, and stroke (Keely, 1998).

Due to the disease's rarity and vague symptoms, diagnosing pheochromocytomas and paragangliomas before delivery may be challenging. Hypertension is frequently linked to pre-eclampsia or gestational hypertension. Given that an inherited genetic mutation accounts for nearly 40% of paraganglioma cases, a thorough family history can raise suspicions. Genetic tumor syndromes frequently include phenochromocytoma. Paradoxical hypertension, orthostatic hypotension, palpitations, dizziness, and hypertension without proteinuria or ankle edema are other related symptoms. The diagnosis of pheochromocytoma or paraganglioma is not ruled out in the presence of persistent hypertension, as these conditions can cause paroxysmal or continuous hypertension.

Catecholamine levels remain constant throughout a healthy pregnancy, with the exception of the start of labor and the second postpartum day. Hospitalized pre-eclamptic patients have elevated urinary catecholamine levels by 1 to 2.6; however, plasma catecholamine levels typically remain normal or lower. When pheochromocytomas and paragangliomas are present, the body continuously produces metabolites of epinephrine and norepinephrine, which are normetanephrine and methenephrine, respectively. These tumors are best diagnosed in non-pregnant patients as well as during pregnancy. The diagnosis can be established using either plasma or 24-hour urine metanephrine testing. Due to its excellent specificity of 97.5%, plasma metanephrine is preferred in patients for whom there is a high degree of suspicion. The diagnosis is essentially ruled out if it is negative.

Like in the non-pregnant population, false positive elevations in catecholamine and metanephrine measurements are frequent and can be brought on by medications that interfere with normal functioning or by incorrect sample collection. Tandem mass spectrometry (LC-MS/MS) assays can be used to resolve interference caused by labetalol and methyldopa, which are commonly used for hypertension in pregnancy. These drugs can cause falsely elevated catecholamines and metanephrines when measured by older liquid chromatography assays. Tricyclic antidepressants are among the drugs that can also result in a slight physiological increase in catecholamines and metanephrines. When measuring plasma catecholamines or metanephrine levels, it is optimal to have the patient in the supine position. This is because sitting upright without having first had supine rest can result in a 30% increase in plasma metanephrine levels. Provocative testing is not recommended during pregnancy due to potential risks to the developing foetus, although it can be used on non-pregnant patients (e.g., the clonidine suppression test).

Similar to the non-pregnant population, false positive elevations in measurements of catecholamines and metanephrine are frequent and can be caused by medications that interfere with normal functioning or by incorrectly collected samples. When measured by older liquid chromatography assays, labetalol and methyldopa, which are commonly used for hypertension in pregnancy, can cause falsely elevated catecholamines and metanephrines. This interference can be eliminated, though, by employing tandem mass spectrometry (LC-MS/MS) assays. Certain drugs, like tricyclic antidepressants, can also result in a slight physiological increase in catecholamines and metanephrines. The ideal way to measure plasma catecholamines or metanephrine levels in a patient is in a supine position. This is because sitting upright without first having a supine rest can cause a 30% increase in plasma metanephrine levels. Provocative testing, like the clonidine suppression test, is safe to use in non-pregnant patients but should not be administered to pregnant women due to potential risks to the developing foetus (Wilson et al., 1980).

Once a biochemical diagnosis of catecholamine excess due to a pheochromocytoma or paraganglioma is made, imaging is required for localization. Radionuclide imaging agents such as [^{123}I]- or [^{131}I]-metaiodobenzylguanidine (MIBG) or [^{68}Ga]-DOTATATE are contra-indicated during pregnancy, and so ultrasound and MRI without contrast are the preferred imaging studies. While abdominal ultrasound is safe and accessible, it often misses small lesions, and visualization might be compromised by the gravid uterus in the third trimester. Unlike aldosterone-producing adenomas, symptomatic pheochromocytomas are typically several cm wide and have well-defined imaging characteristics, such as no signal loss on out-of-phase images and high signal on T2-weighted images. Consequently, MRI has sensitivity of 100% in lesions that are greater than 1.5 cm. Biopsy is contra-indicated due to concern that a catecholamine surge may initiate a hypertensive crisis.

The best course of treatment, once the pheochromocytoma or paraganglioma has been identified, is surgery. A multidisciplinary team, comprising skilled surgeons and anesthesiologists, is needed for surgical planning. According to the research that is currently available, surgical resection should either take place before 24 weeks of pregnancy or wait until delivery. Cesarean delivery with concurrent tumor removal is the recommended delivery method if surgery cannot be completed before 24 weeks.

Patients need to be pre-operatively prepared pharmacologically to avoid cardiovascular collapse from the massive release of catecholamines during surgery. The cornerstone of pre-operative care is doxazosin or phenoxybenzamine alpha-blockade. Although the safety of these drugs has not been thoroughly studied in pregnant patients, the advantages of treatment exceed the hazards. Fetal mortality decreases from 55% to 6% and maternal mortality drops from 95% to 0% with appropriate alpha blockade. Doxazosin and phenoxybenzamine both pass through the placenta. While doxazosin has not been linked to adverse fetal outcomes, phenoxybenzamine, which unlike doxazosin irreversibly blocks the alpha receptors, has been linked to neonatal hypotension and respiratory distress. To treat the tachycardia that may result from using alpha-blockade alone, beta-blockade is frequently required in addition to alpha-blockade. Labetalol, which offers both alpha- and beta-blockade, can be used during pregnancy; however, it is best to start labetalol a few days after starting alpha-blocking medication. Alpha-blockade may worsen orthostatic hypotension in patients with paragangliomas and pheochromocytomas, who are volume-contracted and may require aggressive hydration (Eguchi et al., 2014).

A Closer Look

Diabetes and Pregnancy

Diabetes during pregnancy, encompassing both pregestational diabetes (pre-existing type 1 or type 2 diabetes) and gestational diabetes mellitus (GDM), presents significant health challenges for both the mother and the developing fetus. Pregestational diabetes involves women who already have diabetes before becoming pregnant, while GDM refers to diabetes that is first diagnosed during pregnancy, typically manifesting in the second or third trimester. The prevalence of diabetes in pregnancy is rising globally, mirroring the increasing rates of obesity and type 2 diabetes. This condition necessitates careful management to mitigate risks such as congenital anomalies, preeclampsia, preterm birth, and macrosomia (large birth weight), which can lead to complications like shoulder dystocia during delivery.

Women with pregestational diabetes face the dual challenge of managing their condition while adapting to the physiological changes of pregnancy, which can exacerbate glycemic instability. Elevated blood glucose levels during the first trimester are particularly concerning, as they are associated with a higher risk of congenital malformations, including neural tube defects and cardiac anomalies. Strict glycemic control before and during early pregnancy is crucial to minimize these risks. Additionally, these women are at higher risk for diabetic ketoacidosis, hypertensive disorders, and progression of diabetes-related complications such as retinopathy and nephropathy. Continuous glucose monitoring and frequent insulin dose adjustments are often required to maintain optimal blood sugar levels.

Gestational diabetes, which affects about 7-10% of pregnancies worldwide, is diagnosed through glucose tolerance tests typically conducted between 24 and 28 weeks of gestation. Risk factors for GDM include obesity, advanced maternal age, a family history of diabetes, and certain ethnic backgrounds. GDM results from a combination of insulin resistance, which naturally increases during pregnancy, and an inadequate insulin response. If not properly managed, GDM can lead to adverse outcomes such as fetal overgrowth, increased cesarean delivery rates, neonatal hypoglycemia, and a higher likelihood of developing type 2 diabetes later in life for both the mother and child.

Management of diabetes in pregnancy requires a multidisciplinary approach involving obstetricians, endocrinologists, dietitians, and diabetes educators. For women with pregestational diabetes, preconception counseling and optimization of glycemic control are paramount. During pregnancy, treatment goals include maintaining blood glucose levels within target ranges, monitoring for complications, and adjusting treatment as necessary. Insulin therapy is commonly used, as it does not cross the placenta and allows for precise control of blood glucose levels. For women with GDM, lifestyle modifications such as dietary changes and increased physical activity are first-line treatments. If these measures are insufficient, insulin or oral hypoglycemic agents may be prescribed.

Regular monitoring of fetal growth and maternal health is essential. Ultrasound assessments help in detecting macrosomia and monitoring amniotic fluid levels, while non-stress tests and biophysical profiles evaluate fetal well-being. Postpartum, women with GDM should be re-evaluated for glucose intolerance and provided with counseling on lifestyle changes to reduce the risk of developing type 2 diabetes. Long-term follow-up is important for both mothers and their offspring, who are at increased risk of metabolic disorders. Effective management of diabetes during pregnancy is crucial for ensuring favorable outcomes and minimizing risks, thereby supporting the health and well-being of both mother and child.

Summary

- Hypertensive disorders during pregnancy may result in substantial short-term maternal morbidity ranging from 10-15% worldwide whereas chronic hypertension and an increase in lifetime cardiovascular risk as to the long-term consequences.
- Medical treatment of chronic hypertension in pregnancy, that is, hypertension present before 20 weeks' gestation, is recommended at 160 mm Hg systolic or 110 mm Hg diastolic with labetalol or extended-release nifedipine, treating to 120 to 159 mm Hg systolic and 80 to 109 mm Hg diastolic.
- Low-dose aspirin is recommended in patients with chronic hypertension in pregnancy from between 12 and 28 weeks' gestation to delivery.
- Blood pressure control in pregnancy is challenging because of the uncertain risks of mild hypertension and potential uteroplacental insufficiency with overtreatment. Pregnant women with chronic hypertension should start antihypertensive medication when their blood pressure reaches 160 mm Hg systolic or 110 mm Hg diastolic, although it may be initiated earlier if the patient has concerning comorbidities or impaired renal function.
- Women with chronic hypertension should undergo an evaluation before becoming pregnant to evaluate for end-organ damage or comorbidities that will need to be managed before and during the pregnancy. It also may be beneficial to assess for secondary hypertension, which occurs in 11% to 14% of pregnant women with chronic hypertension.
- Fetal growth restriction is more frequent with chronic hypertension and is usually associated with superimposed preeclampsia. Another risk associated with chronic hypertension in pregnancy is the exposure to antihypertensive medications in utero that may cause growth restriction and fetal malformations; this has been extensively evaluated.
- The risk of fetal growth restriction is higher in pregnant women with chronic hypertension. In patients with mild chronic hypertension, the incidence of SGA infants is 8–15.5%, but in women with severe chronic hypertension, the incidence may be as high as 40%.
- Clinical trials that have evaluated antihypertensive therapy that included women with chronic hypertension have not specifically addressed lowering BP once the diagnosis of superimposed preeclampsia is established.
- Eclampsia is associated with maternal mortality in the range of 0.3–1% and serious morbidity, including renal failure, pulmonary edema, aspiration pneumonia, stroke, and cardiopulmonary arrest.
- Women with chronic hypertension before and during pregnancy will usually require treatment with antihypertensive medications in the postpartum period, even if they were not treated during pregnancy.
- Good clinical practice suggests that women with chronic hypertension should be encouraged to breastfeed, although the task force is not aware of clinical trials that have assessed either maternal or fetal outcomes in this patient population.

- PA has a variable course during pregnancy, with some patients diagnosed before pregnancy demonstrating clinical improvement due to the anti-mineralocorticoid activity of progesterone.
- Catecholamine excess can occur either due to pheochromocytoma, which arises from the chromaffin cells in the adrenal gland, or due to paraganglioma, which arises from sympathetic ganglia.

References

1. Affinati, A. H., & Auchus, R. J. (2020). Endocrine causes of hypertension in pregnancy. *Gland Surgery, 9*(1), 69–79. https://doi.org/10.21037/gs.2019.11.01.
2. Ananth, C. V., Savitz, D. A., Bowes, W. A. Jr., & Luther, E. R. (1997). Influence of hypertensive disorders and cigarette smoking on placental abruption and uterine bleeding during pregnancy. *British Journal of Obstetrics and Gynaecology, 104*(5), 572–578. https://doi.org/10.1111/j.1471-0528.1997.tb11523.x.
3. Arias, F., & Zamora, J. (1979). Antihypertensive treatment and pregnancy outcome in patients with mild chronic hypertension. *Obstetrics & Gynecology, 53*(4), 489–494.
4. Blumenthal, J. A., Babyak, M. A., Sherwood, A., Craighead, L., Lin, P. H., Johnson, J., et al. (2010). Effects of the dietary approaches to stop hypertension diet alone and in combination with exercise and caloric restriction on insulin sensitivity and lipids. *Hypertension, 55*(5), 1199–1205. https://doi.org/10.1161/HYPERTENSIONAHA.109.149153.
5. Duley, L., Meher, S., & Jones, L. (2013). Drugs for treatment of very high blood pressure during pregnancy. *Cochrane Database of Systematic Reviews, 2013*(7), CD001449. https://doi.org/10.1002/14651858.CD001449.pub3.
6. Eguchi, K., Hoshide, S., Nagashima, S., et al. (2014). An adverse pregnancy-associated outcome due to overlooked primary aldosteronism. *Internal Medicine, 53*(23), 2499–2504. https://doi.org/10.2169/internalmedicine.53.2762.
7. Fardella, C. E., Mosso, L., Gómez-Sánchez, C., et al. (2000). Primary hyperaldosteronism in essential hypertensives: Prevalence, biochemical profile, and molecular biology. *Journal of Clinical Endocrinology & Metabolism, 85*(5), 1863–1867. https://doi.org/10.1210/jcem.85.5.6563.
8. Ferrer, R. L., Sibai, B. M., Mulrow, C. D., Chiquette, E., Stevens, K. R., & Cornell, J. (2000). Management of mild chronic hypertension during pregnancy: A review. *Obstetrics & Gynecology, 96*(5), 849–860. https://doi.org/10.1016/S0029-7844(00)01012-0.
9. Keely, E. (1998). Endocrine causes of hypertension in pregnancy: When to start looking for zebras. *Seminars in Perinatology, 22*(6), 471–484. https://doi.org/10.1016/S0146-0005(98)80027-X.
10. Lawler, J., Osman, M., Shelton, J. A., & Yeh, J. (2007). Population-based analysis of hypertensive disorders in pregnancy. *Hypertension in Pregnancy, 26*(1), 67–76. https://doi.org/10.1080/10641950601147912.
11. Leather, H. M., Humphreys, D. M., Baker, P., & Chadd, M. A. (1968). A controlled trial of hypotensive agents in hypertension in pregnancy. *Lancet, 292*(7564), 488–490. https://doi.org/10.1016/S0140-6736(68)90252-9.

12. Martin, C. L., & Brunner Huber, L. R. (2010). Physical activity and hypertensive complications during pregnancy: Findings from 2004 to 2006 North Carolina Pregnancy Risk Assessment Monitoring System. *Birth, 37*(3), 202–210. https://doi.org/10.1111/j.1523-536X.2010.00407.x.

13. Pickard, J., Jochen, A. L., Sadur, C. N., et al. (1990). Cushing's syndrome in pregnancy. *Obstetrical & Gynecological Survey, 45*(2), 87–93. https://doi.org/10.1097/00006254-199002000-00002.

14. Rey, E., & Couturier, A. (1994). The prognosis of pregnancy in women with chronic hypertension. *American Journal of Obstetrics & Gynecology, 171*(2), 410–416. https://doi.org/10.1016/0002-9378(94)90053-1.

15. Rossi, G. P., Bernini, G., Caliumi, C., et al. (2006). A prospective study of the prevalence of primary aldosteronism in 1,125 hypertensive patients. *Journal of the American College of Cardiology, 48*(11), 2293–2300. https://doi.org/10.1016/j.jacc.2006.07.059.

16. Sibai, B. M. (2002). Chronic hypertension in pregnancy. *Obstetrics & Gynecology, 100*(2), 369–377. https://doi.org/10.1016/S0029-7844(02)02137-3.

17. Sibai, B. M., & Stella, C. L. (2009). Diagnosis and management of atypical preeclampsia-eclampsia. *American Journal of Obstetrics & Gynecology, 200*(5), 481.e1–481.e7. https://doi.org/10.1016/j.ajog.2008.07.048.

18. Sibai, B. M., Lindheimer, M., Hauth, J., Caritis, S., VanDorsten, P., Klebanoff, M., et al. (1998). Risk factors for preeclampsia, abruptio placentae, and adverse neonatal outcomes among women with chronic hypertension. *The New England Journal of Medicine, 339*(10), 667–671. https://doi.org/10.1056/NEJM199809033391003.

19. Taguchi, N., Rubin, E. T., Hosokawa, A., Choi, J., Ying, A. Y., Moretti, M. E., et al. (2008). Prenatal exposure to HMG-CoA reductase inhibitors: Effects on fetal and neonatal outcomes. *Reproductive Toxicology, 26*(2), 175–177. https://doi.org/10.1016/j.reprotox.2008.08.009.

20. Vanek, M., Sheiner, E., Levy, A., & Mazor, M. (2004). Chronic hypertension and the risk for adverse pregnancy outcome after superimposed pre-eclampsia. *International Journal of Gynaecology and Obstetrics, 86*(1), 7–11. https://doi.org/10.1016/j.ijgo.2004.02.008.

21. Williams, M. A., Mittendorf, R., & Monson, R. R. (1991). Chronic hypertension, cigarette smoking, and abruptio placentae. *Epidemiology, 2*(6), 450–453. https://doi.org/10.1097/00001648-199111000-00006.

22. Wilson, M., Morganti, A. A., Zervoudakis, I., et al. (1980). Blood pressure, the renin-aldosterone system, and sex steroids throughout normal pregnancy. *American Journal of Medicine, 68*(1), 97–104. https://doi.org/10.1016/0002-9343(80)90178-3.

23. Zetterstrom, K., Lindeberg, S. N., Haglund, B., & Hanson, U. (2005). Maternal complications in women with chronic hypertension: A population-based cohort study. *Acta Obstetricia et Gynecologica Scandinavica, 84*(5), 419–424. https://doi.org/10.1111/j.0001-6349.2005.00610.x.

Chapter 9

IMAGING FOR PATIENTS WITH ENDOCRINE HYPERTENSION

Contents

INTRODUCTION

Disorders of the adrenal gland, such as primary aldosteronism, glucocorticoid excess, and the pheochromocytoma-paraganglioma syndromes, are commonly associated with endocrine hypertension. Hypertension can also result from uncommon conditions in individuals with glucocorticoid resistance (Chrousos syndrome) and congenital adrenal hyperplasia. Hypertension is also associated with nonadrenal endocrine disorders, including growth hormone excess or deficiency, thyroid dysfunction, primary hyperparathyroidism, testosterone deficiency, poor vitamin D intake, obesity-related hypertension, insulin resistance, and metabolic syndrome (Smith and Vale, 2006).

Because of the overproduction of hormones by different endocrine glands, endocrine hypertension makes up about 3% of secondary hypertension. The fact that endocrine or hormone-mediated hypertension has a known cause and is typically treatable with surgery makes it significant. There may be a full recovery from the surgery, negating the need for ongoing antihypertensive medication. In determining whether hypertension is primary or essential, imaging has very little bearing. Imaging is clearly necessary for patients with secondary hypertension, and it may play a crucial role in clinical decision-making. Furthermore, the secondary form of hypertension is more common in younger age groups. For this reason, it is wise to pursue diagnostic imaging in young hypertensive patients.

Imaging of hypertension is changing paradigmatically with the introduction of more advanced diagnostic imaging techniques. The pituitary, thyroid, and adrenal glands can all be examined using nuclear medicine imaging techniques, magnetic resonance imaging (MRI), and computed tomography (CT). Imaging is required in the problematic case where endocrine hypertension appears to be a possibility based on clinical and laboratory data.

Orientation and Directional Terms

Term	Definition	Illustration
Magnetic resonance imaging	Magnetic resonance imaging, or MRI, is a noninvasive medical imaging test that produces detailed images of almost every internal structure in the human body, including the organs, bones, muscles and blood vessels. MRI scanners create images of the body using a large magnet and radio waves.	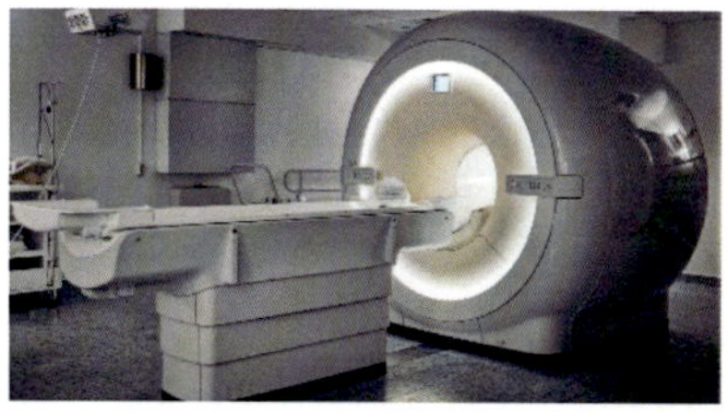
Scintigraphy	Scintigraphy is a diagnostic test in nuclear medicine, where radioisotopes attached to drugs that travel to a specific organ or tissue (radiopharmaceuticals) are taken internally and the emitted gamma radiation is captured by gamma cameras, which are external detectors that form two-dimensional images in a process similar to the capture of x-ray images.	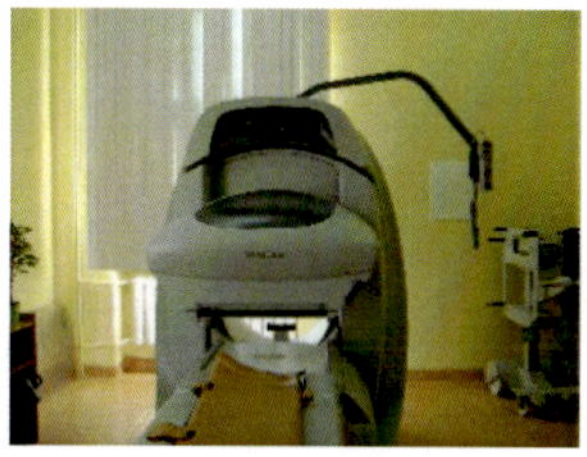
Pheochromocytoma	A pheochromocytoma is a tumor in the adrenal gland. It causes the gland to make too much of the hormones epinephrine and norepinephrine. This tumor often occurs when you are in your 30s, 40s, or 50s. It happens to both men and women.	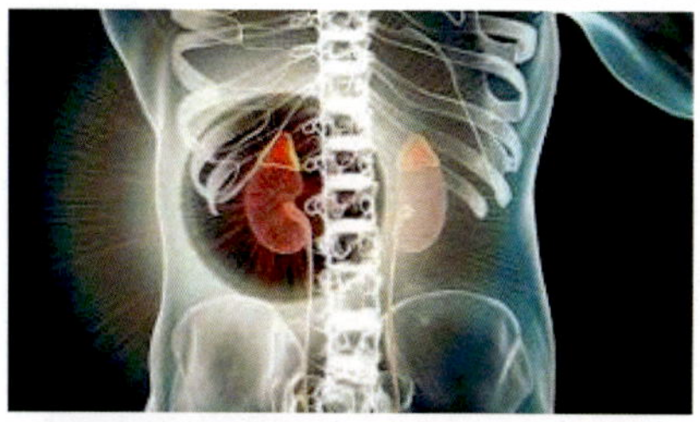
Neurofibromatosis type 1	Neurofibromatosis type 1 (NF1) is a genetic condition that causes tumours to grow along your nerves. The tumours are usually non-cancerous (benign) but may cause a range of symptoms. Neurofibromatosis type 2 (NF2) is much less common than NF1. It is covered separately as it has different symptoms and causes.	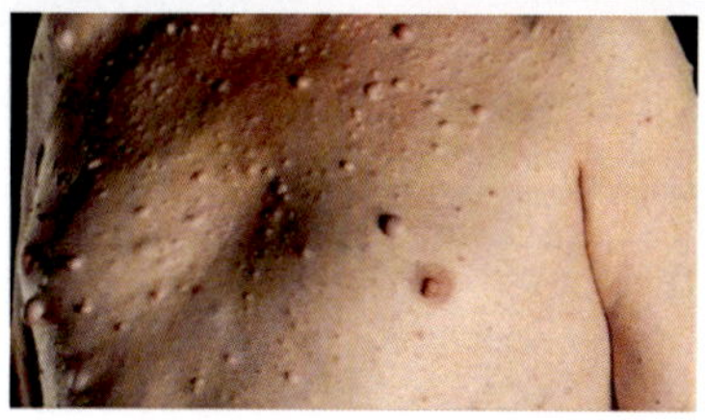

9.1. IMAGING IN THE CAUSES OF SECONDARY HYPERTENSION: UNVEILING THE HIDDEN CULPRITS

About 10% of all cases of hypertension are classified as secondary hypertension, which is defined as hypertension with a particular underlying cause. Endocrine and nonendocrine causes of secondary hypertension can be further separated. Acute elevation of blood pressure in a patient under 30 years of age, accelerated hypertension resulting in end-organ damage, or the onset of hypertension in a patient under 30 years of age are indicators of secondary hypertension. Imaging is essential to the assessment of a patient with hypertension because it helps diagnose the majority of secondary hypertension cases, evaluates its consequences, and determines how much strain it puts on the heart and large blood vessels (Figure 9.1) (Newell-Price, 2009).

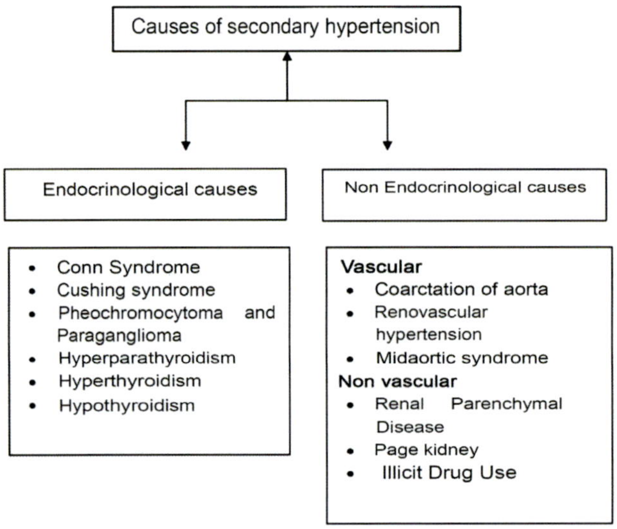

Figure 9.1. *Common causes of secondary hypertension.*

Source: Gopinath Periaswamy, et al., Imaging in the Causes of Secondary Hypertension: Unveiling the Hidden Culprits, DOI https://doi.org/ 10.1055/s-0044-1782596.

9.1.1. Endocrinological Causes of Secondary Hypertension

Roughly 3% of cases of secondary hypertension are caused by endocrinological factors. These can usually be treated and are characterized by an increase in hormone output. The initial clinical sign of many endocrine disorders can be hypertension. Endocrine hypertension is most common in children and young adults under 40 years of age. Diseases of the pituitary gland, adrenal glands, or sympathetic and parasympathetic ganglia that run from the base of the skull to the pelvis can all be the cause of this condition.

9.1.1.1. Conn Syndrome

The most common cause of secondary hypertension is primary hyperaldosteronism, also known as Conn syndrome, which is characterized by increased autonomous aldosterone production without renin-angiotensin-aldosterone axis activation. It is commonly observed in cases of hyperplasia and adrenal adenoma. Less common causes include ectopic aldosterone production (from an ovarian or renal source), familial hyperaldosteronism syndrome, and adrenal cortical cancer (Walther et al., 1999).

A high aldosterone-to-renin ratio, hypokalemia, and a blood sodium level greater than 140 mEq/L are found in laboratory testing results. Oval or round masses with an average attenuation value of 10 Hounsfield units (HU) or less in non-enhanced CT, which has a high sensitivity and specificity of 79 and 96%, respectively, are imaging features of adrenal adenoma in computed tomography (CT). Additional features that set contrast-enhanced CT apart include absolute washout of 60% or greater and relative washout of 40% or more. Where HU1min is the attenuation value at one minute, HU_{15minD} is the attenuation value at fifteen minutes at the delayed phase, and HUnon is the attenuation value at nonenhanced CT, the absolute washout is defined as $[(HU_{1min} - HU_{15minD})/(HU_{1min} - H_{Unon})] \times 100$, and the relative washout is defined as $[(HU_{1min} - HU_{15minD})/HU_{1min}] \times 100$. Chemical shift magnetic resonance (MR) can be used to differentiate an adenoma from other lesions when CT results are unclear. The adenoma's intracellular fat will cause a reduction in the signal in out-of-phase imaging. A decline in signal strength of more than 16.5% is required for the diagnosis of an adenoma (Figure 9.2).

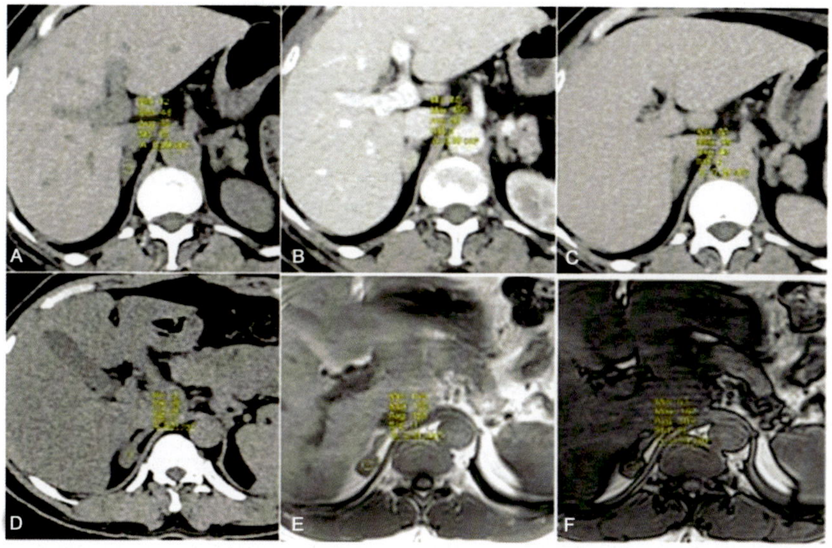

Figure 9.2. *Adrenal adenoma. Axial noncontrast (A), venous phase (B), and 15 minutes delayed phase (C) images show a well-defined nodule in right adrenal gland with mean attenuation of 30 Hounsfield unit (HU) on noncontrast scan, with absolute contrast washout of 75%, suggestive of adrenal adenoma. (D) Axial noncontrast computed tomography image of another patient shows a well-defined nodule in right adrenal gland with mean attenuation of 29 HU. (E, F) Axial in-phase (A) and out-of-phase (B) magnetic resonance imagings of the same patient as in (D) show that there signal drop on out-of-phase image with signal intensity index of 33%, suggestive of adrenal adenoma.*

Source: *Gopinath Periaswamy, et al., Imaging in the Causes of Secondary Hypertension: Unveiling the Hidden Culprits, DOI https://doi.org/ 10.1055/s-0044-1782596.*

9.1.1.2. Cushing Syndrome

Cushing syndrome patients, 70% to 80% have hypertension, even though Cushing syndrome is an uncommon cause of hypertension. This is a result of the body producing too much cortisol, and it shows up clinically as pigmented striae, moon facies, and a cervical fat pad. Laboratory results for dexamethasone suppression testing reveal hypokalemia, hyperglycemia, and an inability to lower morning cortisol levels. The differentiation of ACTH-dependent and ACTH-independent causes is aided by plasma levels of the hormone adrenocorticotropic hormone (ACTH).

An excess of ACTH produced by a pituitary tumor—typically a pituitary adenoma—causes Cushing disease. Rare causes include adrenal adenoma, adrenal cortical carcinoma, thymic carcinoid, medullary thyroid carcinoma, pancreatic neuroendocrine tumor, pheochromocytoma, and ovarian steroid cell tumor. Paraneoplastic syndrome is typically brought on by small cell lung cancer.

There are two types of pituitary adenoma: microadenoma, which is less than 10 mm in size, and macroadenoma, which is larger than 10 mm. Pituitary adenoma is a neuroendocrine tumor of the pituitary gland. When diagnosing pituitary adenoma, magnetic resonance imaging (MRI) is the preferred test because it shows the infundibulum's deviation away from the tumor and the pituitary gland's asymmetric bulkiness. A particular thin slice, dynamic contrast acquisition is needed for microadenoma identification. When compared to normal pituitary gland enhancement (60–80 seconds), the microadenoma showed delayed enhancement (90–120 seconds) in dynamic MRI. On delayed imaging, the nodule exhibits variable enhancement, giving rise to a nodule that is hypo-, iso-, or hyperenhancing. It is possible that the MRI is normal in about half of the patients. Due to its lower sensitivity, CT is not recommended as a routine treatment for pituitary adenoma; however, it can be utilized in situations where MRI is not an option. If the MRI results are normal, inferior petrosal sampling (IPS) may be performed to verify if an ACTH-secreting microadenoma is present. It is also possible to lateralize the microadenoma using IPS (Figure 9.3).

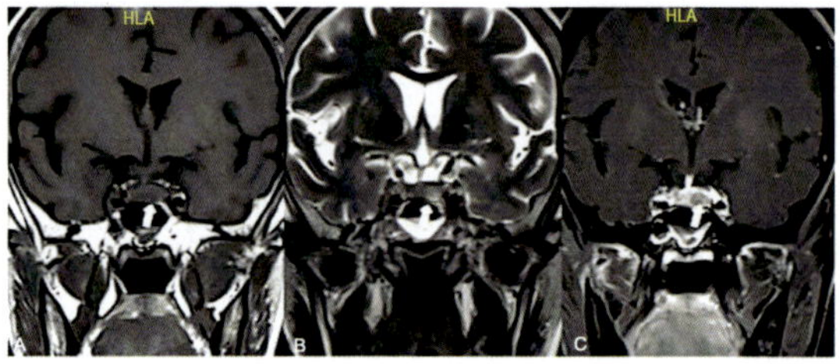

Figure 9.3. *Pituitary microadenoma. Coronal T1-weighted (T1W) (A), T2W (B), and dynamic postcontrast T1W (C) images show a well-defined T1 hypointense and T2 hyperintense lesion in the left half of pituitary gland, with hypoenhancement compared to the pituitary gland parenchyma in the early arterial phase image (arrow), suggestive of pituitary microadenoma.*

Source: *Gopinath Periaswamy, et al., Imaging in the Causes of Secondary Hypertension: Unveiling the Hidden Culprits, https://doi.org/10.1055/s-0044-1782596.*

9.1.1.3. Pheochromocytoma and Paraganglioma

Less than 5% of all cases of hypertension are caused by the rare tumors pheochromocytoma and paraganglioma. However, over 90% of people with these lesions have hypertension as a result of excessive catecholamine excretion. Higher 24-hour urine fractionated metanephrine and catecholamine levels, as well as plasma metanephrine levels, have been observed in laboratory studies.

While paragangliomas arise from chromaffin cells outside the adrenal glands, such as parasympathetic ganglia at the base of the brain or along vagal or glossopharyngeal nerves, pheochromocytomas arise from chromaffin cells within the adrenal glands (Lenders et al., 1995).

Malignant pheochromocytomas and paragangliomas can occur in about 10% to 17% of cases. Usually sporadic, but 15%–20% could be linked to congenital conditions like familial pheochromocytoma–paraganglioma syndrome, neurofibromatosis I, tuberous sclerosis, von Hippel-Lindau disease, or MEN-2A and 2B. When it comes to imaging assessments, CT works best for examining the chest, abdomen, and pelvis, while MRI works best for examining the base of the skull, the neck, and any suspected metastases. If tumors are invisible on CT or MRI, nuclear medicine tests, such as iodine 123-MIBG scintigraphy, may be used.

Typically, pheochromocytomas and paragangliomas appear as spherical or oval soft tissue masses measuring 3 to 5 cm, although they can also exceed 10 cm in size. Hemorrhage, calcifications, cystic changes, necrosis, or fibrosis can all be seen in tumorous regions. Malignant tumors are more likely to spread locally to nearby structures or to metastasize distantly. Lesions measure more than 10 HU on non-contrast CT, and during the arterial or portal phases of contrast-enhanced CT, lesions are markedly enhanced. T2-weighted images may occasionally show the MRI appearance of a "light bulb–bright" mass with a signal resembling cerebrospinal fluid. On T1-weighted images, the majority of tumors appear hypointense to the liver and isointense to the muscle. The lesions do not show the signal drop seen in adenomas on out-of-phase contrast images because they do not contain intracellular lipids. Comparable to contrast-enhanced CT, MRI contrast enhancement has been observed. Certain paragangliomas may exhibit pepper and salt because of flow voids.

9.1.1.4. Hyperparathyroidism

Nearly half of patients with primary hyperparathyroidism experience hypertension. Elevated serum parathyroid hormone and hypercalcemia are detected by laboratory screening tests. The most frequent cause of hyperparathyroidism is parathyroid adenoma, followed by parathyroid hyperplasia. Multiple parathyroid adenomas and parathyroid carcinoma are two other less common causes. For preoperative localization of parathyroid, the preferred imaging investigations are technetium 99m-sestamibi scintigraphy and ultrasonography (USG), which exhibit higher sensitivity when performed in tandem. An oval hypoechoic nodule located in the parathyroid region, usually inferior or posterior to the thyroid gland, is the typical appearance of a parathyroid adenoma on USG. It is characterized by an extrathyroidal feeding vessel that enters the parathyroid from its pole and exhibits an arc or rim of vascularity.

It is possible to identify ectopic adenomas and confirm nonectopic adenoma using technetium 99m-sestamibi scintigraphy. When compared to thyroid tissue, the majority of adenomas exhibit avid tracer uptake and delayed washout. When compared to thyroid tissue, the majority of adenomas exhibit avid tracer uptake and delayed washout. If ectopic glands are suspected or a previous parathyroidectomy has not been successful, CT and MRI scans may be conducted.

9.1.1.5. Hyperthyroidism

Hypertension, which primarily presents as elevated systolic blood pressure because of heightened heart rate, cardiac output, and lowered systemic vascular resistance, affects about one-third of patients with hyperthyroidism. Clinical signs and symptoms include hyperhidrosis, muscle weakness, heat intolerance, increased appetite but weight loss, and hyperadrenergic symptoms.

Thyroiditis, toxic multinodular goiter, toxic adenoma, and Graves' disease are the most frequent causes of hyperthyroidism. Thyroid-related ophthalmopathy is another possible presentation of Graves' disease. Thyroid-stimulating hormone levels in the serum have decreased, according to laboratory testing. Thyromegaly with heterogeneous echo texture and increased vascularity, displaying a "thyroid inferno" pattern of vessels, are USG imaging features associated with Graves' disease. MRI and CT scans are inconclusive, displaying only a slightly enlarged gland. Iodine-131 and sodium pertechnetate scintigraphy reveal elevated activity in the enlarged gland. There can be one or more toxic adenomas. These are benign monoclonal tumors that naturally secrete too much thyroid hormone. These nodes have a less than 1% chance of being malignant. USG may reveal one or more nodules. The nodules exhibit both intraparenchymal and peripheral vascularity on color Doppler. A hot (hyperactive) nodule is a common finding in toxic thyroid adenoma using thyroid scintigraphy (Lenders et al., 2005).

9.1.1.6. Hypothyroidism

Roughly 1% of diastolic hypertension cases are caused by hypothyroidism. Thyroid-stimulating hormone levels are higher in laboratory tests. Lethargy, slurred speech, hoarse voice, cold intolerance, periorbital edema, constipation, enlarged tongue, brittle hair, and bradycardia are some of the clinical signs of hypothyroidism. Thyroiditis caused by Hashimoto's is the most frequent cause. Additional conditions include iodine deficiency, pregnancy, pituitary disorders, thyroid surgery, radiation therapy, thyroiditis, and congenital hypothyroidism. Hashimoto's thyroiditis manifests on USG as a diffusely enlarged thyroid gland with variable vascularity, heterogeneous echoes, and echogenic septa. Hypoechoic micronodules are a common occurrence. Particularly at level VI, reactive cervical lymphadenopathy is frequent.

9.1.2. Nonendocrinological Causes of Secondary Hypertension

Coarctation of Aorta: This narrowing of the aorta, which accounts for approximately 0.2% of cases of hypertension, occurs next to the left subclavian artery and ligamentum arteriosum. It can result in mechanical obstruction or renal ischemia, both of which can cause hypertension. Patients may continue to experience hypertension even after their coarctation is repaired. Clinical manifestations include blood pressure in the thigh that is lower than in the upper arm, persistent murmur over the back, and claudication pain in the lower extremities.

Because CT angiography can provide high spatial resolution and accurately depict the location and severity of the coarctation, it is the preferred study method. The location and degree of stenosis can also be precisely described by MR angiography, which is useful for long-term follow-up, particularly in kids and young adults. To measure collateral flow within the remaining portion of the aorta and to evaluate flow velocity and turbulence throughout the coarctation, phase-contrast MR and four-dimensional flow techniques can be employed (Lenders et al., 2002).

9.1.2.1. Renovascular Hypertension

About 1% to 2% of cases of hypertension are related to renal disease; the most common causes are atherosclerotic disease and fibromuscular dysplasia. Renal injury, dissection, arterial embolism, stent migration, and cancer surrounding the renal artery are less frequent causes. Laboratory tests reveal hypokalemia, elevated serum creatinine, and elevated serum creatinine when angiotensin II receptor blockers or angiotensin-converting enzyme inhibitors are used. USG and renal Doppler may be the first line of investigation that demonstrates increased peak systolic velocity (PSV) above 180 cm/s, increased renal–interlobar ratio, that is, $PSV_{renal\ artery\ (intrastenotic)}/PSV_{interlobar\ (distal)}$: greater than 5, increased renal–aortic ratio, that is, $PSVrenal/PSV_{aorta}$: more than 3.5, turbulent flow in a poststenotic area, pulsus parvus et tardus waveform due to stenosis, decreased (interlobar) renal arterial resistive index: less than 0.55 in severe stenosis, resistive index difference between kidneys more than 5%, intraparenchymal acceleration time more than 0.07 s and acceleration index: lower than 3 m/s^2.

MR and CT angiography are advised forms of imaging. When atherosclerotic disease occurs, the proximal renal artery narrows focally, and in fibromuscular dysplasia, the middle renal artery narrows and becomes irregular, giving the appearance of a string of beads. When diagnosing a stenosis of 50% or more, CT angiography has a sensitivity and specificity of 94% and 99%, respectively. When detecting a stenosis of 60% or more, MR angiography has a sensitivity and specificity of 90% and 86%. For the detection of 60% or more stenosis, duplex USG has a sensitivity and specificity of 81% and 87%, respectively.

9.1.2.2. Midaortic Syndrome

A progressive narrowing of the abdominal aorta and its major branches is known as midaortic syndrome. It is typically observed in young adults and children. The three most typical symptoms are kidney failure, claudication pain, and elevated blood pressure. Segmental narrowing of the thoracic or abdominal aorta is one of the imaging findings. This narrowing usually occurs in the inter-renal segment, which is where the bilateral renal arteries originate. The iliac arteries and aortic bifurcation are spared when dilated splanchnic arteries are observed. Color Doppler displays a tardus-parvus pattern in the distal segments and an increased PSV in narrow vessels (typically between 230 and 480 cm/s).

9.1.2.3. Renal Parenchymal Disease

Renal parenchymal disease, associated with over 75% of patients with acute glomerulonephritis and most patients with autosomal dominant polycystic kidney disease, is another common cause of secondary hypertension.

People with diabetic nephropathy are also at an increased risk of developing hypertension. Hypertension is brought on by an increase in intravascular volume or activation of the renin-angiotensin system. Laboratory tests reveal hyper- or hypokalemia, elevated serum creatinine levels, and anemia. On USG, the renal parenchyma is thinned and echogenic, and there are also papillary calcifications, reduced renal length, cortico-medullary distinction loss, and poor visibility of the renal sinus and pyramids.

Because subcapsular hematoma compresses the renal parenchyma and activates the renin-angiotensin-aldosterone axis, Page kidney causes hypertension. Patients usually develop subcapsular collections as a consequence of an initiating event, like trauma or surgery. Sometimes the cause is a spontaneous rupture of a mass, aneurysm, or cyst. USG, CT, or MRI images may reveal subcapsular collection with a mass effect in the underlying renal parenchyma. With Doppler USG, renal artery high resistive index can be determined. The collection could include hematomas, urinomas, or seromas (Lenders et al., 2002).

9.2. PHEOCHROMOCYTOMA: THE RANGE OF APPEARENCES ON ULTRASOUND, CT, MRI, AND FUNCTIONAL IMAGING

Pheochromocytomas are extremely uncommon neuroendocrine tumors that release catecholamines and originate from the extra-adrenal paraganglia or the chromaffin cells of the adrenal medulla. Because of the variability in symptoms and geographic distribution of these tumors, imaging and biochemical markers are necessary to confirm the diagnosis. Enhancing diagnostic accuracy requires knowledge of both typical and atypical multimodality imaging findings because the radiographic appearances of pheochromocytomas can vary greatly.

9.2.1. Epidemiology

Pheochromocytomas range in prevalence from 0.1% to 0.6% in hypertensive adults, and an autopsy series found that their incidence in the general population was 0.05%. A female-to-male ratio of 1:4 indicates a slight preference for females in pheochromocytomas. Patients' average age at presentation varies. The mean age of patients with sporadic pheochromocytomas at presentation is approximately 44 years, which is older than that of patients with a genetic predisposition. The mean age of patients with a genetic predisposition is usually about 25 years old at presentation. Pheochromocytomas are extremely uncommon in children, and to our knowledge, no data for a sizable pediatric population have been reported. On the other hand, compared to adults with pheochromocytoma, pediatric patients have a higher genetic predisposition and a higher incidence of malignancy (47% vs. 10% in adults).

9.2.2. Associations

In most cases, sporadic pheochromocytomas are the cause of diagnosis. The belief that 10% of pheochromocytomas are inherited has been refuted in the last ten years due to advancements in molecular diagnostics. The protooncogene RET, the tumor suppressor gene linked to von Hippel-Lindau (VHL) disease, the succinate dehydrogenase subunit D gene, SDHD, and the succinate dehydrogenase subunit B gene, SDHB, are among the approximately 25% of patients with pheochromocytomas that appear to be sporadic. Furthermore, there is a higher likelihood of a genetic predisposition in patients under the age of eighteen who present with pheochromocytomas, multifocal tumors, extra-adrenal tumors, and bilateral tumors. 10% of sporadic cases, 50% to 80% of cases of multiple endocrine neoplasia type II (MEN2), and 40% to 80% of cases of VHL have bilateral pheochromocytomas.

9.2.2.1. von Hippel–Lindau Disease

An autosomal-dominant disorder called VHL disease is brought on by a mutation in the tumor suppressor gene VHL. It causes a variety of benign and malignant tumors, such as pancreatic cysts and tumors, including serous tumors and islet cell tumors, pheochromocytomas, renal cysts and renal cell carcinomas, hemangioblastomas, and papillary cystadenoma of the epididymis. 10% to 26% of patients with VHL, whose mean age at presentation is about thirty, develop pheochromocytomas (Walther, Reiter, Keiser, et al., 1999).

9.2.2.2. Multiple Endocrine Neoplasia Type II

The MEN2 gene mutation causes autosomal-dominant disorders known as MEN2 syndromes. Pheochromocytoma is more common in patients with MEN2A than in those with MEN2B, and patients with MEN2 syndromes are predisposed to it. Additional clinical characteristics linked to the MEN2 syndromes include hyperparathyroidism (MEN2A), neuromas and marfanoid habitus (MEN2B), and medullary thyroid carcinoma (MEN2A and 2B). About 50% of patients with MEN2 develop pheochromocytomas.

9.2.2.3. Neurofibromatosis Type 1

A variety of benign and malignant tumors, such as cutaneous and plexiform neurofibromas, optic nerve gliomas, peripheral nerve sheath tumors, and gastrointestinal stromal tumors, can manifest as symptoms of neurofibromatosis type 1 (NF1), an autosomal-dominant disorder. Pheochromocytomas are caused by NF1, a comparatively uncommon cause that affects about 1% of patients.

9.2.2.4. Pheochromocytoma-Paraganglioma Syndromes Associated with SDHB and SDHD Mutations

Pheochromocytoma-paraganglioma syndromes are now known to be significantly influenced by genetic mutations of the succinate dehydrogenase gene family (SDHB and SDHD). Approximately 10% of patients with pheochromocytoma have these gene mutations. Individuals with head and neck paragangliomas and extraadrenal tumors are more likely to carry the SDHB mutation. Furthermore, malignant pheochromocytomas can be up to 50% more likely in patients with the SDHB mutation.

9.2.3. Clinical Features

When present, pheochromocytomas can have a wide range of clinical symptoms and indicators that are frequently nonspecific. Sweating, palpitations, and headaches are the most typical symptoms. The triad is rare, occurring in 10–36.5% of patients with pheochromocytomas, despite being 90% specific for the presence of a pheochromocytoma. Pallor, nausea, flushing, weight loss, exhaustion, psychologic symptoms like anxiety and panic, sustained hypertension, paroxysmal hypertension, orthostatic hypotension, and hyperglycemia are some additional symptoms and indicators.

The clinical presentation of pheochromocytomas is influenced by the variability of their hormone production. The most common presentation patterns for dopamine-producing tumors are either normotension or hypotension. It has even been reported that tumors secreting epinephrine can appear as shock. Of pheochromocytomas, incidentally found adrenal tumors account for roughly 23%–58%.

The most concerning clinical characteristic of pheochromocytoma is hypertensive crises. Certain medications, foods, or tumor manipulation may cause these crises. There has been debate regarding the role that iodinated IV contrast material plays in the onset of a hypertensive crisis in pheochromocytoma patients. In one of the first studies, six patients treated with α-adrenergic blockade before receiving ionic iodinated contrast material had their catecholamine levels measured. Catecholamine levels in five out of the six patients were high enough to cause a hypertensive crisis. Two more studies that followed patient cohorts not receiving α-adrenergic blocker treatment before nonionic IV contrast material administration revealed no negative reaction. There have never been any instances of an adrenergic crisis following the intravenous administration of nonionic iodinated contrast material in our institution's experience. To avoid a hypertensive crisis, contrast medium injections should not be made directly into the renal or adrenal arteries. Nonetheless, preoperative administration of an α-adrenergic blocker is a standard procedure to avert intraoperative hypertensive crises (Anderson et al., 1994).

Clinical features to distinguish benign pheochromocytomas from malignant pheochromocytomas have been studied because malignant pheochromocytomas indicate a much worse prognosis. In a single study of 10 malignant and 85 benign tumors, high preoperative 24-hour urinary dopamine levels, extraadrenal tumor location, high tumor weight (> 80 g), tumor dopamine concentration, and persistent postoperative hypertension increased the risk of malignant pheochromocytoma.

9.2.4. Biochemical Features

Pheochromocytoma patients usually experience symptoms due to catecholamines secreted by the tumor, which are mainly metabolized intratumorally into metanephrines. Biochemical measurements of catecholamines or their metabolites (metanephrines) are usually carried out if there is a clinical suspicion of pheochromocytoma. Urinary catecholamines, total plasma metanephrines (metanephrine and normetanephrine), plasma concentration of free metanephrines, and 24-hour fractionated urine metanephrines (with or without vanillylmandelic acid) are among these tests. To the best of our knowledge, there is no universal agreement among institutions regarding the preferred biochemical test.

The preferred initial biochemical test is a 24-hour urine-fractionated metanephrine evaluation. This test quantifies the total concentration of metanephrines as well as the 24-hour urinary excretion of normetanephrine, a norepinephrine metabolite, 3-methoxy tyramine, a dopamine metabolite, and metanephrine, a metabolite of epinephrine. For pheochromocytoma, urinary-fractionated metanephrines have a high sensitivity, ranging from 90% to 97%. There is a range of 69%% to 98% specificity (Lenders et al., 1995).

Compared to urinary metanephrines, plasma-fractionated metanephrines have been reported to have a lower specificity (77%–89%) but a higher sensitivity (96%–100%). The negative predictive value of plasma metanephrines for pheochromocytomas is high (95%–100%). Pheochromocytoma has a low incidence and prevalence, which makes it difficult to determine the positive predictive value with precision given the range of pretest probabilities. Due to the low specificity and low positive predictive value of plasma-fractionated metanephrines, there is a significant likelihood of false-positive results, which calls for further testing. If the biochemical analysis is positive, imaging is needed for additional assessment.

9.2.5. Pathologic Features: Macro- and Microscopic Criteria

9.2.5.1. Macroscopy

The gross pathology of phéochromocytomas shows a variety of appearances. Small, well-circumscribed, yellow-tan lesions limited to the adrenal glands can be found among them, as can large, hemorrhagic, cystic-necrotic masses weighing as much as 4 kg.

9.2.5.2. Microscopy

Pheochromocytomas also have a range of histologic appearances. Usually, the tumors are primarily composed of chromaffin cells, but on rare occasions, spindle cells may predominate.

9.2.6. Malignancy

Researchers have found that no single pheochromocytoma histologic characteristic can reliably forecast clinical outcome. No single histologic feature could predict malignancy in a large retrospective study of 100 pheochromocytomas, 50 of which were benign and the remaining 50 malignant. While some characteristics, like tumor necrosis and tumor cell spindling, are more frequently observed in malignant pheochromocytomas, benign tumors can also exhibit these characteristics. Consequently, the "Pheochromocytoma of the Adrenal Gland Scaled Score," or "PASS," a 12-feature histologic scoring system, was developed. All malignant tumors with metastatic disease had a PASS of 4 or higher, which was deemed indicative of a potentially aggressive clinical course. On the other hand, at a mean follow-up of 14 years, tumors with a PASS of 3 or less did not metastasize; this finding implies that if these tumors did metastasize, it would happen much later than for those with a PASS of 4 or higher. The accuracy of PASS in predicting malignancy is variable, making it a controversial tool even after some encouraging studies. Therefore, the presence of metastatic disease alone ultimately serves as the basis for the final pathologic diagnosis of malignancy. Imaging cannot identify malignancy in a pheochromocytoma unless metastatic disease is discovered. Therefore, to conclude that the pheochromocytoma is malignant, the radiologist plays a crucial role in determining whether metastatic spread of the tumor is present (Omura et al., 2004).

9.2.7. Imaging Appearances

The size of phenochromocytomas varies; one study found that the tumors ranged in size from 1.2 to 15 cm, with a mean of 5.5 cm. Larger lesions tend to be more heterogeneous, while smaller lesions are usually more homogeneous.

9.2.7.1. Ultrasound

Pheochromocytomas can appear solid (75% in one case series), mixed cystic, solid, or cystic on ultrasonography.

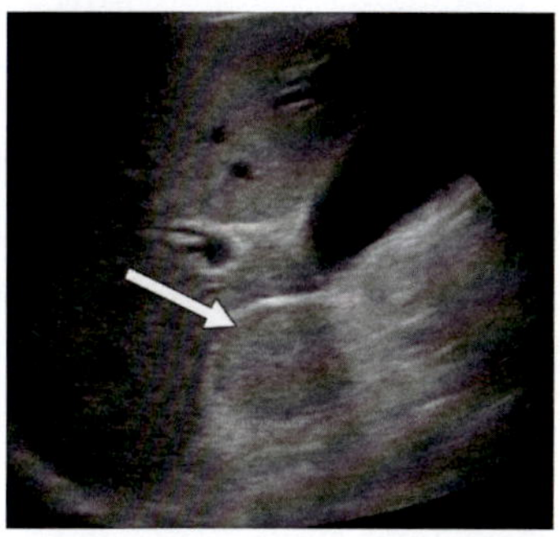

Figure 9.4. *20-year-old man with hypertension, diaphoresis, headache, and palpitations. Sagittal gray-scale ultrasound image shows 4-cm solid right adrenal pheochromocytoma (arrow) that is iso- to hyperechoic compared with liver.*

Source: https://ajronline.org/doi/full/10.2214/ajr.12.9126.

When confirming a cystic-necrotic change within a pheochromocytoma, gray-scale ultrasonography can be useful. There could be an accompanying feature of posterior acoustic enhancement along with the cyst fluid being anechoic or containing echogenic debris. In a pheochromocytoma, acute hemorrhage may have an echogenic appearance (Figures 9.4 and 9.5).

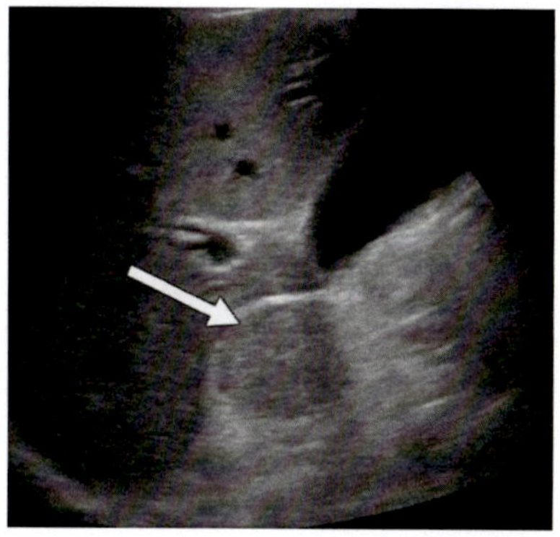

Figure 9.5. *54-year-old woman with headache, palpitations, pain, and diaphoresis.*

Source: https://ajronline.org/doi/full/10.2214/ajr.12.9126.

9.2.7.2. CT

Pheochromocytomas appear differently on unenhanced CT. They vary in soft-tissue attenuation to low density. Pheochromocytomas are classified as solid in about two thirds of cases, complex or cystic in the remaining cases. The majority of pheochromocytomas have attenuation values greater than 10 HU; however, a small percentage of pheochromocytomas that contain intracellular fat may have attenuation values lower than 10 HU, which is comparable to adenomas. On the other hand, bleeding might make the pheochromocytoma denser. Calcifications are best seen on unenhanced CT and are present in roughly 10% of pheochromocytomas and up to 21% of symptomatic pheochromocytomas (Figures 9.6, 9.7 and 9.8) (McNeil et al., 2000).

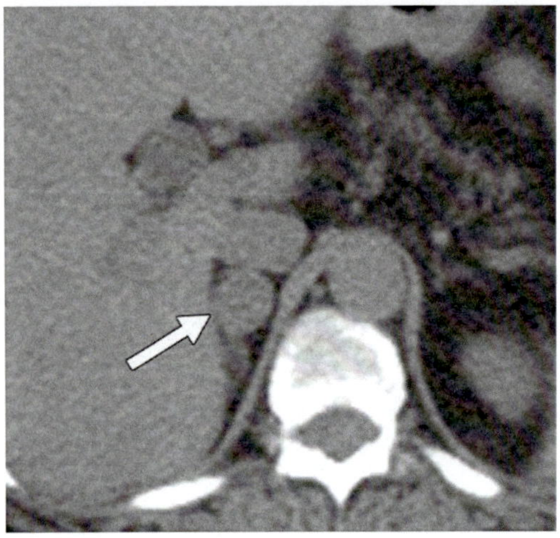

Figure 9.6. *68-year-old woman with hypertension. Axial unenhanced CT image shows homogeneous solid (27 HU) right adrenal pheochromocytoma (arrow). Fatty atrophy of pancreas is incidentally noted.*

Source: https://ajronline.org/doi/full/10.2214/ajr.12.9126.

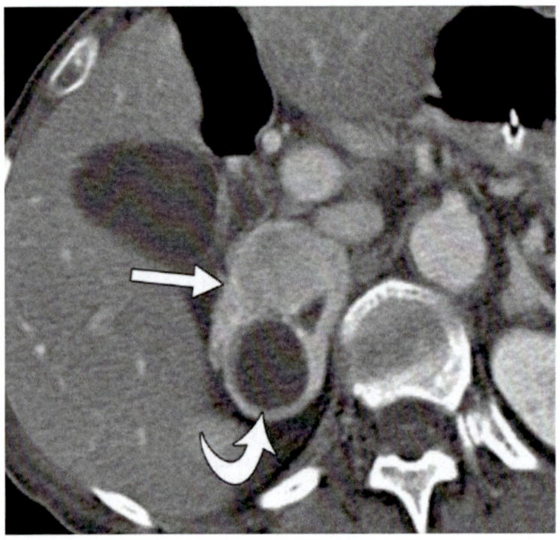

Figure 9.7. *66-year-old woman with incidental right adrenal pheochromocytoma. Axial contrast-enhanced CT image shows bilobed pheochromocytoma consists of solid enhancing anterior component (straight arrow) and cystic posterior component (curved arrow).*

Source: https://ajronline.org/doi/full/10.2214/ajr.12.9126.

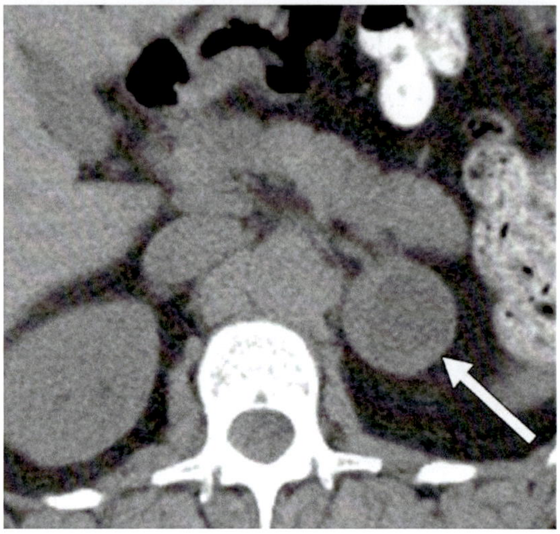

Figure 9.8. *52-year-old woman with hypertension. Axial unenhanced CT image shows low-attenuation left adrenal pheochromocytoma (arrow) with density of 10 HU, which is similar to density of adenoma.*

Source: https://ajronline.org/doi/full/10.2214/ajr.12.9126.

Pheochromocytomas can exhibit homogeneous or variable enhancement on contrast-enhanced CT (CECT), with avid enhancement of the solid components seen in the majority of cases. Pheochromocytomas can have variable contrast washout that can overlap with malignant and benign lesions, including adenomas. Research from the past has indicated that pheochromocytomas have washout characteristics similar to those of adrenocortical carcinomas (ACCs) and metastases, meaning they washout less than 60% of the total and less than 40% of the relative percentage at 15 minutes or less than 50% of the total and less than 40% of the relative percentage at 10 minutes. A study conducted more recently, however, found that a higher percentage of pheochromocytomas had washout patterns similar to those of adenomas (45% vs 32% similar to ACCs and metastases) (Figure 9.9).

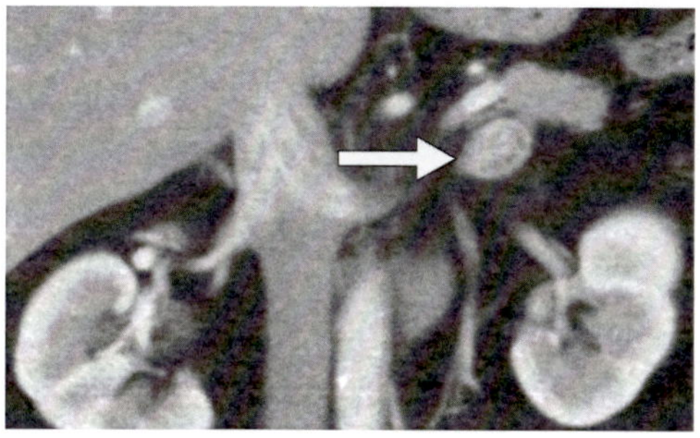

Figure 9.9. *46-year-old woman with incidental left adrenal pheochromocytoma. Adrenal washout characteristics of this pheochromocytoma (calculated relative percentage washout = 59%) simulate adrenal adenoma.*

Source: https://ajronline.org/doi/full/10.2214/ajr.12.9126.

9.2.7.3. MRI

Pheochromocytomas are typically detected by a "light-bulb" bright lesion on T2-weighted imaging, which is similar in signal intensity to CSF. However, the prevalence of this classic appearance varies in reported case series, with 11% to 65% of pheochromocytomas having it. Increased water content in the cystic or liquefactive necrotic tumor is the cause of this variability. Pheochromocytomas may show low signal intensity on T2-weighted imaging in about 35% of cases. Pheochromocytomas are usually isointense to muscle and hypointense to liver on T1-weighted imaging. The presence of necrosis or hemorrhage can cause quite variable appearances on T1-weighted imaging. Rarely, microscopic fat may be present in pheochromocytomas, which can mimic adenomas by causing signal loss on chemical-shift MRI (dual-echo in and opposed-phase T1-weighted imaging). The presence of cystic-necrotic areas, which do not enhance, can affect the degree of gadolinium enhancement seen in phenochocytomas, which usually show avid enhancement (Figure 9.10) (Stenström et al., 1986).

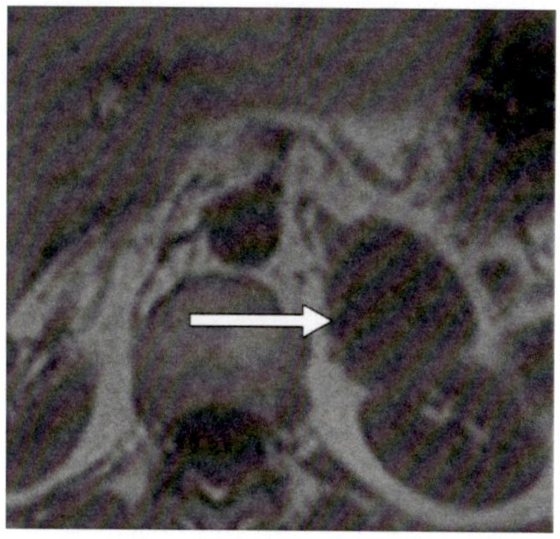

Figure 9.10. *69-year-old woman with incidentally detected left adrenal pheochromocytoma.*

Source: https://ajronline.org/doi/full/10.2214/ajr.12.9126.

9.2.8. Functional Imaging

To maximize sensitivity and specificity for the detection of pheochromocytomas, functional imaging is frequently necessary due to the variable clinical presentation of pheochromocytomas, the lack of specific biochemical tests, and the generally nonspecific imaging appearances. When conducting a comprehensive assessment of the body, functional imaging plays a crucial role in identifying extraadrenal pheochromocytomas, metastatic disease, and tumor recurrence. Functional imaging examinations are performed using ^{131}I- and ^{123}I-metaiodobenzylguanidine (MIBG), ^{111}In-pentetreotide (Octreoscan, Covidien), and several PET ligands including ^{18}F-fluorodopamine, ^{18}F-dihydroxyphenylalanine (DOPA), and ^{18}F-FDG (FDG).

9.2.8.1. ^{131}I- and ^{123}I-Metaiodobenzylguanidine

The most widely used and accessible functional imaging method for evaluating pheochromocytomas is MIBG imaging. MIBG is a norepinephrine analog that enters cytoplasmic storage vesicles after first localizing to sympathomedullary tissue and presynaptic adrenergic nerves via an active amine transport system. The characteristic appearance of a pheochromocytoma is unilateral focal uptake within the tumor, which is proportionate to the number of neurosecretory granules within the tumor. Due to its superior imaging quality and lower radiation dose, ^{131}I-MIBG imaging has mostly been replaced by ^{123}I-MIBG imaging. With a specificity of 95–100%, the sensitivity of ^{123}I MIBG has been reported to range from 77% to 90%. The varying amount of cytoplasmic storage granules, the loss of the amine transport system in dedifferentiated tumors, and the variable affinity of MIBG to the amine transport system all contribute to the lower sensitivity (McNeil et al., 2000). Many drugs also obstruct MIBG absorption. The combination of anatomic and functional imaging with CT and MIBG improves sensitivity and specificity with the introduction of hybridized SPECT/CT technology; in one case series, MIBG SPECT/CT was shown to increase diagnostic certainty in 89% of discordant CT and planar MIBG cases (Figure 9.11).

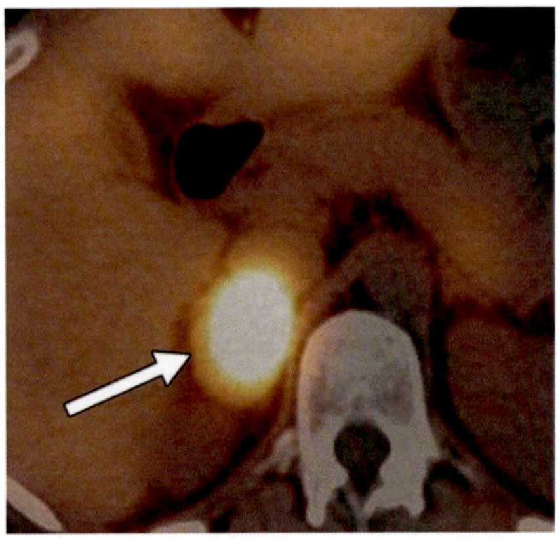

Figure 9.11. *46-year-old woman with right adrenal pheochromocytoma. Axial 123I-MIBG fused CT image shows intense radiotracer uptake within tumor (arrow).*

Source: *https://ajronline.org/doi/full/10.2214/ajr.12.9126.*

9.2.8.2. ^{111}In-Pentetreotide

The compound indium-111 pentetreotide is a somatostatin analog. Pentetreotide can be used in the diagnostic procedure because phenochromocytomas have the ability to express somatostatin receptors. Given its lower sensitivity (25% in one case series) for nonmetastatic pheochromocytomas and its reduced specificity for pheochromocytomas—granulomas, autoimmune disorders, and other tumors being sources of false-positives—penetreotide is not recommended as a first-line diagnostic tool. Its primary applications are in metastasis detection and the evaluation of dedifferentiated pheochromocytomas that are MIBG-negative, meaning they no longer express the amine transporter system (Kearney et al., 2005).

9.2.8.3. PET

There are currently many PET ligands under development, some of which are being used for pheochromocytoma diagnostic workup. The production process is challenging and their limited availability prevents their widespread use. Currently, research settings are the main applications for the majority of PET ligands. Compared to SPECT, PET offers the advantages of higher signal-to-noise ratio and higher resolution images.

9.2.8.4. ^{18}F-Fluorodopamine, ^{18}F-Dihydroxyphenylalanine

The use of DOPA, a dopamine precursor, in pheochromocytoma imaging has been studied. It is believed that fluorine-18-fluorodopamine is a more effective substrate for the amine transport system than DOPA and norepinephrine. It can also result in higher sensitivity when evaluating pheochromocytomas than MIBG. These PET agents are more sensitive to metastatic disease; 100% sensitivities for DOPA and ^{18}F-fluorodopamine have been documented. Fluorine-18-fluorodopamine has been shown to show pheochromocytomas that have negative MIBG imaging results, and it has a sensitivity of up to 100% for primary pheochromocytomas. The widespread use of ^{18}F-fluorodopamine has been limited due to its unavailability.

9.2.8.5. ^{18}F-FDG

An analog of glucose called FDG gets stuck in cells. Tumors exhibit increased intracellular metabolism, which is reflected in its concentration, making tumor detection possible. Given that PET's main function is to differentiate between benign and malignant adrenal lesions, it should not be used as a first-line imaging method. When examining dedifferentiated tumors that are devoid of the amine transport system, PET may be useful.

9.2.9. Benign Versus Malignant

In the absence of metastatic disease, the diagnosis of malignant pheochromocytoma is particularly challenging to establish on imaging. Even though it is more frequently observed in malignant pheochromocytomas, the presence of vascular or capsular invasion does not indicate malignancy (Figure 9.12).

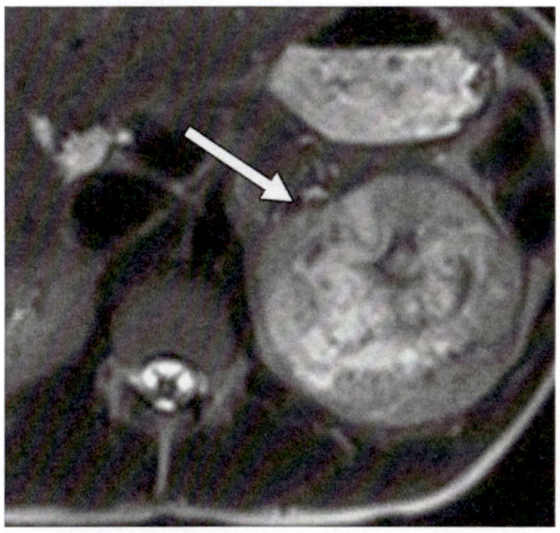

Figure 9.12. *18-year-old man who presented with hypertensive crisis and palpitations.*

Source: https://ajronline.org/doi/full/10.2214/ajr.12.9126.

9.3. CUSHING SYNDROME: DIAGNOSTIC WORKUP AND IMAGING FEATURES

Harvey W. The endocrinologic syndrome of hypercortisolism brought on by a pituitary gland malfunction was initially described by Cushing, the father of modern neurosurgery, in the early 1900s. He called this condition "polyglandular syndrome." This illness, which is now known by its own name, Cushing disease, is characterized by elevated cortisol levels brought on by a pituitary adenoma. On the other hand, hypercortisolism resulting from a variety of sources other than a pituitary adenoma is represented by Cushing syndrome (CS).

9.3.1. Normal Hypothalamic-Pituitary-Adrenal Axis Function

The production of cortisol, a glucocorticoid steroid hormone, occurs in the zona fasciculata of the adrenal cortex and is crucial for maintaining homeostasis when stressors are present. It is produced by a sequence of enzymatic processes from cholesterol. Stressors that are both psychological and physical serve as the primary triggers for the hypothalamus to release corticotropin-releasing hormone (CRH). Adrenocorticotropic hormone (ACTH) is released into the systemic circulation by corticotrophs in the anterior lobe of the pituitary gland in response to CRH transported via the hypothalamic-pituitary tract. This, in turn, stimulates the zona fasciculata of the adrenal cortex to synthesize and secrete glucocorticoids. Numerous organs and systems are impacted by cortisol, such as the immune system (particularly anti-inflammatory and immunosuppressive processes), the liver (particularly gluconeogenesis), the kidneys (particularly electrolyte and water balance), the stomach (particularly increased gastric acid secretion), and the bones (particularly decreased bone formation). Through its negative feedback on hypothalamic-pituitary-adrenal axis activation, cortisol regulates blood cortisol levels at the hypothalamic (decreased CRH secretion) and pituitary gland (decreased ACTH secretion) levels. Urine contains the metabolites of cortisol's breakdown, which occurs in the liver. Long-term exposure to excessive cortisol is the cause of CS, which manifests as a constellation of clinical symptoms (Stelios et al., 2006).

9.3.2. Epidemiology

Population-based studies indicate that endogenous CS is a rare disorder, with an incidence of 0–2 cases per million people annually. With the exception of the subtype of ectopic ACTH syndrome, which is equally common in male patients, the ratio of female to male patients is 3:1. Subclinical CS, which affects 5%–20% of patients with an incidental finding of an adrenal mass (adrenal incidentaloma), is defined as the presence of autonomous mild cortisol hypersecretion in a patient who does not exhibit the classic or overt signs of CS.

9.3.3. Clinical Features of Cushing Syndrome

The age of the patient as well as the length and severity of the hypercortisolism all affect the clinical presentation of CS. CS is linked to a five-fold excess mortality, morbidity, and a low quality of life. Patients with florid cases may have a variety of symptoms, including fatigue, proximal muscle weakness, hypertension, glucose intolerance, hirsutism, acne, menstrual irregularities, thinned skin with wide purple striae, and central obesity with accumulation of dorsocervical and supraclavicular fat. Neuropsychological symptoms are common and include emotional instability, depression, sleep issues, and cognitive impairments. Growth retardation in children is a common observation. Since CS manifests in a variety of ways, it can be difficult to diagnose the condition when signs and symptoms are mild. Therefore, without a definitive diagnosis of CS, a patient may receive treatment for another systemic disease that shares symptoms, such as diabetes mellitus or hypertension. When several symptoms, such as glucose intolerance and hypertension, occur together in the context of recent weight gain, or when symptoms that are unusual for the patient's age appear, it may be possible to diagnose mild hypercortisolism in clinical phenotypes. Subclinical CS patients lack overt hypercortisolism symptoms like wide purple striae or proximal muscle weakness, but they do have higher rates of obesity, hypertension, dyslipidemia, diabetes mellitus, and osteoporosis (Figure 9.13) (Newell-Price, 2009).

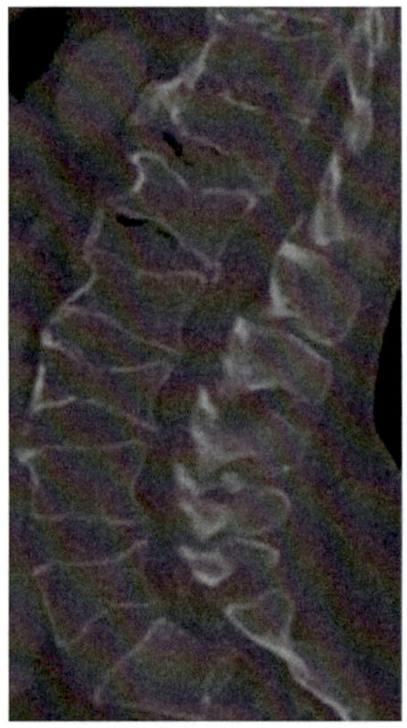

Figure 9.13. *Clinical features of Cushing syndrome in various patients.*

Source: https://ajronline.org/doi/full/10.2214/AJR.16.17290.

9.3.4. Classification of Cushing Syndrome

Exogenous glucocorticoid administration or excessive endogenous cortisol production can both cause CS. Endogenous cortisol production is typically categorized as either ACTH independent, when the adrenal glands secrete excessive amounts of cortisol on their own, or ACTH dependent, when pathologic ACTH secretion drives cortisol production. Confirmation of hypercortisolism, distinction between ACTH-dependent and ACTH-independent causes, and distinction between pituitary and ectopic sources of ACTH in ACTH-dependent CS are necessary for the diagnosis of CS (Shilpan et al., 2007).

9.3.4.1. Exogenous Cushing Syndrome

More often than endogenous CS, exogenous or iatrogenic CS is brought on by the administration of supraphysiologic doses of glucocorticoids. Glucocorticoids are administered exogenously to treat neoplastic, inflammatory, and autoimmune diseases. These days, prescriptions for synthetic ACTH administration are less common.

9.3.4.2. Endogenous Cushing Syndrome: Adrenocorticotropic Hormone–Dependent Cushing Syndrome

About 80% of the endogenous causes of CS are ACTH-dependent, which includes CRH-producing tumors, ectopic ACTH syndrome, and ACTH-secreting pituitary adenomas (Cushing disease).

About 80% of cases of ACTH-dependent CS are caused by Cushing disease, which is caused by a pituitary adenoma making ACTH. The adrenal glands are stimulated to release cortisol by the pituitary adenoma, which secretes ACTH. Cushing disease can affect children and young adolescents as well, but it usually manifests in the third or fourth decade of life. The incidence of Cushing disease is considerably greater in the female population (Figures 9.14 and 9.15) (Lockhart et al., 2002).

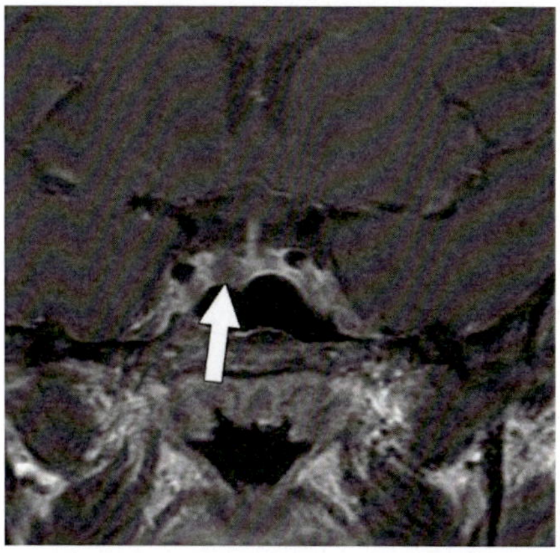

Figure 9.14. *51-year-old man with Cushing disease. Coronal contrast-enhanced T1-weighted MR image of pituitary gland shows hypoenhancing microadenoma of right aspect of pituitary gland (arrow).*

Source: https://ajronline.org/doi/full/10.2214/AJR.16.17290.

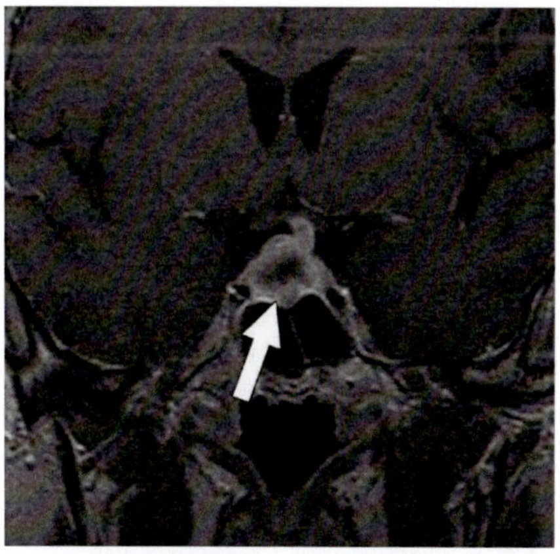

Figure 9.15. *56-year-old man with Cushing disease. Contrast-enhanced coronal T1-weighted image of sella shows peripherally enhancing macroadenoma (arrow) with nonenhancing central necrotic area and its relation to cavernous sinus and carotid arteries, with no evidence of invasion or encasement.*

Source: https://ajronline.org/doi/full/10.2214/AJR.16.17290.

- **Ectopic Adrenocorticotropic Hormone Syndrome:** Of ACTH-dependent CS cases, ectopic ACTH syndrome (caused by ACTH production from nonpituitary tumors) accounts for about 20% of cases. Differentiating ectopic ACTH syndrome from the more common Cushing disease and identifying the source of ectopic ACTH secretion are critical because the extrapituitary tumors are often malignant and surgical removal of the primary lesion has a high chance of cure (complete remission in up to 80% of cases). The most common cause of ectopic ACTH is lung tumors; roughly half of ectopic ACTH-secreting tumors are small cell lung cancer and bronchial carcinoid tumors. Additional causes of ectopic ACTH syndrome include medullary thyroid carcinomas (7.5%); pheochromocytoma (2.5%); and nonlung neuroendocrine tumors (22.5%), including gastrointestinal, pancreatic, and thymic carcinoids (Figures 9.16 to 9.19) (Blake et al., 2006).

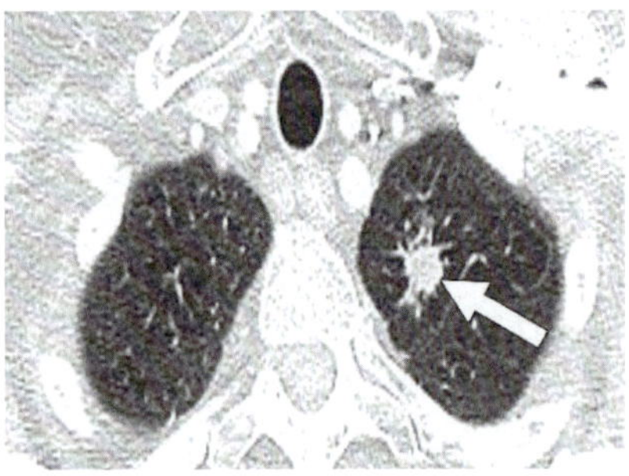

Figure 9.16. *55-year-old woman with adrenocorticotropic hormone (ACTH)–dependent Cushing syndrome and ectopic secretion of ACTH resulting from small cell lung cancer.*

Source: https://ajronline.org/doi/full/10.2214/AJR.16.17290.

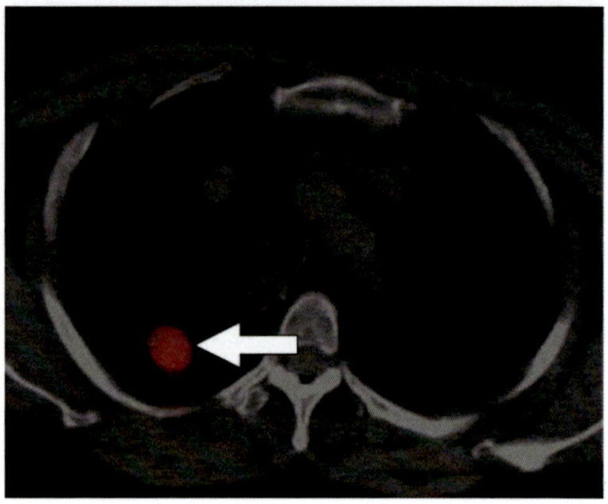

Figure 9.17. *57-year-old woman with bronchial neuroendocrine tumor and ectopic adrenocorticotropic hormone (ACTH) syndrome. Axial SPECT/CT octreotide scan through upper chest localized ectopic source of ACTH to 2-cm bronchial neuroendocrine tumor (arrow) in right upper lobe.*

Source: https://ajronline.org/doi/full/10.2214/AJR.16.17290.

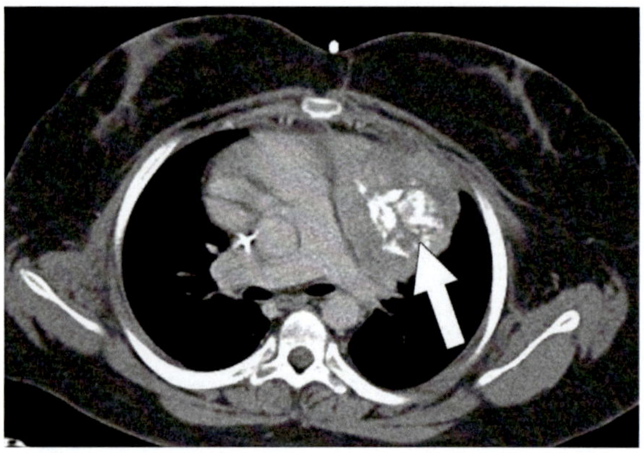

Figure 9.18. *12-year-old girl with adrenocorticotropic hormone (ACTH)–dependent Cushing syndrome and ectopic secretion of ACTH from thymic neuroendocrine tumor.*

Source: https://ajronline.org/doi/full/10.2214/AJR.16.17290.

Because locating the ectopic source of ACTH can be challenging and take months or years, there will likely be a higher rate of morbidity and mortality. In 12.5% of cases, despite numerous clinical and imaging assessments as well as extended follow-up, the cause of ectopic ACTH syndrome remains unidentified. Tumors that produce corticotropin-releasing hormone (CRH) are incredibly rare; they cause less than 1% of cases of ACTH-dependent CS. Twenty cases were published in the literature; of these, five cases had single cases of sellar choristoma and gangliocytoma. The isolated CRH-producing tumors included medullary thyroid carcinoma (33%), pheochromocytoma (19%), carcinoma of the prostate (14%), small cell lung carcinoma (95%), and carcinoid (5%). Ectopic CRH syndrome is an extremely rare cause of CS, but it should be considered in the differential diagnosis.

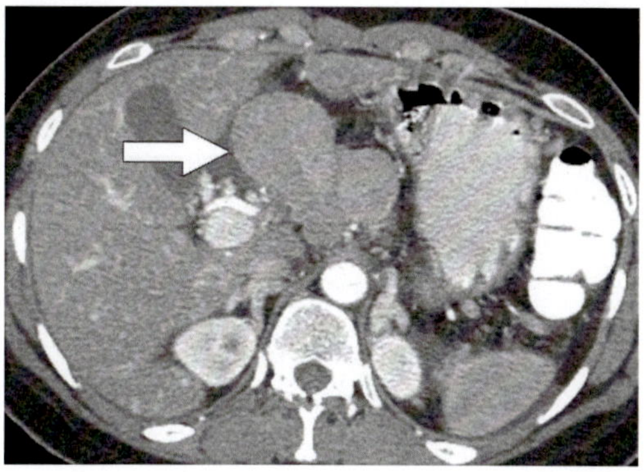

Figure 9.19. *23-year-old man with adrenocorticotropic hormone (ACTH)–dependent Cushing syndrome and ectopic ACTH secretion from pancreatic neuroendocrine tumor.*

Source: https://ajronline.org/doi/full/10.2214/AJR.16.17290.

9.3.4.3. Endogenous Cushing Syndrome: Adrenocorticotropic Hormone–Independent Cushing Syndrome

Adenomas and adrenocortical carcinomas (ACC) are the most common adrenal gland lesions that cause autonomous cortisol secretion in ACTH-independent CS. Less frequently, ACTH-independent macronodular adrenal hyperplasia or primary pigmented nodular adrenal disease (PPNAD) cause CS. About 20% of all endogenous causes are caused by this condition.

- **Adrenal Adenoma:** About 60% of adrenal causes of CS are benign neoplasms of adrenocortical cells called adrenal adenomas. Adrenal adenomas can cause clinical syndromes of hypercortisolism (CS), hyperaldosteronism, or, in rare cases, virilization or feminization. They can also be hormonally silent. They are frequently found by accident during abdominal imaging tests, or they may be sought out when patients exhibit symptoms of excess hormone production (Figure 9.20). (Smith and Vale, 2007)

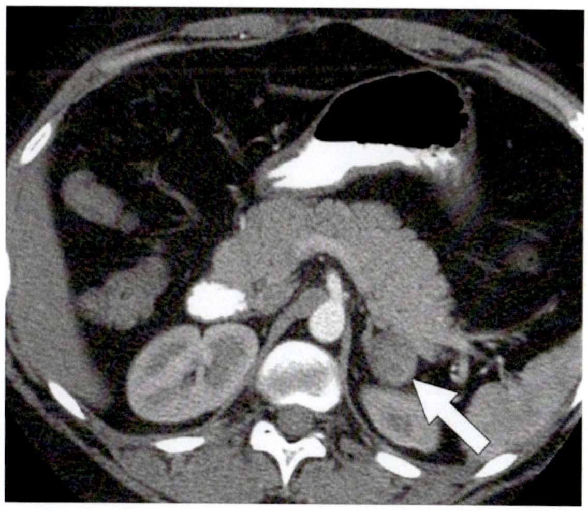

Figure 9.20. *35-year-old woman with adrenal adenoma causing Cushing syndrome. Contrast-enhanced axial CT image shows small well-defined ovoid nodule (arrow) arising in left adrenal gland that proved to be hormonally active adrenal adenoma.*

Source: https://ajronline.org/doi/full/10.2214/AJR.16.17290.

- **Adrenocortical Carcinoma:** About 40% of adrenal causes of CS are ACCs, which are uncommon and frequently aggressive tumors. With an estimated 5-year overall survival rate of 15%–44%, ACCs are thought to occur twice a million people annually. ACC typically strikes in the fourth or fifth decade of life and very infrequently in childhood. In addition to being linked to Li-Fraumeni syndrome, Lynch syndrome, familial adenomatous polyposis, and Beckwith-Wiedemann syndrome, ACC can also occur sporadically or be syndromic. Children with ACC may have up to 80% of the germline TP53 mutation associated with Li-Fraumeni syndrome. Roughly 40% of ACCs have functional hormones and can secrete androgens, aldosterone, or cortisol, the most common hormone. Compared to nonfunctioning tumors, functioning tumors are linked to higher morbidity and lower survival rates.
- **Primary Pigmented Nodular Adrenal Disease:** Less than 1% of adrenal causes of CS are caused by PPNAD, a rare cause of ACTH-independent CS. The most common age groups for PPNAD are newborns, kids, and young adults. Atypical clinical presentation is possible, with common features including short stature, asthenic body habitus, severe muscle wasting, and advanced osteoporosis. A Carney complex, which includes PPNAD, testicular tumors, growth hormone-secreting pituitary tumors, cardiac and cutaneous myxomas, lentigines, and patchy skin pigmentation, is responsible for the majority of PPNAD cases. The PRKAR1A gene mutation causes the Carney complex (Pena et al., 2000).
- **Adrenocorticotropic Hormone – Independent Macronodular Adrenal Hyperplasia:** ACTH-independent macronodular adrenal hyperplasia accounts for fewer than 1% of adrenal causes of CS. In contrast to the predominantly female distribution of most cases of CS, ACTH-independent macronodular adrenal hyperplasia affects both male and female patients equally. It also has a higher mean patient age compared to adenomas, Cushing disease, or PPNAD, most often presenting in the fifth or sixth decades of life. The majority of cases of sporadic ACTH-independent macronodular adrenal hyperplasia can be found during the workup of adrenal oversecretion syndrome or as a result of an accidental imaging finding. Patients may exhibit overt or subclinical CS.

9.3.5. Imaging Evaluation of Cushing Syndrome

9.3.5.1. Adrenocorticotropic Hormone–Dependent Cushing Syndrome

- **Adrenocorticotropic Hormone–Independent Macronodular Adrenal Hyperplasia:** ACTH-independent macronodular adrenal hyperplasia accounts for fewer than 1% of adrenal causes of CS.
- **Pituitary MRI:** Following

confirmation of the diagnosis of ACTH-dependent CS, all patients should undergo a high-resolution pituitary MRI using a gadolinium-based contrast agent. This is done to confirm the existence or absence of a pituitary lesion and to distinguish between ectopic lesions and pituitary adenomas as the source of ACTH. Without using ionizing radiation, MRI offers excellent soft-tissue contrast, anatomic detail, and multiplanar imaging capacity. Thin-section (2 or 3 mm) T1-weighted spin-echo coronal images are obtained through the sella turcica at 10-second intervals following an IV injection of the gadolinium-based contrast agent. Spoilt gradient recalled acquisition in the steady state offers superior sensitivity and better spatial resolution for pituitary adenoma detection when compared to standard contrast-enhanced T1-weighted spin-echo techniques. However, this comes at a slightly higher false-positive rate. It has been demonstrated that pituitary microadenomas can be better localized using volume interpolated 3D spoiled gradient-echo MRI sequences than with dynamic contrast-enhanced spin-echo MRI sequences, especially when the latter is negative or unclear.

In as many as 60% of patients with ACTH-dependent CS, an MRI shows a distinct pituitary adenoma. A pituitary adenoma is typically a microadenoma, which is defined as having a mean size of 6 mm as determined by MRI and being smaller than 10 mm in the longest dimension. However, due to the small size of these adenomas, it should be noted that in up to 40–50% of patients with documented ACTH-secreting pituitary adenomas, MR images may be interpreted as normal. Compared to unenhanced MRI, dynamic contrast-enhanced pituitary MRI improves detection; nevertheless, not all possible adenomas will be detected (Pena et al., 2000).

In the early dynamic phase of an MRI, a pituitary adenoma is visible as a focal hypoenhancing nodule in contrast to the surrounding homogeneously enhanced gland. One potential problem is that 10% of the population may have incidentally discovered focal lesions resembling microadenomas during an MRI; therefore, more testing is required to determine whether the pituitary gland is the source of ACTH. These lesions are typically less than 5 mm in diameter. Additional tests include additional biochemical testing (e.g., CRH stimulation test) or bilateral inferior petrosal sinus sampling, which can confirm the pituitary gland as the source of ACTH excess. It may be challenging to identify normal glandular tissue when a pituitary macroadenoma (> 10 mm) is present; in these situations, any mass effect on the nearby structures (such as the optic chiasm and cavernous sinus) should be evaluated. Due to its lower sensitivity than MRI, CT is not recommended for initial evaluation of the pituitary gland; however, it may be utilized in situations where MRI is not appropriate, such as in the presence of an aneurysm clip.

- **Bilateral Inferior Petrosal Sinus Sampling:** Bilateral inferior petrosal sinus sampling, with its high sensitivity (95%–99%), specificity for Cushing disease, and diagnostic accuracy of over 90%, is performed as the reference standard to confirm the pituitary gland as the source of excess ACTH and to help exclude an ectopic source of ACTH. This is because transsphenoidal surgery is widely accepted as the primary treatment option for pituitary adenoma. Patients with ACTH-dependent CS whose clinical, biochemical, or radiologic results are unclear or contradictory should consider bilateral inferior petrosal sinus sampling. However, due to the serious complications that can arise from this procedure—such as brainstem vascular damage, deep vein thrombosis, pulmonary emboli, and cranial nerve palsies—it should only be carried out in specialized facilities by highly qualified radiologists. When the tumor is actively secreting ACTH, as indicated by elevated cortisol measurements, the procedure should be carried out. Following the radiologist's catheterization of both inferior petrosal sinuses, blood samples are taken simultaneously from both sides for ACTH measurements. Additionally, a peripheral vein sample is taken in the basal state and at specific intervals (three, five, and ten minutes) following the intravenous injection of 100 μg of CRH.

Cushing disease is diagnosed by an inferior petrosal sinus-to-peripheral ACTH ratio greater than 2.0 in the basal state or greater than 3.0 following CRH injection. With a specificity of 95–99%, lower inferior petrosal sinus–to–peripheral ACTH ratios are strongly suggestive of an ectopic ACTH-secreting tumor.

9.3.5.2. Ectopic Adrenocorticotropic Hormone–Secreting Tumors

- **Thoracic Sources of Ectopic Adrenocorticotropic Hormone:** When bilateral inferior petrosal sinus sampling or pituitary MRI rule out Cushing disease, the ectopic source of ACTH is sought in cases of ACTH-dependent CS. Since the chest is the most common body region for ectopic ACTH-secreting tumors, the next study obtained to evaluate for intrathoracic tumors that could be the source of ACTH is a contrast-enhanced CT scan of the chest. Roughly 20% to 50% of these cases are lung small cell carcinomas. ACTH may also be secreted by other thoracic tumors, including medullary thyroid carcinoma and bronchial and thymic carcinoids. Because locating the ectopic source of ACTH can be challenging and take months or years, there is a higher risk of morbidity and mortality. Selective pulmonary arterial sampling with measurement of ACTH has been reported to be helpful in identifying and verifying ectopic production of ACTH by small bronchial carcinoid tumors when noninvasive techniques such as 18F-FDG PET or somatostatin receptor scintigraphy were unable to confirm the diagnosis. While MRI is not very useful for identifying bronchial carcinoids in the chest, it may be useful for identifying lesions in the mediastinum, such as thymic tumors (Blake et al., 2006).
- **Abdominal Sources of Ectopic Adrenocorticotropic Hormone:** A CT or MRI scan of the abdomen is done to check for intraabdominal ACTH-secreting neoplasms after more common intrathoracic sources of ACTH-secreting tumors have been ruled out. These tumors include pheochromocytomas, pancreatic islet

cell tumors, gastrointestinal carcinoids, and gastroenteropancreatic neuroendocrine tumors. Pancreatic islet cell tumors are typically small and exhibit intense enhancing in the early arterial phase. The tumor markers and hormonal profile suggest a particular diagnosis. When a calcified mesenteric mass is observed, usually in conjunction with mesenteric fibrotic changes, it is suspected that the tumor is an intestinal carcinoid. Mesenteric ischemia and vascular compromise may be linked to these tumors.

Multiple imaging techniques (e.g., MRI plus octreotide scan or whole body PET scan) should be used to identify the ectopic source of ACTH if one of these modalities is unable to identify the ectopic focus. Selective venous sampling, which includes pancreatic, portal, systemic, and transhepatic intestinal sampling, may aid in the localization of occult endocrine tumors. When surgical planning is requested, certain cases might require confirmation through image-guided biopsy.

9.3.6. Nuclear Medicine Tests

When hormone-secreting tumors in CS are difficult to detect, nuclear medicine functional imaging tests such as octreotide scan, FDG PET, and ^{68}Ga-somatostatin receptor PET/CT can increase the sensitivity of conventional CT and MRI. About 80% of tumors that are missed by traditional radiology can be found through molecular imaging.

9.3.6.1. Octreotide Scan (^{111}In-Pentetreotide Scintigraphy)

When CT and MRI are unable to identify the source of ACTH, octreotide scan, also known as octreoscan, is a scintigraphy test that can be used to detect occult ectopic ACTH-secreting neuroendocrine tumors. Synthetic somatostatin analog octreotide is conjugated with diethylenetriamine pentaacetic acid (pentetreotide), which is injected intravenously (IV) and labeled with ^{111}In. Many different kinds of neuroendocrine tumor cells have somatostatin receptors (subtypes 2 and 5) on their cell membranes, which the pentetreotide binds to. Small cell lung carcinoma, adrenal medullary tumors (such as pheochromocytomas), bronchial carcinoids, and gastroenteropancreatic neuroendocrine tumors (such as intestinal carcinoid) can all be located with an octreotide scan.

9.3.6.2. Gallium-68 Somatostatin Receptor PET/CT

Somatostatin-analogs radiolabeled with ^{68}Ga for PET are useful for detecting ectopic ACTH-secreting tumors and offer higher spatial resolution and improved pharmacokinetics compared with somatostatin-analog scintigraphy. Gallium-68 somatostatin receptor PET/CT, which includes ^{68}Ga-1, 4, 7, 10-tetraazacyclododecane-1, 4, 7, 10-tetraacetic acid (DOTA)-(Tyr^3)-octreotate, ^{68}Ga-DOTA-(Tyr^3)-octreotide, and ^{68}Ga-DOTA-1-Nal^3-octreotide, shows the highest sensitivity among molecular imaging tests for detecting neuroendocrine tumors in ectopic CS.

9.3.7. Imaging for Adrenocorticotropic Hormone–Independent Cushing Syndrome

9.3.7.1. Adrenal CT or MRI

Patients with ACTH-independent CS do not require adrenal imaging studies, but those with ACTH-dependent CS do. Since CT always detects adrenal adenoma, carcinoma, and ACTH-independent macronodular adrenal hyperplasia, it is the best noninvasive imaging modality for diagnosing adrenal lesions in ACTH-independent CS. Thin (2–5–3 mm) CT slices should be used for an adrenal CT both before and after 100–150 mL of iodinated contrast agent is injected intravenously. Excellent delineation of adrenal anatomy and the anatomic relationship of an adrenal lesion is possible with MDCT scanners equipped with collimation of 1 mm or less and multiplanar reconstruction capabilities. When viewed on CT, normal adrenal glands have a similar soft-tissue attenuation to the kidney and appear homogeneous and symmetric. Analogous to CT, adrenal MRI can offer a comparable evaluation.

9.3.7.2. Adrenal Adenoma

Adrenal adenomas are typically round or ovoid nodules that are well-defined and relatively small, with homogeneous or slightly heterogeneous attenuation, typically measuring 1-2 cm. Although adrenal venous sampling can distinguish between the two, conventional imaging is unable to separate hyperfunctioning cortisol-producing adenomas that cause CS from one another due to their overlap with incidental nonfunctioning adenomas' imaging features at CT.

Compared to the vast majority of malignant lesions, about 70% of adrenal adenomas are lipid rich, meaning they contain abundant intracellular lipid (fatty acids, cholesterol, and neutral fat). An ROI drawn over the nodule with attenuation measuring less than 10 HU allows for the differentiation of adenomas from nonadenomas at unenhanced CT because most adenomas have intracellular lipid content that lowers the lesion's CT attenuation. With a sensitivity of 71% and a specificity of 98%, this threshold value of 10 HU is very high. Larger adenomas, typically larger than 3 cm, may show internal areas of liquefaction and bleeding along with heterogeneous attenuation. Like most malignant lesions, about 30% of adrenal adenomas have attenuation values greater than 10 HU on unenhanced CT images and are lipid poor. Consequently, additional assessment, such as CT wash-out, is required for a lesion whose unenhanced CT attenuation exceeds 10 HU to identify the cause (Mayo-Smith et al., 1995).

Two phases are involved in IV contrast-enhanced CT of the adrenal glands: the early phase happens one minute after the contrast agent is injected intravenously, and the delayed phase usually happens fifteen minutes later. Contrast washout is the term for the rapid enhancement and deenhancement that adrenal adenomas typically exhibit. Malignant lesions, on the other hand, exhibit slower contrast washout but comparable rapid enhancement. It has been demonstrated that adenomas can be distinguished from nonadenomas with accuracy using the ratio of the lesion's attenuation values at the 15-minute delayed phase compared to the 1-minute early phase.

The following equations are used to measure washout in an adrenal lesion on an adrenal CT image: absolute washout = 100% × (attenuation in early phase − attenuation in delayed phase) / (attenuation in early phase − unenhanced attenuation), and relative wash-out = 100% × (attenuation in early phase − attenuation in delayed phase) / attenuation in early phase. An absolute enhancement wash-out of more than 60% or a relative enhancement washout of more than 40% is diagnostic for adrenal adenoma with high sensitivity (> 86% for absolute washout and > 96% for relative washout) and high specificity (> 92% for absolute washout and 100% for relative washout).

Because chemical-shift imaging (CSI), a critical step in the MRI evaluation of adrenal lesions, and magnetic resonance imaging (MRI) have intrinsic tissue-characterizing capabilities, MRI is helpful in the imaging of the adrenal glands. When compared to the liver, normal adrenal glands show low to intermediate signal on T1-weighted imaging and similar or slightly lower signal on T2-weighted imaging. Adenomas typically show up as smooth-bordered, round, or ovoid lesions that are well-defined. They also show uniform early contrast enhancement, homogeneously relatively low signal at T1-weighted imaging, and isointense signal at T2-weighted imaging in comparison to the liver. Larger adenomas may have hemorrhaging, cystic degeneration, and necrosis areas. When signal dropout on opposed-phase T1-weighted gradient-recall echo sequences is present compared with the in-phase sequence, chemical-shift images can be used to detect the presence of intracellular lipid. While most lipid-rich adenomas can be diagnosed with just visual inspection, a signal dropout of more than 11.2% on the opposed-phase sequence allows for 100% accuracy in differentiating adenomas from metastatic adrenal tumors. The diagnostic performance of CT and MRI for lipid-rich adrenal adenomas is nearly identical. However, because CT can evaluate for enhancement washout, it is thought to be more effective in identifying lipid-poor adenomas that CSI MRI was unable to identify.

9.3.7.3. Adrenocortical Carcinoma

About 40% of adrenal-related cases of CS are caused by ACC, which typically manifests as a unilateral large (mean size, 9 cm; range, 2–25 cm) heterogeneously enhancing soft-tissue mass. In 30% of cases, ACC may also have microscopic or coarse calcifications present, as well as small areas of intracytoplasmic lipid or macroscopic fat. In 9–19% of cases, adjacent structures may be invaded by ACC, exhibiting venous extension into the renal vein or inferior vena cava. Even though ACC exhibits intense early enhancement, it does not exhibit the same degree of contrast washout as an adenoma on the 15-minute delayed phase, which permits differentiation in cases where the lesion is homogeneous and small, potentially mimicking an adenoma at imaging. Bilateral ACC occurs in 2–10% of cases. At presentation, metastatic disease is often discovered, usually to the lungs, liver, bone, and lymph nodes in the area. Because of the necrosis and bleeding in certain areas, the signal intensity of ACC is typically heterogeneous at MRI. Generally, the T1-weighted imaging signal is isointense to hypointense in the liver; however, hemorrhage may cause areas of high T1 signal. Generally, the T2-weighted imaging signal is hyperintense to the liver, with necrotic regions showing varying degrees of increased signal. In contrast to lipid-rich adenomas, which exhibit uniform signal loss on CSI, small areas of intracytoplasmic lipid may cause small, nonuniform areas of signal decrease over less than 30% of the lesion area.

9.3.7.4. Primary Pigmented Nodular Adrenal Disease

Multiple small nodules, typically smaller than 6 mm, with atrophy of the intervening adrenal cortex as a result of the nodules' autonomous function and subsequent suppression of pituitary ACTH, are the hallmark appearance of the adrenal glands in PPNAD. This may result in an uneven or knobby adrenal gland shape. The size of the adrenal glands can range from normal to slightly enlarged.

The normal appearance of the adrenal glands should prompt a search for supporting features of the Carney complex, such as cardiac myxomas, which can be asymptomatic but potentially fatal, when evaluating a case of established ACTH-independent CS. The adrenal glands may even appear normal on CT. Genetic testing for PRKAR1A gene mutations may be beneficial in these cases to ascertain the presence of the Carney complex. When compared to the surrounding atrophic cortex on T1- and T2-weighted MRI images, the adrenal nodules show a lower signal. Larger than 1 cm macronodules are an uncommon occurrence in PPNAD (Shilpan et al., 2007).

9.3.7.5. Adrenocorticotropic Hormone–Independent Macronodular Adrenal Hyperplasia

When it comes to imaging, ACTH-independent macronodular adrenal hyperplasia is different from PPNAD in that it appears pathological. The contours of both adrenal glands are usually distorted by nodules and are greatly enlarged. Nodules usually measure between 0.1 to 5.5 cm on a CT scan, appearing hypodense due to a matrix rich in lipids. The diaphragm to the level of the renal hila is often covered in enlarged adrenal glands. When compared to the liver on T1-weighted MRI images, the adrenal nodules are hypointense; on T2-weighted images, they are iso- to hyperintense. Due to the high lipid content, CSI shows a signal dropout.

A Closer Look

A Delayed Diagnosis of Endocrine Hypertension

With a history of bilateral adrenal hypertrophy, a 43-year-old woman was referred to an endocrinologist for treatment of resistant arterial hypertension. The patient and the medical staff first interacted in 2012 when the patient was admitted to the urology department. A small left kidney, bilateral adrenal masses, and liver hypodens lesions were discovered on an abdominal CT scan. Similar results were obtained from additional MRI imaging. Hemangiomas were the diagnosis made for the liver lesions. The patient was transferred to nephrology due to elevated tensions during their hospital stay. Low ACTH, elevated PAC/ARC ratio, and high to normal serum cortisol were all indicators of an imbalance in hormones. Urine collected for a full day did not support the presence of a pheochromocytoma. Hyperaldosteronism was not correlated with an oral salt loading test. A mass at the right kidney lower pole was discovered during a renal artery CT angiography six months following the initial imaging. After additional MRI imaging, the enlarged mass that had initially been diagnosed as a hemorrhagic cyst was thought to be cancerous. Additionally, a lesion in the fourth liver lobe that had previously been diagnosed as focal hepatic steatosis was also thought to be cancerous. The patient was lost in follow-up and never showed up for a consultation.

The patient's family doctor didn't refer them to cardiology until four years later because of resistant arterial hypertension. A repeat CT scan of the abdomen revealed new bilateral adrenal nodules next to previously reported bilateral nodules and a new renal mass next to the known right kidney under pole mass. An endocrinologist saw the patient five years after the initial visit. A recent hormonal balance revealed low ACTH and elevated serum cortisol. An increased HbA1C (8.4%) and deterioration of renal function were also observed in the control blood sample. The patient was brought into the department of endocrinology. Serum cortisol levels were not suppressed in a 48-hour low dose dexamethasone suppression test. To sum up, there are three major issues with this case.

Resistant hypertension is the first issue. Cushing syndrome, hyperdeoxycorticosteronism, and primary hyperaldestoronism are adrenocortical causes of hypertension. An oral salt loading test was utilized to rule out primary hyperaldosteronism. A 48-hour low-dose dexamethasone suppression test, an elevated late-night salivary cortisol, and an elevated free cortisol on a 24-hour urine collection all supported the diagnosis of Cushing syndrome. We diagnosed macronodular hyperplasia after finding bilateral macronodular adenoma on the abdomen using CT and MRI scans. Second, the patient is in stage four chronic renal failure. In terms of metabolism, we observe elevated PTH and high to normal calcium. Thirdly, a PET-CT scan was carried out since two kidney masses and a liver lesion are thought to be cancerous. This showed that the lesion in the fourth liver lobe had increased tracer uptake. A liver biopsy did not reveal any evidence of cancer. The suggestion was for a partial right nephrectomy. An ACTH-independent Cushing syndrome characterized by bilateral adrenal adenoma larger than one centimeter is called macropodular hyperplasia. It is an uncommon reason behind Cushing syndrome. Macrodular hyperplasia is a rare condition, but over 50% of patients have an ARMC5 gene mutation. Two significant discoveries—a paracrine secretion of ACTH and aberrant expression of hormone receptors—have been made, though the pathophysiology is still unclear. Imaging and hormone balance are used to make the diagnosis. It is recommended to screen for luteinizing hormone (LH), human chorionic gonadotropin (hCG), and beta-adrenergic receptor abnormalities. Since most patients only have a mild form of Cushing syndrome, treatment may only need a unilateral adrenalectomy. For patients with aberrant beta-adrenergic, hCG, or LH receptors in macronodular hyperplasia, medication treatment may be an alternative to surgery.

Summary

- Endocrine hypertension typically refers to disorders of the adrenal gland including primary aldosteronism, glucocorticoid excess, and the pheochromocytoma-paraganglioma syndromes.
- Endocrine hypertension accounts for approximately 3% of secondary hypertension due to the excess production of hormones from various endocrine glands.
- Primary hyperaldosteronism (or Conn syndrome) is the most prevalent cause of secondary hypertension and is defined as increased autonomous production of aldosterone without renin-angiotensin-aldosterone axis activation.
- A pituitary adenoma is a neuroendocrine tumor of the pituitary gland that is classified as microadenoma (less than 10 mm in size) and macroadenoma (more than 10 mm in size).
- Hypertension is seen in almost 50% of patients with primary hyperparathyroidism. Laboratory screening tests reveal hypercalcemia and elevated serum parathyroid hormone. Parathyroid adenoma is the most common cause of hyperparathyroidism and the next common cause is parathyroid hyperplasia.
- CT angiography is the study of choice because it can provide high spatial resolution and accurately depict the location and severity of the coarctation.
- Pheochromocytomas are relatively rare catecholamine-secreting neuroendocrine tumors that arise from the chromaffin cells of the adrenal medulla or extraadrenal paraganglia.
- Pheochromocytomas exhibit variability in size, with one study reporting tumors ranging from 1.2 to 15 cm with a mean size of 5.5 cm. Smaller lesions are typically homogeneous and larger lesions, more heterogeneous.
- Imaging using MIBG is the most common and available technique for functional imaging used in the assessment of pheochromocytomas.
- Cortisol, a glucocorticoid steroid hormone that is produced in the zona fasciculata of the adrenal cortex, is essential to the maintenance of homeostasis in the presence of stressors.
- Nuclear medicine functional imaging tests, including octreotide scan, FDG PET, and 68Ga-somatostatin receptor PET/CT, improve the sensitivity of conventional CT and MRI when hormone-secreting tumors in CS prove difficult to detect.
- The characteristic appearance of the adrenal glands in PPNAD is that they contain multiple small nodules, usually smaller than 6 mm, with atrophy of the intervening adrenal cortex due to the autonomous function of the nodules with resultant suppression of pituitary ACTH.

References

1. Anderson, G. H. Jr., Blakeman, N., & Streeten, D. H. (1994). The effect of age on the prevalence of secondary forms of hypertension in 4429 consecutively referred patients. *Journal of Hypertension, 12*(5), 609–615. https://doi.org/10.1097/00004872-199405000-00009.

2. Blake, M. A., Kalra, M. K., Sweeney, A. T., Lucey, B. C., Maher, M. M., & Sahani, D. V., et al. (2006). Distinguishing benign from malignant adrenal masses: Multi-detector row CT protocol with 10-min delay. *Radiology, 238*(2), 578–585. https://doi.org/10.1148/radiol.2382050213.
3. Kearney, P. M., Whelton, M., Reynolds, K., Muntner, P., Whelton, P. K., & He, J. (2005). Global burden of hypertension: Analysis of worldwide data. *The Lancet, 365*(9455), 217–223. https://doi.org/10.1016/S0140-6736(05)17741-1.
4. Lenders, J. W., Eisenhofer, G., Mannelli, M., & Pacak, K. (2005). Phaeochromocytoma. *The Lancet, 366*(9486), 665–675. https://doi.org/10.1016/S0140-6736(05)67139-5.
5. Lenders, J. W., Keiser, H. R., Goldstein, D. S., et al. (1995). Plasma metanephrines in the diagnosis of pheochromocytoma. *Annals of Internal Medicine, 123*(2), 101–109. https://doi.org/10.7326/0003-4819-123-2-199507150-00003.
6. Lenders, J. W., Pacak, K., Walther, M. M., et al. (2002). Biochemical diagnosis of pheochromocytoma: Which test is best? *JAMA, 287*(11), 1427–1434. https://doi.org/10.1001/jama.287.11.1427.
7. Lockhart, M. E., Smith, J. K., & Kenney, P. J. (2002). Imaging of adrenal masses. *European Journal of Radiology, 41*(2), 95–112. https://doi.org/10.1016/S0720-048X(01)00435-0.
8. Mayo-Smith, W. W., Lee, M. J., McNicholas, M. M., Hahn, P. F., Boland, G. W., & Saini, S. (1995). Characterization of adrenal masses (< 5 cm) by use of chemical shift MR imaging: Observer performance versus quantitative measures. *AJR American Journal of Roentgenology, 165*(1), 91–95. https://doi.org/10.2214/ajr.165.1.7785550.
9. McNeil, A. R., Blok, B. H., Koelmeyer, T. D., Burke, M. P., & Hilton, J. M. (2000). Phaeochromocytomas discovered during coronial autopsies in Sydney, Melbourne, and Auckland. *Australian and New Zealand Journal of Medicine, 30*(6), 648–652. https://doi.org/10.1111/j.1445-5994.2000.tb01174.x.
10. Newell-Price, J. (2009). Diagnosis/differential diagnosis of Cushing's syndrome: A review of best practice. *Best Practice & Research Clinical Endocrinology & Metabolism, 23*(Suppl 1), S5–S14. https://doi.org/10.1016/j.beem.2009.04.003.
11. Omura, M., Saito, J., Yamaguchi, K., Kakuta, Y., & Nishikawa, T. (2004). Prospective study on the prevalence of secondary hypertension among hypertensive patients visiting a general outpatient clinic in Japan. *Hypertension Research, 27*(3), 193–202. https://doi.org/10.1291/hypres.27.193.
12. Peña, C. S., Boland, G. W., Hahn, P. F., Lee, M. J., & Mueller, P. R. (2000). Characterization of indeterminate (lipid-poor) adrenal masses: Use of washout characteristics at contrast-enhanced CT. *Radiology, 217*(3), 798–802. https://doi.org/10.1148/radiology.217.3.r00nv19798.
13. Shilpan, M. P., Ravi, K. L., Tina, I. B., Tan, L. T., & Beata, B. (2007). Role of radiology in the management of primary aldosteronism. *Radiographics, 27*(4), 1145–1157. https://doi.org/10.1148/rg.274065120.
14. Smith, S. M., & Vale, W. W. (2006). The role of the hypothalamic-pituitary-adrenal axis in neuroendocrine responses to stress. *Dialogues in Clinical Neuroscience, 8*(4), 383–395. https://doi.org/10.31887/DCNS.2006.8.4/ssmith.
15. Stelios, F., & Agathocles, T. (2006). Molecular genetic aspects and pathophysiology of endocrine hypertension. *Hormones, 5*(2), 90–106. https://doi.org/10.14310/horm.2002.11039.

16. Stenström, G., & Värdsudd, K. (1986). Pheochromocytoma in Sweden 1958–1981: An analysis of the National Cancer Registry Data. *Acta Medica Scandinavica, 220*(3), 225–232. https://doi.org/10.1111/j.0954-6820.1986.tb02868.x.

17. Walther, M. M., Reiter, R., Keiser, H. R., et al. (1999). Clinical and genetic characterization of pheochromocytoma in von Hippel-Lindau families: Comparison with sporadic pheochromocytoma gives insight into natural history of pheochromocytoma. *Journal of Urology, 162*(3), 659–664. https://doi.org/10.1016/S0022-5347(05)68674-2.

Chapter 10

SYSTEMATIC APPROACH FOR THE DIAGNOSIS AND MANAGEMENT OF ENDOCRINE HYPERTENSION

Contents

INTRODUCTION

Primary aldosteronism, glucocorticoid excess, and the pheochromocytoma-paraganglioma syndromes are among the adrenal gland disorders that are commonly associated with endocrine hypertension. In rare cases, hypertension can also result from glucocorticoid resistance (Chrousos syndrome) and congenital adrenal hyperplasia. Additionally linked to hypertension are nonadrenal endocrine disorders, including growth hormone excess or deficiency, thyroid dysfunction, primary hyperparathyroidism, testosterone deficiency, vitamin D deficiency, obesity-associated hypertension, insulin resistance, and metabolic syndrome.

Finding and treating an endocrine cause of hypertension that is specifically treatable can have significant advantages, such as improving quality of life, reducing morbidity and mortality, and curing or at least controlling hypertension. For most hypertensives, screening for primary aldosteronism is recommended due to its prevalence and the well-established positive outcomes of targeted treatment. Although screening for renovascular hypertension is less common and requires more expensive imaging techniques, intervention may also have a significant positive impact, particularly when directed by functional testing.

Even though pheochromocytoma is far less common, failing to diagnose it could have serious consequences, and biochemical screening is a simple and affordable method. Given the low prevalence of other endocrine conditions like Cushing syndrome and acromegaly, screening for them should be based on clinical suspicion. This chapter outlines a method for managing and diagnosing different types of endocrine hypertension with an emphasis on useful clinical features (Arnaldi et al., 2003).

Orientation and Directional Terms

Term	Definition	Illustration
Primary aldosteronism	Primary aldosteronism, also called Conn's syndrome, is a disorder in which your adrenal glands make too much of a hormone called aldosterone. Aldosterone helps regulate your blood pressure by balancing sodium and potassium levels in your body.	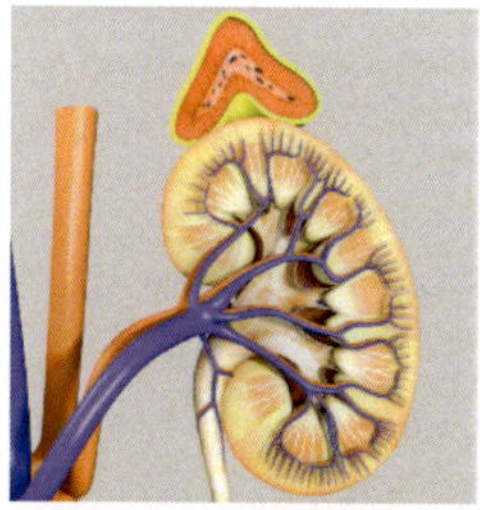
Cushing syndrome	Cushing's syndrome occurs when your body makes too much of the hormone cortisol.	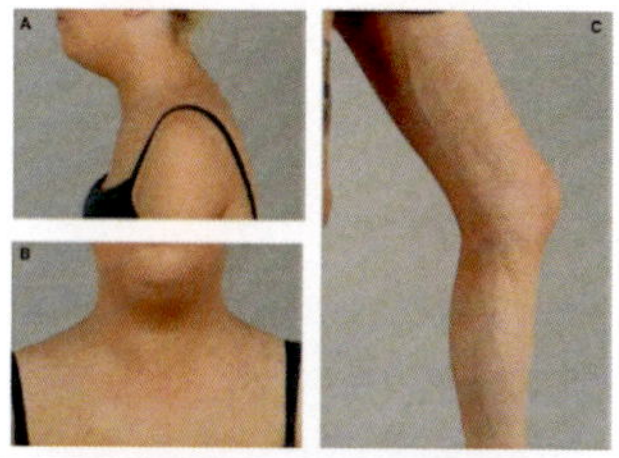
Acromegaly	Acromegaly is a hormonal disorder that develops when your pituitary gland produces too much growth hormone during adulthood.	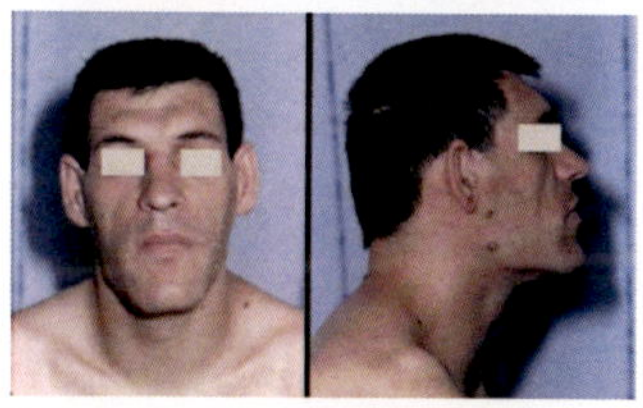
Hypothyroidism	Hypothyroidism (underactive thyroid) is a condition where the thyroid gland doesn't release enough thyroid hormone into the bloodstream.	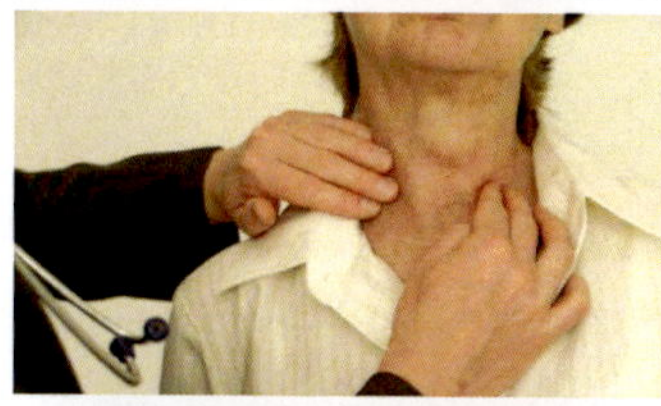
Primary Hyperparathyroidism	Primary hyperparathyroidism is a disorder of the parathyroid glands, four pea-sized glands located on or near the thyroid gland in the neck. "Primary" means this disorder begins in the parathyroid glands, rather than resulting from another health problem such as kidney failure.	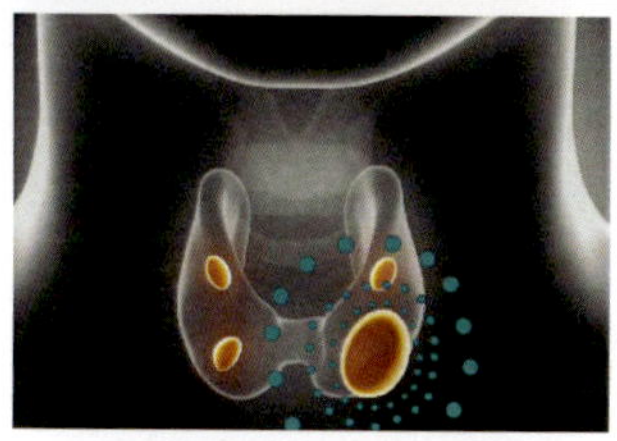
Renal Artery Stenosis	Renal artery stenosis is the narrowing of one or more arteries that carry blood to your kidneys (renal arteries).	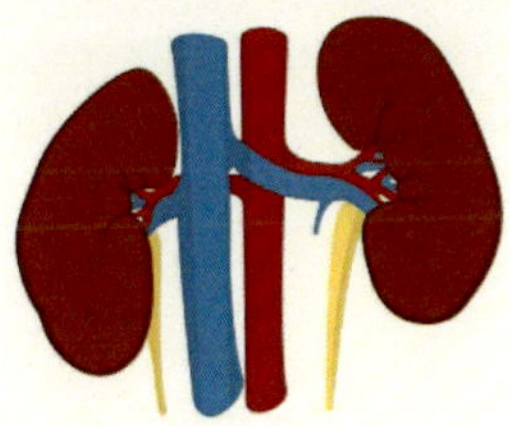

10.1. PRIMARY ALDOSTERONISM

With an estimated prevalence of 4% among hypertensive patients in primary care and roughly 10% among referred patients, primary aldosteronism (PA) is the most prevalent type of secondary hypertension (HTN). Compared to age- and sex-matched patients with essential hypertension and the same degree of blood pressure elevation, patients with PA have higher cardiovascular morbidity and mortality. Autonomous aldosterone production in PA results in sodium retention, plasma renin suppression, hypertension, cardiovascular damage, and increased potassium excretion, which causes hypokalemia to vary in severity. About 40% of cases of PA are caused by aldosterone-producing adenomas (APAs), and approximately 60% are caused by idiopathic hyperaldosteronism. The most accurate way to screen for PA is with the aldosterone-to-renin ratio.

Numerous confirmatory tests exist. Adrenal CT should be performed on all PA patients as the first step in subtype testing after case confirmation to rule out adrenocortical carcinoma. Although it is not always necessary, bilateral adrenal vein sampling (AVS) is the gold standard technique for determining the PA subtype. AVS must be carried out by a qualified radiologist. For patients with APAs, bilateral laparoscopic adrenalectomy is the preferred course of action, and mineralocorticoid antagonists (spironolactone or eplerenone) should be used to treat bilateral hyperplasia. One of two treatments for aldosterone excess-related cardiovascular morbidity is unilateral adrenalectomy or mineralocorticoid antagonist (Bakris et al., 2020).

10.1.1. Pathophysiology

Although all or most body cells are impacted by testosterone, the kidney's late distal convoluted tubule and medullary collecting duct cells are the most significantly affected clinically. Aldosterone stimulates basolateral membrane sodium-potassium ATPase, apical epithelial sodium channels (ENaC), and potassium channels (ROMK) in the main cells. Both potassium secretion and sodium reabsorption are boosted by these processes. Because potassium is secreted in smaller amounts than sodium is reabsorbed, the lumen becomes more electrically negative, which causes chloride to follow sodium. Then, by osmosis, water follows sodium and chloride. These processes result in decreased extracellular potassium and an increase in extracellular sodium and fluid volume in Conn syndrome. Additionally, aldosterone stimulates an apical proton ATPase in intercalated cells, resulting in proton secretion that alkalizes extracellular fluid and acidifies urine. In conclusion, metabolic alkalosis, hypokalemia, and hypernatremia are brought on by hyperaldosteronism.

More detailed information about aldosterone reveals that it increases intracellular potassium by stimulating sodium-potassium ATPase in muscle cells. It also increases sodium reabsorption throughout the intestine and nephron, possibly as a result of this widespread stimulation of ATPase. Lastly, the principal cells of the nephron respond precisely the same way as the epithelial cells in the ducts of sweat glands and the distal surface of the colon. These reactions have a role in both aldosterone-induced constipation and climate adaptation.

Blood pressure rises and plasma volume expands as a result of the sodium retention. Renin released from the granular cells of the kidney's juxtaglomerular apparatus decreases sodium reabsorption and returns sodium renal excretion to nearly normal levels as a result of elevated blood pressure, which causes sodium to "escape" the effects of mineralocorticoids (also known as aldosterone escape mechanism in primary hyperaldosteronism also contributed to by increased ANP level). Reduced renin (and consequently reduced angiotensin II) will not cause a drop in aldosterone levels if primary hyperaldosteronism is present. This is a very useful clinical tool in the diagnosis of primary hyperaldosteronism.

10.1.2. Epidemiology

Less than 1% of patients with hypertension were thought to have primary aldosteronism in previous times. Primary aldosteronism is far more common than previously thought, with rates as high as 12.7% in primary care and 29.8% in referral centers, according to more recent research. Underdiagnosis of primary aldosteronism occurs when screening guidelines are not followed at very high rates.

10.1.3. Diagnosis – Screening and Confirmatory Tests

By measuring plasma aldosterone (PA), plasma renin activity (PRA), or direct renin concentration, primary aldosteronism is screened for. Aldosterone can be measured using a variety of assays, which can present challenges (Stowasser and Gordon, 2006). It is difficult to measure PRA because it involves producing angiotensin from endogenous angiotensinogen. The conversion of angiotensinogen to angiotensin by renin is quantified using radioimmunoassays for PRA, which vary amongst laboratories. It is also possible to measure the direct renin concentration by using an automated chemiluminescence immunoassay to measure plasma renin molecules. For primary aldosteronism, a PA/PRA ratio > 30 and a concurrent PA > 20 ng/dl have a sensitivity of 90% and specificity of 91%, respectively. An upright plasma aldosterone of at least 15 ng/dl may be beneficial because low renin hypertension can be challenging to differentiate from PA (Seiler et al., 2004).

Before pursuing additional diagnostic testing, hypokalemia should be treated because it can lower aldosterone secretion. Furthermore, primary aldosteronism is likely if a patient with hypertension who is receiving treatment with an ACE inhibitor or ARB, calcium channel blocker, and a diuretic—all of which are supposed to raise PRA and decrease the PA/PRA-ratio or ARR—still exhibits suppressed renin and a 2-digit plasma aldosterone level. Premenopausal women who are taking estrogen-containing contraceptive medication or who are in the luteal phase of their menstrual cycle may experience false-positive ARRs (Young et al., 2017). It is frequently advised to stop taking betablockers, ACE inhibitors, renin inhibitors, dihydropyridine calcium channel blockers, ARBs (angiotensin receptor blockers), nonsteroidal anti-inflammatory drugs, and central alpha 2-agonists approximately due to medication interference. roughly hold spironolactone, eplerenone, amiloride, triamterene, and loop diuretics for two weeks before PA/PRA-ratio or ARR testing. four weeks before the ARR exam. Additionally, four weeks before testing, licorice root products should be avoided (Palermo et al., 2004). Several methods can be used for confirmatory testing (Streeten et al., 1979) (Vaidya and Dluhy, 2000) Table 10.1. A new overnight diagnostic test using pharmaceutical renin-angiotensin-aldosterone system blockade with dexamethasone, captopril, and valsartan has been found to be easy to perform, safe, and inexpensive. The test included 148 hypertensive patients and had an estimated sensitivity of 98% and specificity of 100% (Tsiavos et al., 2016).

CT and magnetic resonance imaging are useful in imaging to help clinically distinguish unilateral adenoma from hyperplasia.

Table 10.1. *Confirmatory Tests*

Confirmation Method	Protocol	Interpretation of Results
Oral Salt Suppression Test	·Increase sodium intake for 3-4 days via supplemental tablets or dietary sodium to >200 mmol/day · Monitor blood pressure · Provide potassium supplementation to ensure normal serum levels · Measure 24h urinary aldosterone excretion and urinary sodium on 3rd or 4th day	· PA confirmed: if 24h urinary aldosterone excretion >12 mcg in setting of 24h sodium balance >200 mmol · PA unlikely: if 24h urinary aldosterone excretion <10mcg
Intravenous Saline Infusion Test	· Being infusion of 2L of normal saline after patient lies supine for 1 hour. · Infuse 2L of normal saline over 4 hours (500 mL/h) · Monitor blood pressure, heart rate, potassium · Measure plasma renin and serum aldosterone at time=0h and time=4h	· PA confirmed: 4h aldosterone level > 10 ng/dL · PA unlikely: 4h aldosterone level < 5 ng/dL
Captopril Challenge Test	· Administer 25-50mg of captopril in the seated position · Measure renin and aldosterone at time=0h and again at time=2h · Monitor blood pressure	· PA confirmed: serum aldosterone high and renin suppressed* · PA unlikely: renin elevated and aldosterone suppressed* *varying interpretations without specific validated cut-offs
Fludrocortisone Suppression Test	· Administer 0.1 mg fludrocortisone q6h for 4 days · Supplement 75-100 mmol of NaCl daily to ensure a urinary sodium excretion rate of 3 mmol/kg/body weight · Monitor blood pressure · Provide potassium supplementation to ensure normal serum levels · Measure plasma renin and serum aldosterone in the morning of day 4 while seated	· PA confirmed: Seated serum aldosterone > 6 ng/dL on day 4 with PRA< 1ng/mL/h · PA unlikely: suppressed aldosterone < 6 ng/dL

Oral Salt Suppression Test	·Increase sodium intake for 3-4 days via supplemental tablets or dietary sodium to >200 mmol/day · Monitor blood pressure · Provide potassium supplementation to ensure normal serum levels · Measure 24h urinary aldosterone excretion and urinary sodium on 3rd or 4th day	· PA confirmed: if 24h urinary aldosterone excretion >12 mcg in setting of 24h sodium balance >200 mmol · PA unlikely: if 24h urinary aldosterone excretion <10mcg
Intravenous Saline Infusion Test	· Being infusion of 2L of normal saline after patient lies supine for 1 hour. · Infuse 2L of normal saline over 4 hours (500 mL/h) · Monitor blood pressure, heart rate, potassium · Measure plasma renin and serum aldosterone at time=0h and time=4h	· PA confirmed: 4h aldosterone level > 10 ng/dL · PA unlikely: 4h aldosterone level < 5 ng/dL

Source: *Koch C, Papadopoulou-Marketou N, Chrousos GP. Overview of Endocrine Hypertension. [Updated 2020 Feb 4]. In: Feingold KR, Anawalt B, Blackman MR, et al., editors. Endotext [Internet]. South Dartmouth (MA): MDText.com, Inc.; 2000-. Available from: https://www.ncbi.nlm.nih.gov/books/NBK278980/.*

10.1.4. Management

The decision between medical and surgical treatment depends on many factors, including the patient's preference, surgical candidacy, and the unilateral or bilateral nature of the aldosterone overproduction source. Adrenal computed tomography aids in the planning of procedures, but it is not very good at identifying micronodules or differentiating between nonfunctioning adrenal adenomas and aldosterone-producing adenomas, unless the patient is young (≤35 years) and has a unilateral adenoma >10 mm along with severe primary aldosteronism (i.e., spontaneous hypokalemia and plasma aldosterone concentration >30 ng/dL [>831 pmol/L]) (Lenders et al., 2009). Therefore, the gold standard for determining the laterality of aldosterone secretory autonomy in most patients is adrenal venous sampling (Kempers et al., 2009).

Adrenal venous sampling is a complex and costly procedure that is not widely accessible and should only be carried out in centers with a track record of success and on surgical candidates (Young and Stanson, 2009). To measure aldosterone and cortisol and calculate the lateralization index, adrenal venous sampling involves cannulating the adrenal veins using a percutaneous femoral approach. Venous samples are then collected from the external iliac vein and the adrenal veins (Young and Stanson, 2009). Unilateral aldosterone overproduction is indicated by an aldosterone lateralization index of 4 or higher when cosyntropin is infused, or by an index greater than 2 in the absence of cosyntropin infusion (Funder J. W. Carey RdotM. Mantero F. et al., 2016).

Technically difficult, successful cannulation of the adrenal vein—particularly on the right side—is determined by measuring the cortisol gradient between the adrenal vein and the external iliac vein. Point-of-care cortisol assays can enhance success in centers with limited experience with adrenal venous sampling by offering a dependable evaluation of cannulation within minutes of sample collection (Yoneda et al., 2016).

10.1.4.1. Surgical Management

For patients with unilateral aldosterone overproduction, unilateral laparoscopic adrenalectomy performed by a skilled adrenal surgeon is the preferred treatment when it is possible. Because of the possibility of hyperkalemia following surgery, potassium-sparing drugs (such as ACEI, ARB, MR antagonist, and ENaC inhibitor) and potassium supplements are discontinued right away, and serum potassium concentration is checked once a week for four weeks (Chiang et al., 2013). After surgery, hypertension usually improves one to three months later. Close observation and antihypertensive medication adjustments are necessary.

10.1.4.2. Medical Therapy

Targeted pharmacotherapy with an MR antagonist (spironolactone or eplerenone) should be started when surgery is not practical, including in cases of bilateral aldosterone overproduction. The dose should be adjusted every one to two weeks to achieve a high-normal serum potassium concentration (without the need for potassium supplementation) and unsuppressed renin (signaling adequate MR blockade). When renin is consistently suppressed even after taking the maximum amount of MR antagonist that is safe, it indicates that there is too much sodium in the diet. This needs to be taken into consideration. Up to 20% of patients may experience gynecomastia, female mastodynia, or irregular menstruation as a result of spirolactone, a strong, long-acting, nonselective MR antagonist with progestational and antiandrogenic effects (Parthasarathy et al., 2011). In contrast, eplerenone is a selective MR antagonist with a significantly better adverse effect profile due to its low affinity for androgen and progesterone receptors; however, due to its shorter half-life, it requires twice daily dosing, is 50% less potent than spironolactone, and is not readily available or subsidized in many countries (Parthasarathy et al., 2011). Both spironolactone and eplerenone are effective when titrated to optimal dosages; patient preference, adverse effect profile, availability, and cost should all be taken into consideration when selecting an agent.

Two new nonsteroidal MR antagonists are finerenone and esaxerenone. Based on the findings of the FIDELIO-DKD study (Bakris et al., 2020), finerenone is authorized for use in the United States and the European Union for the treatment of patients with diabetic kidney disease to lower the risk of cardiovascular events and the progression of chronic kidney disease. (Anker et al., 2020). In the same trial, the rate of hyperkalemia was relatively high (22%), but the effect of finerenone on systolic blood pressure was modest (−3.1 and −2.1 mm Hg at 1 month and 12 months, respectively). However, the latter is complicated by the presence of underlying kidney disease (Bakris et al., 2020). Due to finerenone's brief half-life (2 to 3 hours), repeated dosages (every 4 to 6 hours) may be necessary for long-term blood pressure control (Lentini et al., 2016). In Japan, esaxerenone is licensed for the management of hypertension and has a longer half-life (12 hours) (Rakugi et al., 2019). In patients with primary aldosteronism, more research is required to fully comprehend the antihypertensive efficaciousness, safety, and outcome profile of this novel class of MR antagonists.

A promising new drug on the horizon is baxdrostat, a selective inhibitor of aldosterone synthase, the terminal enzyme in the aldosterone biosynthesis pathway. Baxdrostat showed a significant dose-dependent reduction in blood pressure (systolic blood pressure, −20 mm Hg; diastolic blood pressure, −14 mm Hg) at 12 weeks in a recent multicenter, placebo-controlled, phase 2 trial of patients with treatment-resistant hypertension, and hyperkalemia only developed in 3% of patients (Freeman et al., 2023).

10.2. CUSHING'S SYNDROME

Prolonged exposure to high cortisol levels in the blood can result in Cushing syndrome. Iatrogenic corticosteroid use is the most common cause of cushingoid features; however, some herbal preparations can also raise corticosteroid levels in the blood, which can result in Cushing syndrome.

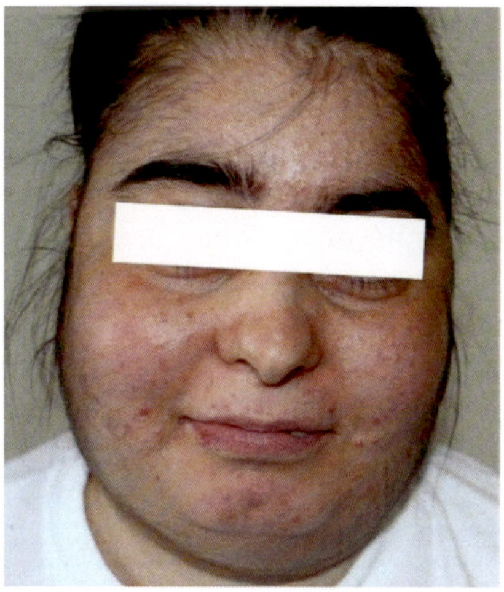

Figure 10.1. *Patient's facial appearance 3 months after therapy with inhaled fluticasone propionate and antidepressants.*

Source: By Ozlem Celik, Mutlu Niyazoglu, Hikmet Soylu and Pinar Kadioglu – http://mrmjournal.biomedcentral.com/articles/10.1186/2049-6958-7-26, CC BY 2.5, https://commons.wikimedia.org/w/index.php?curid=47877333.

It is also referred to as hypercortisolism. 80% of endogenous Cushing syndrome is caused by Cushing disease, which is defined as an ACTH-dependent cortisol excess resulting from a pituitary adenoma (Figure 10.1).

10.2.1. Pathophysiology

The brain's hypothalamus is located above the pituitary gland. Adrenocorticotropin (ACTH) is released by the pituitary gland in response to stimulation by corticotropin-releasing hormone (CRH) released by the paraventricular nucleus (PVN) of the hypothalamus. Through the bloodstream, ACTH reaches the adrenal gland and triggers the release of cortisol. In reaction to ACTH, the cortex of the adrenal gland secretes cortisol from a location known as the zona fasciculata. The hypothalamus's CRH is negatively impacted by elevated cortisol levels, which lowers the amount of ACTH secreted by the anterior pituitary gland.

As a syndrome is a collection of symptoms, Cushing's syndrome strictly refers to excess cortisol of any etiology. A cortisol-secreting adenoma in the adrenal glands cortex (primary hypercortisolism/hypercorticism) is one of the causes of Cushing's syndrome. The adenoma raises blood cortisol levels, which in turn lowers ACTH levels due to the pituitary's negative feedback loop caused by elevated cortisol.

Only hypercortisolism secondary to excess ACTH production from a corticotroph pituitary adenoma (secondary hypercortisolism/hypercorticism) or resulting from excess hypothalamic CRH (corticotropin releasing hormone) production (tertiary hypercortisolism/hypercorticism) is referred to as Cushing's disease. As a result, there is an increase in blood ACTH levels as well as adrenal gland cortisol levels. Because the tumor is resistant to the negative feedback caused by elevated cortisol levels, the ACTH levels stay elevated. Ectopic Cushing syndrome is the term used to describe

Cushing's syndrome caused by excess ACTH. An example of this would be a paraneoplastic syndrome (Colao et al., 2004).

Either a 24-hour urinary measurement for cortisol or a dexamethasone suppression test—which involves administering dexamethasone and frequently monitoring cortisol and ACTH levels—offers comparable detection rates when Cushing's syndrome is suspected. As a glucocorticoid, dexamethasone mimics the actions of cortisol, including the pituitary gland's negative feedback loop. If a blood sample is tested after dexamethasone is given, cortisol levels greater than 50 nmol/L (1.81 µg/dL) would suggest Cushing's syndrome because there is an ectopic source of cortisol or ACTH (adrenal adenoma, for example) that is not suppressed by the dexamethasone. Since late-night salivary cortisol levels are elevated in cushingoid patients, a novel method that was recently approved by the US FDA involves sampling cortisol in saliva over a 24-hour period. This method may be equally sensitive. There may be more pituitary hormone levels that need to be found. If a pituitary lesion is suspected, a physical examination may be required to rule out any visual field defect since a pituitary lesion has the potential to compress the optic chiasm and cause typical bitemporal hemianopia.

In the event that any of these tests yield positive results, incidentalomas - the unintentional discovery of benign lesions - as well as pituitary and adrenal adenomas are detected using MRI and CT scanning of the glands. Sometimes an iodocholesterol scan is required for adrenal gland scintigraphy. Periodically, venous catheterization is required to measure the levels of ACTH in the body's veins, progressing towards the pituitary through petrosal sinus sampling. The tumors that cause Cushing's disease are frequently smaller than 2 mm, making it challenging to find them with MRI or CT imaging. In a study involving 261 patients with confirmed pituitary Cushing's disease, MRI was only able to identify 48% of pituitary lesions before surgery.

Due to peripheral dilution and binding to CRHBP, plasma CRH levels are insufficient at diagnosis (perhaps except for tumors secreting CRH).

10.2.2. Epidemiology

The most prevalent type of Cushing's syndrome is brought on by corticosteroid treatment. According to a Danish study, the yearly incidence of Cushing's disease is less than one case per million individuals. However, approximately one in six people have pituitary microadenomas (less than 10 mm in size) that are asymptomatic. Venous thrombosis is a risk factor for 0.09 to 1% of people with Cushing's syndrome. Obesity and other medical conditions raise the risk of thrombosis as well.

10.2.3. Diagnosis

A history is taken and the presenting signs and symptoms are evaluated physically to diagnose CS. As of right now, there are two first-line screening tests available for CS, and a third screening test is undergoing validation. The low-dose dexamethasone suppression test (DST) and the 24-hour urine free cortisol (UFC) test are the first-line screening methods (Orth, 1995).

10.2.3.1. Confirmation of CS

- **UFC Test:** Cortisol levels in free plasma are correlated with UFC levels. Three 24-hour urine samples are collected by the patient for analysis (Arnaldi G, Angeli A, Atkinson AB, et al., 2003). Under 100 mcg/24 h is considered normal for urine cortisol tests (Pagana and Pagana, 2009). Seldom occurring results exceeding four times the upper limit of normal (usually 440 mcg/24 h) are indicative of CS (Arnaldi et al., 2003). Because of their decreased excretion of cortisol, patients with renal impairment—defined as a glomerular filtration rate less than 30 mL/min—should not undergo the UFC test. The sensitivity of the screening prevents the identification of preclinical or subclinical CS.

- **DST:** The medication dexamethasone lowers plasma cortisol levels in healthy individuals. In CS, the underlying illness may take precedence over this mechanism. Between 2300 and 2400 hours, the patient receives 1 mg of dexamethasone for the DST. Cortisol concentrations are measured the next morning. As in CS, a measurement greater than 5 mcg/dL suggests inhibition of a negative feedback loop. The detection of pseudo-CS, cyclic CS, or early stages of CS is possible at a level of 1.8 mcg/dL, but it may also lead to false-positive results (Giraldi et al., 2007). In clinical practice, a two-day 2-mg DST may be utilized; however, its use is constrained by cost and the potential for increased hospitalization.
- **Late-Night Salivary Cortisol Test (LST):** A new screening instrument called LST is being assessed for CS. Although salivary cortisol concentration and free plasma are closely correlated, salivary flow rate has no effect on it. This screening has assay-dependent normal ranges. High specificity and sensitivity are suggested by current studies, but more investigation is required to support the use of LST as a screening tool (Arnaldi et al., 2003).

10.2.3.2. Differential Diagnosis

After CS is diagnosed, additional testing is required to identify the underlying cause and facilitate appropriate treatment. The CRH stimulation test, high-dose DST, and ACTH measurement are the current second-line tests. An ACTH-dependent CS patient should have a pituitary MRI. Blood surrounding the pituitary gland can be sampled using the bilateral inferior petrosal sinus sampling (BIPSS) test, which enables precise identification of the pituitary origin of elevated ACTH. BIPSS is advised for patients who have CS that is dependent on ACTH as well. However, the advantages and disadvantages must be weighed due to uncommon but serious complications. BIPSS can achieve a sensitivity of 95% to 99% when conducted at "experienced centers." Research is presently being done on many novel differential diagnosis tests, one of which uses desmopressin.

10.2.3.3. Complications of CS

It is critical to treat CS accurately to prevent the many complications that can arise from the disease's progression. Hypertension, poor glucose tolerance, obesity, hyperlipidemia, hypercoagulability, metabolic syndrome, and osteoporosis are major cardiovascular complications. Psychosis, mania, suicidal thoughts, obsessive-compulsive disorder, altered cognition, and anxiety are examples of psychiatric complications that may arise. The gonadal axis, which can negatively impact reproductive organs, the thyroid axis, which can cause hypothyroidism or hyperthyroidism, the somatotrophic axis, which can slow down growth in younger patients or change the distribution of fat in adults, and other areas of the endocrine system may all be affected by high cortisol levels. Even in cases where a patient has subclinical CS, these complications may still exist.

10.2.4. Management

The goal of Cushing syndrome treatments is to reduce the body's cortisol levels. Your individual treatment plan will be determined by the syndrome's etiology. Options include:

10.2.4.1. Reducing Glucocorticoid Use

In the event that long-term glucocorticoid medication use is the cause of Cushing syndrome, your doctor may be able to manage your symptoms by reducing your dosage. This is done gradually and with caution, all the while managing the ailment you are taking it for. Don't stop taking glucocorticoids on your own or lower the dosage. Only accomplish this with your healthcare provider's assistance. If you stop taking these medications too soon, your body may produce insufficient amounts of cortisol. Reducing the dosage gradually enables your body to produce a sufficient level of cortisol (Fitzgerald, 2009).

10.2.4.2. Surgery

If a tumor is the cause of your Cushing syndrome, your doctor might advise surgery to remove the tumor. Neurosurgeons frequently remove pituitary tumors; they may even perform the procedure through your nose. Tumors that produce ACTH in other body parts can be removed through standard surgery or through less invasive methods involving smaller incisions.

In the event that an ACTH-producing tumor is not detected or cannot be completely excised and Cushing syndrome persists, your physician may suggest adrenal gland excision. We refer to this as a bilateral adrenalectomy. This process instantly prevents the body from producing excessive amounts of cortisol. You might require lifelong medication to replace cortisol and another adrenal hormone called aldosterone following the removal of both adrenal glands. It is possible to remove adrenal gland tumors by making a back or midsection incision. Noncancerous adrenal gland tumors can frequently be removed using a minimally invasive procedure (Funder et al., 2016).

Your body won't produce enough ACTH following surgery for Cushing syndrome. To provide the proper amount of cortisol to your body, you will need to take a cortisol replacement medication. Your body usually regains its ability to produce enough cortisol, at which point your doctor can reduce the dosage of the replacement medication. To determine whether you require cortisol medication and when it can be discontinued, your endocrinologist may perform blood tests. This procedure may require six months to a year or longer. Cushing syndrome sufferers may require replacement medication for the rest of their lives.

10.2.4.3. Radiation Therapy

In addition to surgery, radiation therapy might be required if the surgeon is unable to completely remove a pituitary tumor. For those who are not candidates for surgery, radiation therapy is another option. Radiation can be administered as a single, high dose or in small doses spread out over six weeks. Your medical professional can arrange your surgery to minimize radiation exposure to surrounding tissues in both situations.

10.2.4.4. Medications

In cases where surgery and radiation are not effective or are not an option, cortisol levels can be regulated with medication. Before surgery, medications may also be administered to individuals with severe Cushing syndrome. This can lessen the need for surgery while also improving the disease's symptoms. Medical treatment for Cushing syndrome may not fully alleviate all symptoms of excessive cortisol and is not a cure.

Ketoconazole, osilodrostat (Isturisa), mitotane (Lysodren), levoketoconazole (Recorlev), and metyrapone (Metopirone) are medications that regulate the adrenal gland's ability to produce cortisol. Mifepristone (Korlym, Mifeprex) is authorized for use in individuals with Cushing syndrome who have elevated blood sugar levels or type 2 diabetes. Mifepristone inhibits the effects of cortisol on tissues, but it does not decrease the body's production of cortisol (Kelly, 2009).

Two shots of pasireotide (Signifor) are administered daily. It functions by reducing the tumor's production of ACTH, which lowers cortisol levels. There are more medications being developed. These medications may cause fatigue, emesis, headaches, muscle aches, low potassium, high blood pressure, and swelling in addition to other side effects. Some have more serious side effects, like damage to the liver and brain and nervous system. Sometimes the pituitary or adrenal gland produces too few other hormones due to the tumor or the treatment for it. Your healthcare provider may suggest hormone replacement therapy if this occurs.

10.2.4.5. Lifestyle and Home Remedies

Cushing syndrome recovery is typically a gradual, slow process. Before you feel better, it may take some time. You might find these suggestions useful as you return to health.

- **Increase Activities Slowly:** Without going overboard, increase your exercise or activity level to a comfortable level. Avoid engaging in activities that put you at risk of injury, like high-impact exercise. Over time, with perseverance and dedication, your skills will gradually get better.
- **Eat Sensibly:** Your body can get good fuel from nutrient-rich foods while it heals. They can also aid in the loss of any weight that the Cushing syndrome caused you to gain. Ensure that you are getting adequate calcium and vitamin D. Together, these nutrients aid in the body's absorption of calcium, potentially strengthening your bones. This can mitigate the loss of bone mass brought on by Cushing syndrome.
- **Keep an Eye on your Mental Health:** In addition to being a potential side effect of Cushing syndrome, depression can develop or worsen after treatment is initiated. Don't try to ignore or endure depression. If you find yourself feeling down, overwhelmed, or struggling to cope with your recuperation, get help as soon as possible from your medical professional or a therapist.
- **Gently Soothe Aches and Pains:** A portion of the muscle and joint pain experienced during Cushing syndrome recovery can be lessened with hot baths, massages, and low-impact activities like tai chi and water aerobics.

10.3. ACROMEGALY

Approximately 46% of patients with growth hormone excess also have hypertension, which is more common in this population than it is in the general population (Colao et al., 2004).

Growth hormone may cause volume expansion and sodium retention due to its antinatriuretic properties. Congestive heart failure may result from hyperkinetic syndrome symptoms such as elevated heart rate and systolic output. Compared to individuals with normal glucose tolerance, those with acromegaly associated with reduced glucose tolerance or diabetes have higher blood pressure values. Patients with growth hormone excess appear to have a pathophysiology of hypertension that involves the RAAS system. Even with partial biochemical control of growth hormone excess, comorbidities in acromegalics, such as hypertension, hyperlipidemia, diabetes mellitus, and cardiomyopathy, may improve. Even after attempting a biochemical cure or remission, hypertension and diabetes mellitus may still exist in certain patients.

10.3.1. Etiology

Acromegaly has three main causes: excess growth hormone-releasing hormone (GHRH), ectopic or iatrogenic GH excess, and primary GH excess. A somatotroph GH-secreting adenoma of the anterior pituitary gland is the most common cause of amegaly. Activating the guanine nucleotide stimulatory protein gene's alpha subunit is the most frequently found associated mutation (Kempers et al., 2009).

GH-cell carcinomas and pituitary adenomas that secrete several hormones are two additional causes of primary GH excess. Key familial syndromes linked to acromegaly are Carney complex, McCune-Albright syndrome, familial acromegaly, and Multiple Endocrine Neoplasia Type 1. GH excess can also be ectopic, meaning it can be produced by tumors other than pancreatic-islet cell tumors or lymphomas. Additionally, GH excess resulting from over-administered GH may be iatrogenic.

Less common reasons for acromegaly are linked to an abundance of GHRH. These can be categorized into central and peripheral causes. Central causes consist of hypothalamic hamartomas, choristoma, and ganglioneuroma. Peripheral causes include the release of GHRH by bronchial carcinoid tumors, small cell lung cancer, adrenal adenoma, and in some cases, by certain medullary thyroid cancer or pheochromocytoma.

10.3.2. Epidemiology

Acromegaly affects approximately 4,600 out of every million people worldwide, with around 116.9 new cases per million each year, and the number of cases is rising. The average age of diagnosis is 40 for men and 45 for women, usually occurring in the third decade of life.

10.3.3. Diagnosis

Along with a physical examination, your doctor will inquire about your medical history. Next, he or she might advise taking the subsequent actions:

- **IGF-1 measurement:** Following an overnight fast, your doctor will draw blood to test for elevated IGF-1 levels, which may indicate the presence of acromegaly.
- **Growth Hormone Suppression Test:** This is the most effective way to validate a diagnosis of acromegaly. Your GH blood level is measured before and after you consume a sugar preparation (glucose) during this test. The glucose drink generally lowers the GH level in individuals without acromegaly. However, if you have acromegaly, your GH level is likely to remain elevated.
- **Imaging:** If your doctor suspects a tumor on your pituitary gland, they may suggest conducting an imaging

test like magnetic resonance imaging (MRI) to determine the location and size. If no pituitary tumors are detected, additional imaging tests may be ordered to investigate the presence of nonpituitary tumors.

10.3.4. Management

Treatment for amegaly varies from person to person. The location and size of your tumor, the intensity of your symptoms, your age, and your general health will probably all have an impact on your treatment plan. Treatment options usually involve surgery or radiation to remove or reduce the size of the tumor causing your symptoms, and medication to help normalize your hormone levels. This will help lower your GH and IGF-1 levels. Your doctor might suggest extra treatments if your acromegaly is causing your health issues to help manage your complications.

10.3.4.1. Surgery

Transsphenoidal surgery is a commonly used method to remove the majority of pituitary tumors. In this procedure, the surgeon accesses the tumor through the nose, removing it from the pituitary gland. If the tumor is not located on the pituitary gland, a different type of surgery will be recommended by the doctor.

When a tumor is removed, your GH levels usually return to normal, especially if the tumor is small. Removing the tumor also helps relieve headaches and changes in vision if it was pressing on the tissues surrounding your pituitary gland. Your surgeon might not always be able to remove the entire tumor. If so, following surgery, you might continue to have high GH levels. Your physician might suggest more surgery, drugs, or radiation therapy (Lentini et al., 2016).

10.3.4.2. Medications

To help your hormone levels return to normal, your doctor might advise taking any one of the following drugs, or a mix of them:

- Medications that lower the production of growth hormone (analogues of somatostatin). Somatostatin is a brain hormone that prevents the body from producing growth hormone. Synthetic versions of somatostatin are found in the medications lanreotide (Somatuline Depot) and octreotide (Sandostatin). Using one of these medications causes the pituitary gland to release less growth hormone and may even cause a pituitary tumor to shrink. These medications are usually injected by a medical professional once a month into the gluteal muscles in your buttocks.
- Dopamine agonists, such as cabergoline and bromocriptine, can lower hormone levels in some individuals, including GH and IGF-1. These medications may also reduce tumor size. However, for the treatment of acromegaly, high doses of these drugs are typically necessary, which can raise the likelihood of experiencing side effects. Nausea, vomiting, congestion, fatigue, dizziness, insomnia, and mood swings are common side effects associated with these medications.
- Medication that inhibits GH production (growth hormone antagonist). Pegvisomant (Somavert) is a medication that inhibits growth hormone's effects on bodily tissues.

For those who have not responded well to previous treatments, pigvisomant may be especially beneficial. This drug, when administered as a daily injection, can help reduce IGF-1 levels and alleviate symptoms; however, it has no effect on GH levels or tumor size.

10.3.4.3. Radiation

Your doctor might advise radiation therapy if the surgeon was unable to remove the entire tumor during surgery. Radiation therapy gradually lowers GH levels while destroying any remaining tumor cells. The symptoms of acromegaly may not significantly improve for years after starting this treatment. In addition to GH, radiation therapy frequently reduces the levels of other pituitary hormones. You'll probably need to see your doctor for follow-up appointments to ensure that your pituitary gland is functioning normally and to have your hormone levels checked if you receive radiation treatment. You might need this follow-up care for the rest of your life (Table 10.2).

Types of radiation therapy include:

- **Conventional Radiation Therapy:** This radiation therapy regimen typically involves treatment sessions on weekdays for four to six weeks. The full impact of conventional radiation therapy may not be realized until 10 years or more after completing treatment.
- **Stereotactic Radiosurgery:** By limiting the amount of radiation that reaches healthy surrounding tissues, stereotactic radiosurgery delivers a high dose of radiation to the tumor cells. This is achieved through the use of 3D imaging. Typically, a single dose can be given. In five to ten years, GH levels may return to normal under this kind of radiation.

Table 10.2. Management Options for Acromegaly[a]

Treatment Modality	Mechanism of Action	Advantages	**Limitations**
Transsphenoidal surgery	Not applicable	Rapid control of GH excess in most patients with microadenomas Decompression of the optic chiasm in patients with macroadenomas Tumor control	Less effective in achieving biochemical control in patients with macroadenomas Recurrence risk (low probability) Complications (low risk in experienced hands): epistaxis, bleeding, CSF leak, meningitis, stroke, hypopituitarism, hyponatremia
Medical therapy			

Somatostatin receptor ligands	SSTR agonists[b]	Can be effective in achieving both biochemical and tumor control	Adverse effects: diarrhea, dyspepsia, cholelithiasis, hair loss, sinus bradycardia, diabetes mellitus, hyperglycemia
Cabergoline	D2 receptor agonist	More effective in patients with lower baseline IGF-1 levels; orally active	Adverse effects: nausea, orthostasis, headache, nasal congestion, constipation, digital vasospasm, (possibly) cardiac valvulopathy, impulse control disorders
Pegvisomant	GHR antagonist	Rapid control of IGF-1 levels in most patients	No tumor control Adverse effects: injection site reactions, rash, transaminitis
Radiation therapy	Not applicable	Tumor control is achieved in most patients	Biochemical control is slowly achieved in some patients in the absence of medical therapy Risks of anterior hypopituitarism (high probability), cranial neuropathies (low probability); possible risks of secondary tumors or stroke (low probability)

[a] CSF, cerebrospinal fluid; D2, dopamine receptor 2; GH, growth hormone; GHR, growth hormone receptor; IGF-1, insulin-like growth factor 1; SSTR, somatostatin receptor.

[b] First-generation somatostatin receptor ligands (octreotide acetate, octreotide LAR, lanreotide depot, oral octreotide) activate SSTR2 and, to a lesser extent, SSTR5; second-generation somatostatin receptor ligands (pasireotide LAR) activate SSTR1, 2, 3, and 5 (activation of SSTR2 and SSTR5 is considered to be central to drug effectiveness).

Source: Nazanin Ershadinia, Nicholas A. Tritos, Diagnosis and Treatment of Acromegaly: An Update, DOI: https://doi.org/10.1016/j.mayocp.2021.11.007.

10.4. THYROID DISORDERS

A medical condition that prevents your thyroid from producing the proper amount of hormones is commonly referred to as thyroid disease. Individuals of all ages may be affected. The thyroid is a tiny gland beneath the skin that resembles a butterfly and is situated at the front of your neck. As a component of your endocrine system, it produces and releases thyroid hormones, such as triiodothyronine (T3) and thyroxine (T4), which regulate many vital bodily processes. The primary function of your thyroid is to regulate your metabolic rate, or how quickly you burn food. This is the mechanism through which your body converts the food you eat into energy. Your body's cells all require energy to function. An underactive thyroid can have an effect on every part of your body (Palermo et al., 2004).

10.4.1. Pathophysiology

The majority of thyroid diseases in the US are caused by a disorder in which the immune system of the body targets itself. In other cases, the body tries to adjust to new physiological circumstances, such as pregnancy, or to environmental factors, such as an iodine shortage, resulting in thyroid disease.

10.4.1.1. Autoimmune Thyroid Disease

A broad class of diseases known as autoimmune thyroid disease arises when the body is attacked by the immune system. Although the exact cause of this is unknown, given that these illnesses frequently run in families, it is believed to be partly hereditary. The most prevalent kind, Graves' Disease, is characterized by the production of antibodies by the body against the TSH receptor on thyroid cells. This results in the thyroid producing and releasing too much thyroid hormone (hyperthyroidism) and the receptor activating even in the absence of TSH. Hashimoto's thyroiditis is another prevalent type of autoimmune thyroid disease in which the body develops antibodies directed against various thyroid gland normal constituents, most frequently thyroglobulin, thyroid peroxidase, and the TSH receptor. These antibodies trigger the immune system to target the thyroid cells, resulting in gland destruction (fibrosis) and inflammation (lymphocytic infiltration).

10.4.1.2. Goiter

Goiter is a generalized enlargement of the thyroid that is linked to numerous thyroid conditions. The primary cause of this is the thyroid receiving more signals through TSH receptors in an attempt to stimulate the thyroid's production of thyroid hormone. This results in the gland becoming more vascular and growing larger (hypertrophy). The body realizes it is not producing enough thyroid hormone in hypothyroid states or iodine deficiency, so it begins to produce more TSH to help stimulate the thyroid to produce more thyroid hormone. The gland grows larger as a result of this stimulation, producing more thyroid hormone. Even when thyroid hormone levels are normal, there is excess stimulation of the TSH receptor in hyperthyroidism brought on by toxic multinodular goiter or Graves' disease. Thyroid stimulating immunoglobulins, or autoantibodies, bind to and activate TSH receptors in place of TSH in Graves' disease. In toxic multinodular goiter, on the other hand, a mutation in the TSH receptor often causes it to activate without waiting for a signal from TSH. Rarely, the thyroid may enlarge due to congenital abnormalities, increased iodine intake from supplements or medication, or the thyroid filling up with thyroid hormone or thyroid hormone precursors that it cannot release (Rakugi et al., 2019).

10.4.1.3. Pregnancy

Pregnancy causes the body to undergo numerous changes. Making human chorionic gonadotropin (hCG) is one of the main modifications to aid in the development of the fetus. This hormone, which the placenta produces, can bind to the mother's TSH receptor to produce thyroid hormone. Its structure is similar to that of TSH. The mother produces more thyroxine binding globulin, which is responsible for carrying the majority of the thyroid hormone in the blood, as a result of an increase in estrogen during pregnancy. Trimester-specific ranges for TSH and free T4 are required because these normal hormonal changes frequently give the appearance of a hyperthyroid state, even though they may fall within the normal range for pregnancy. The most common cause of true hyperthyroidism during pregnancy is an autoimmune reaction from Graves' disease. Because hypothyroidism frequently makes it difficult to become pregnant in the first place, new diagnoses of hypothyroidism in pregnancy are uncommon. Pregnancy-related hypothyroidism is typically caused by an individual who already has hypothyroidism and needs to increase their levothyroxine dosage to compensate for the increased levels of thyroxine binding globulin.

10.4.2. Epidemiology

The most common type of thyroid disease worldwide is goiter and hypothyroidism brought on by dietary iodine deficiency, but the most common type in the United States is autoimmune inflammation. In the United States alone, thyroid disease affects about 20 million people, according to the American Thyroid Association in 2015. Three to 10% of adults suffer from hypothyroidism; older people and women are more likely to be affected. Currently, a third of people on the planet are thought to reside in regions with low dietary iodine levels. Up to 80% of people have gone through goiter in areas with a severe iodine shortage. With a prevalence of 1-2%, Hashimoto's thyroiditis is an autoimmune subtype of hypothyroidism that is most common in areas without an iodine deficiency. Regarding hyperthyroidism, Graves' disease—an additional autoimmune disorder—is the most prevalent kind, affecting 0.5% of men and 3% of women. Thyroid cancer is uncommon, despite the prevalence of thyroid nodules. Although thyroid cancer is the most common endocrine tumor and causes more than 90% of all endocrine gland cancers, it represents less than 1% of all cancer cases in the United Kingdom (Rubin et al., 2008).

10.4.3. Diagnosis

Each person may experience hypothyroidism symptoms differently. Additionally, they frequently resemble the signs of other medical issues. As such, a diagnosis of hypothyroidism is not made solely on the basis of symptoms. Usually, the outcomes of blood tests serve as the basis.

Serum TSH is the most sensitive test for thyroid dysfunction in an ambulatory population at risk (Demers and Spencer, in press). These days, serum TSH assays are sensitive and specific enough to detect thyroid dysfunction in the general population in all its forms. However, because a serious illness alone can depress TSH secretion, the serum TSH is less specific for thyroid disease among people with acute, serious illness (to be discussed). In the US and many other countries, TSH screening of the neonatal population is required to identify congenital hypothyroidism before it becomes clinically apparent.

The standard course of action following the detection of an abnormal serum TSH value is to repeat the TSH measurement and measure the serum free T_4. The latter can be done in many ways, and among people who are not in the hospital, the majority of the techniques produce results that are negatively correlated with the serum TSH level. Patients with subclinical thyroid dysfunction who have normal serum free T_4 results but high or low serum TSH values are most commonly the cause of discordance between the TSH and free T_4 results.

Results from serum TSH measurements can be misleading for people whose thyroid hormone levels fluctuate. For instance, patients receiving T_4 treatment for hypothyroidism may experience weeks of elevated serum TSH levels. Similarly, in patients receiving treatment for hyperthyroidism, serum TSH levels may stay low for weeks after serum T_4 levels return to normal.

10.4.3.1. Reference Intervals for Thyroid Function Tests

Table 10.3 displays typical reference intervals for thyroid function tests in healthy adults. The middle blood concentration in the U.S. the upper limit of normal (4.5 µU/ml) reported by most laboratories is significantly higher than the value of 1.49 µU/ml for subjects 12 years and older, as reported from 1988 to 1994 in the

NHANES III study (Hollowell et al., 2002). The conclusion drawn from this research is that a serum TSH level greater than 3 µU/ml might not be normal. Within the same research, subjects over 50 had median serum TSH concentrations that were higher than those of younger subjects: 1.60 µU/ml after 50, 1.79 µU/ml after 60, 1.98 µU/ml after 70, and 2.08 µU/ml after 80 years of age. Age-related declines in concentration are seen in serum total and free T_3 levels, but not in serum total or free T_4 levels (Schirpenbach et al., 2006).

Table 10.3. *Serum TSH and Thyroid Hormone Reference Ranges in Adults*

Hormone	Reference Range
TSH	0.4 – 4.5 µU/ml
Total thyroxine (total T_4)	4.0 – 12.0 µg/dl
Free thyroxine (free T_4)	0.7 – 1.8 ng/dl
Total triiodothyronine (total T_3)	100 – 200 ng/dl
Free triiodothyronine (free T_3)	208 – 596 pg/dl

Source: https://www.ncbi.nlm.nih.gov/books/NBK221541/.

10.4.3.2. Thyroid Function Testing in the Elderly

When serum free T_4 results are normal, the prevalence of both low and high serum TSH levels is higher in older subjects than in younger subjects. As will be discussed, an increased prevalence of autoimmune thyroiditis, particularly in women, is believed to be associated with elevated serum TSH values. Low serum TSH values are more common; this could be because of thyroid nodule disease or an undiagnosed non-thyroid condition.

10.4.3.3. Diagnosis of Hypothyroidism

A low level of T_4 and T_3 causes hypothyroidism, a hypometabolic condition. Fatigue, lethargicness, cold intolerance, slowed speech and cognitive function, slowed reflexes, dry skin, hair loss, weight gain, and constipation are some of its main clinical symptoms. It affects women more often than it does men. Primary hypothyroidism, a thyroid disease, is the most common cause of hypothyroidism.

Hashimoto's disease, a chronic autoimmune thyroiditis in which the thyroid is attacked by lymphocytes or antibodies, is the most common cause of primary hypothyroidism. Thyroid inflammatory disease, iodine deficiency, radioactive iodine, surgical treatment for hyperthyroidism or thyroid cancer, and many medications that prevent the production or availability of thyroid hormone are additional causes.

Rarely (less than 1% of cases), hypothyroidism can also result from a TRH deficiency or from reduced TSH secretion brought on by pituitary or hypothalamic disorders, respectively. Because of the negative feedback relationship between serum T_4 and T_3 levels and TSH secretion, this condition is referred to as secondary or central hypothyroidism (Stowasser and Gordon, 2006).

It is necessary to measure serum free T_4 in individuals with high serum TSH values. Primary hypothyroidism is confirmed by the simultaneous discovery of a low free T_4 level and a high serum TSH concentration. Subclinical hypothyroidism is defined as having a high serum TSH concentration and a normal or low-normal serum free T_4 level. The combination of a low serum free T_4 level and a normal or low serum TSH level is used to diagnose secondary hypothyroidism. Although secondary hypothyroidism is far less common than primary hypothyroidism, it is unlikely to be identified by a screening program based on serum TSH measurements.

10.4.3.4. Diagnosis of Hyperthyroidism

Excess T_4 and T_3 production leads to hypermetabolic states such as hyperthyroidism. Nervousness, anxiety, palpitations, fast heartbeat, fatigue, tremor, muscle weakness, weight loss with increased appetite, heat intolerance, frequent bowel movements, increased perspiration, and frequently enlarged thyroid glands (goiter) are its main clinical manifestations. Women make up the majority of those with hyperthyroidism.

Graves' disease, an autoimmune condition marked by the production of antibodies that activate the TSH receptor, is the most common cause of hyperthyroidism. This condition stimulates the production of T_4 and T_3, which in turn causes the thyroid to enlarge. Multinodular goiter, isolated thyroid adenoma, thyroiditis, iodide- or drug-induced hyperthyroidism, and, extremely infrequently, a pituitary tumor that secretes thyroid-stimulating hormone are other causes of hyperthyroidism.

Diagnosing hyperthyroidism involves identifying a high serum free T_4 level and a low serum TSH concentration. In some cases, individuals with hyperthyroidism may exhibit normal serum free T_4 levels and high serum free T_3 concentrations, known as T_3-hyperthyroidism. An increase in serum thyroid hormone binding protein can elevate the serum total T_4 level but won't affect free T_4 concentrations. In such cases, the serum TSH usually remains normal. Patients with a low serum TSH concentration and normal serum free T_4 and free T_3 levels are classified as having subclinical hyperthyroidism.

10.4.3.5. Effect of Medications on Thyroid Test Results

On thyroid function tests, many drugs can have in vivo or in vitro effects that can lead to inaccurate results. Serum total T_4 is increased by medications, particularly estrogens, that raise serum TBG levels; however, serum free T_4 levels and serum TSH concentrations remain unchanged. High doses of glucocorticoids, or adrenal hormones, can reduce serum T_4 (and T_3) by blocking TSH secretion and decrease serum T_3 concentration by preventing the peripheral conversion of T_4 to T_3. The presence of iodide in skin sterilization solutions and radiopaque contrast media during coronary angiography and various other radiological procedures can result in either hyper- or hypothyroidism, contingent on the presence of an undetected thyroid injury or a nodular goiter in the patient. When administered to patients with cardiac arrhythmias, the iodide-containing medication amiodarone can also induce hypothyroidism or hyperthyroidism in those who are suitably susceptible.

The effects of other medications can directly affect the results of thyroid function tests. Heparin, an anticoagulant, for instance, stimulates the release of free fatty acids from triglycerides in serum, which in turn increases serum-free T_4 concentrations. Fluorescence detection-based thyroid test techniques may be susceptible to the presence of medications containing fluorophores or radiology-specific diagnostic agents.

10.4.3.6. Thyroid Function Testing and Nonthyroidal Illness

Thyroid test results are abnormal in many critically ill patients, but there is no other indication of thyroid dysfunction. People with both acute and chronic illnesses experience these abnormalities, and the severity of the illness tends to increase with time. Therefore, it can be very challenging to diagnose thyroid disease in laboratory-dependent patients, particularly those who require hospitalization. Reduced peripheral conversion of T_4 to T_3, decreased serum concentrations of thyroid hormone-binding proteins, and decreased TSH secretion are among the consequences of illness. These alterations are reversible and don't appear to be the cause of thyroid deficiency's clinical symptoms. Small variations in thyroid test results may occur in some healthier individuals, but these may be the consequence of an undiagnosed nonthyroidal illness rather than thyroid dysfunction (Streeten et al., 1979).

10.4.4. Management

The kind of thyroid disease and its underlying cause will determine how it is treated. Restoring your thyroid hormone levels to a healthy range is the aim.

If you have hyperthyroidism, treatment options include:

- **Methylthiouracil and Methimazole:** They are antithyroid drugs that prevent your thyroid from producing hormones.
- **Radioiodine Therapy:** It is also known as radioactive iodine therapy, causes damage to thyroid cells, which stops the thyroid gland from producing high amounts of thyroid hormone.
- **Beta-blockers:** These drugs help control some symptoms, such as an accelerated heart rate, but they have no effect on the thyroid.
- **Surgery:** Your doctor might advise a thyroidectomy (the removal of the thyroid) as a more long-term course of treatment. It will no longer produce hormones as a result. But for the remainder of your life, you will have to take synthetic (manufactured) thyroid replacement hormones in the form of pills.
- **Thyroid Replacement Therapy:** It is the primary treatment option for hypothyroidism. It is a synthetic method of replenishing your body with thyroid hormones. Levothyroxine is one drug that doctors often prescribe.

10.5. PRIMARY HYPERPARATHYROIDISM

In hypertensive patients, parathyroid hormone levels are typically within normal limits and commensurate with the level of calcium in the serum. On the other hand, individuals with essential hypertension excrete more calcium than those with normotension, which may indicate improved parathyroid gland function. PTH is a vasodilator when infused, but in healthy individuals, long-term PTH infusion causes blood pressure to rise. Consuming a lot of calcium may reduce blood pressure. On the other hand, hypertension is linked to a higher incidence of hypercalcemia. Approximately 40% of patients with primary hyperparathyroidism exhibit hypertension. It is unclear how these observations and associations work.

After a parathyroidectomy, hypertension is typically neither cured nor better controlled. When compared to medical management, surgery or parathyroidectomy did not improve blood pressure or quality of life in patients with asymptomatic primary hyperparathyroidism. Conversely, individuals with primary hyperparathyroidism who have a parathyroidectomy may experience a reduction in their severe hypertension. Patients with mild primary hyperparathyroidism appear to have increased arterial stiffness as measured in the radial artery. Abnormalities in the carotid arteries are present in patients with primary hyperparathyroidism (Tsiavos et al., 2016).

Parathyroidectomy decreases SBP variability in normotensive patients with primary hyperparathyroidism. Furthermore, although ambulatory diastolic blood pressure rises in response to surgery, parathyroidectomy in patients with primary hyperparathyroidism may reduce risk of cardiovascular diseases by lowering total cholesterol levels. Endothelial dysfunction may also be a contributing factor to hypertension in patients with primary HPT. In patients with hyperparathyroidism who have MEN syndromes, hypertension may be associated with primary aldosteronism or an underlying pheochromocytoma. At the Fourth International Workshop on the management of asymptomatic primary hyperparathyroidism, criteria for parathyroidectomy were recently reviewed. These criteria now included skeletal and/or renal involvement (nephrocalcinosis on imaging).

10.5.1. Pathophysiology

10.5.1.1. Parathyroid Hormone

To keep calcium homeostasis in check, PTH is an essential hormone that raises serum calcium levels. It controls three main activities to achieve this.

- Increases the resorption of bone, releasing phosphorus and calcium into the bloodstream.
- Reduces the excretion of calcium in the urine by enhancing its reabsorption in the thick ascending loop of Henle and the distal convoluted renal tubule.
- Increases the amount of calcium and phosphorus absorbed through the gastrointestinal tract by activating vitamin D 1-α-hydroxylase in the renal proximal tubule, which changes relatively inactive 25-hydroxyvitamin D (25-VitD) into active 1,25-dihydroxyvitamin D (1,25-VitD).

Serum calcium levels are raised when all three of these activities are combined. Although its contribution to the physiological control of bone metabolism in humans appears to be negligible, the hormone calcitonin, which is generated by the parafollicular in the thyroid gland, has the opposite effect of PTH in that it reduces bone resorption. PTH increases the amount of phosphorus excreted in the urine by blocking the proximal tubular reabsorption of phosphorus. Additionally, it promotes bone resorption and increases phosphorus absorption through the gastrointestinal tract as a result of its effects on vitamin D metabolism. In summary, the majority of individuals diagnosed with primary hyperparathyroidism exhibit normal serum phosphorus levels; however, the presence of hypercalcemia coupled with hypophosphatemia strongly suggests the presence of hyperparathyroidism.

In individuals with primary hyperparathyroidism, the amount of calcium excreted in the urine is determined by the severity of hypercalcemia, GFR, and the impact of PTH on increasing calcium reabsorption in the renal tubules. Because of this, the amount of calcium excreted in urine over a 24-hour period varies, though it is frequently higher due to increased glomerular filtration. Primary hyperparathyroidism can cause hypercalciuria because PTH typically lowers urinary calcium excretion, but this effect can be countered by severe hypercalcemia. In particular, the thick ascending loop of Henle, where roughly 25% of filtered calcium is reabsorbed, contains the calcium-sensing receptor (CaSR) that is present on the parathyroid gland. By reducing the renal tubular urine concentrating ability, defects in CaSR will result in hypocalciuria, whereas activating mutations in this receptor will cause hypercalciuria.

10.5.1.2. Normal Calcium Homeostasis

The concentration of calcium in the extracellular fluid is kept within a specific range during normal physiological conditions. A complex network of hormonal regulatory mechanisms, including the effects of PTH, vitamin D metabolites, and calcitonin on calcium transport in the kidney, gastrointestinal tract, and bones, are responsible for maintaining normal calcium homeostasis. Both active and passive transport mechanisms are involved in the gastrointestinal tract's absorption of calcium. 1,25-VitD increases calcium's active transport. When serum calcium levels are higher than 10 mg/dL, physiological PTH secretion is minimal, and it reaches its maximum when the level falls below 7.5 mg/dL.

Around half of the total serum calcium is bound to proteins, mainly albumin. 45% is in its ionized form, while a small amount binds to anions like phosphate and citrate. Only the ionized calcium is biologically active, but most labs typically report total serum calcium levels. If needed, ionized calcium measurements can be obtained. To correct for variations in serum albumin levels, the following formula can be used:

- Corrected calcium = Measured calcium + 0.8 x (4.0 – albumin)

It is important to exercise caution when assessing normal total serum calcium levels in patients with hypoalbuminemia. In these cases, patients may actually have elevated ionized calcium levels and be considered hypercalcemic. On the other hand, ionized calcium levels are typically normal when there is a low total calcium concentration in the presence of hypoalbuminemia.

A secondary rise in serum PTH levels is brought on by hypocalcemia from lowered 1,25-VitD in chronic kidney disease. Certain parathyroid assays may also inadvertently increase PTH levels in cases of renal failure. Because the failing kidneys are unable to sustain 1,25-VitD levels, intestinal calcium absorption is reduced and serum calcium is lowered, which in turn stimulates the production of PTH. Serum PTH levels are further elevated in chronic renal failure due to reduced PTH clearance. Diffuse, multiglandular parathyroid hyperplasia is the end result of the parathyroid glands' prolonged stimulation. The majority of individuals with chronic kidney disease exhibit low or normal serum calcium levels and secondary hyperparathyroidism. Nonetheless, a small percentage experience tertiary hyperparathyroidism, which is typified by hypercalcemia and autonomous PTH overproduction (Vaidya and Dluhy, 2000).

10.5.2. Epidemiology

About 1 in 1,000 people (0.1% of the population) have primary hyperparathyroidism, and there are 25–30 new cases per 100,000 people in the US each year. According to estimates, the prevalence of primary hyperparathyroidism is as high as 21 per 1000 in postmenopausal women and as low as 3 per 1000 in the general population. In women compared to men, it is nearly three times more common. An elevated all-cause mortality rate is linked to primary hyperparathyroidism.

10.5.3. Diagnosis

Laboratory studies should be used to check for hyperparathyroidism in all patients with hypercalcemia. While strongly suggestive, the discovery of both hypercalcemia and hypophosphatemia does not rule out hyperparathyroidism. Serum phosphorus levels are typically normal in patients with primary hyperparathyroidism; however, hypercalcemia combined with hypophosphatemia strongly suggests hyperparathyroidism or humoral hypercalcemia related to malignancy. The detection of hypercalcemia (i.e., ionized calcium or corrected serum calcium) along with a concurrent elevation of PTH is the conclusive test for primary hyperparathyroidism. PTH levels that are suppressed or appropriately low are linked to the majority of causes of hypercalcemia. To help rule out vitamin D deficiency as a secondary cause of an elevated PTH level, borderline low vitamin D levels should be treated with supplemental vitamin D to achieve a 25-hydroxyvitamin D value >30 ng/mL. PTH levels in patients with primary hyperparathyroidism and other PTH-dependent hypercalcemia-causing conditions are frequently noticeably elevated; in other cases, the values are within the reference range but not appropriately normal. Patients with PTH-independent hypercalcemia should have very low or undetectable PTH levels. PTH levels usually rise with advancing years. "Normal" PTH levels tend to be higher in populations where vitamin D deficiency is prevalent. Immunochemiluminometric or immunoradiometric assays are suggested serum intact parathyroid tests because they can easily distinguish between primary hyperparathyroidism and hypercalcemia related to cancer. In the intact PTH assays, PTH-related protein—which results in humoral hypercalcemia of malignancy—is not found.

Vitamin B-7 sometimes referred to as biotin, is a dietary supplement that can introduce artifacts into laboratory tests, making it difficult to measure certain hormones accurately, including PTH. In such cases, the PTH level should be retested and the biotin should be stopped. If at all feasible, patients taking medications like lithium and thiazide should stop taking them for three to six months and have their PTH and serum calcium levels checked again. Primary hyperparathyroidism is suggested if PTH levels stay high.

Primary hyperparathyroidism and familial hypocalciuric hypercalcemia can be distinguished by analyzing the 24-hour urine calcium and creatinine levels. In familial hypocalciuric hypercalcemia, the urine calcium excretion is usually below 100 mg calcium. The calcium clearance ratio can be calculated by using the formula (urinary calcium x serum creatinine)/(serum calcium x urinary creatinine). A ratio of l<0.01 is indicative of familial hypocalciuric hypercalcemia, while a ratio of >0.02 suggests primary hyperparathyroidism. Values between 0.01 and 0.02 may be influenced by factors such as vitamin D deficiency or chronic kidney disease, requiring repeat testing after vitamin D repletion. Additionally, a calcium infusion test, although rarely performed, can also help differentiate between the two conditions as a calcium load will increase urinary calcium excretion in primary hyperparathyroidism but not in familial hypocalciuric hypercalcemia (Yoneda et al., 2016).

Examining past medical records is frequently very beneficial. Before a conclusive diagnosis of hyperparathyroidism is made, the majority of patients experience intermittent or persistent hypercalcemia for many years. Except for hyperparathyroidism, very few illnesses can cause a healthy-looking person to be hypercalcemic for longer than a few years without exhibiting any symptoms. Studies like 1,25-dihydroxy vitamin D levels, PTH-related protein levels, serum or urine protein electrophoresis, thyroid tests, or mammography can be tailored to the patient's needs and are typically reserved for those with PTH-independent hypercalcemia.

To assess patients for primary hyperparathyroidism, the diagnostic studies listed below are performed:

- Intact PTH;
- Phosphorus;
- Total and ionized calcium;
- Twenty-four-hour urine calcium and

creatinine, with creatinine clearance;

- Vitamin D level (ie, 25-hydroxyvitamin D);
- Albumin and corrected calcium level;
- Alkaline phosphatase;
- Bone densitometry (DEXA), which preferentially affects patients with hyperparathyroidism, including measurement at the distal one-third radius;
- BUN and creatinine;
- Genetic testing for suspicion of a genetic syndrome;
- Imaging studies (e.g., nuclear medicine and ultrasonography) for surgical candidates;
- Imaging to screen for renal calcifications or urolithiasis;
- Kidney, ureters, bladder (KUB) x-ray or renal ultrasound;
- Noncontrast computed tomography (CT) scan;
- Markers of bone formation and resorption (not routinely recommended).

10.5.3.1. Parathyroid Localization Imaging Studies

To locate hyperfunctioning parathyroid glands, standard imaging tests include neck ultrasonography and parathyroid nuclear medicine (Tc-sestamibi) scans. These tests are generally less helpful in multiglandular parathyroid disease and can yield false-negative results, so they are not thought to be definitive. They are most helpful to the surgeon as a "roadmap" in localizing enlarged, hyperfunctioning parathyroid glands, especially when an ectopic gland is suspected, so they shouldn't be ordered unless surgery is planned. Neck ultrasonography is accurate in centers with experience and expertise, but it depends heavily on the operator. Compared to sestamibi scans, which frequently fail to identify nodules smaller than 500 mg, these are thought to be more sensitive. Single-photon emission computed tomography (SPECT) can be used in conjunction with parathyroid imaging scans to increase their sensitivity.

When surgery is planned and sestamibi scans or neck ultrasonography are unable to identify the abnormal parathyroid glands or produce inconsistent results, parathyroid 4-dimensional multiphase (4D) CT should be taken into consideration. 4D CT has been shown to be superior to sestamibi SPECT/CT. Although implementation, instrumentation, and accurate interpretation remain somewhat challenging, this 4D modality is an emerging method of localizing parathyroid adenomas for presurgical planning. In challenging or ambiguous cases, F-18-Fluorocholine positron emission tomography/CT has demonstrated encouraging results in the localization of parathyroid adenomas, indicating superiority over sestamibi scanning, ultrasound, or CT scans alone.

Infrared thermal scanning is a promising imaging technique for pinpointing hyperactive parathyroid glands. This method is particularly valuable when other imaging methods produce conflicting or insufficient results. It relies on the fact that overactive parathyroid glands are highly vascular and typically around 2 degrees warmer than surrounding tissue, making them detectable through thermal imaging. This approach has successfully detected parathyroid adenomas that may be difficult to visualize using other methods. In cases where noninvasive preoperative localization studies are inconclusive, selective parathyroid venous sampling can be used to identify the specific location of abnormal hyperactive glands, despite the technical challenges involved.

10.5.3.2. Bone Imaging

When assessing patients with primary hyperparathyroidism, bone biopsies are rarely necessary; instead, the amount and quality of bone are determined using DEXA and other methods. The effects of PTH excess on skeletal tissue may be more significant than previously believed, according to newer noninvasive imaging technologies. An indirect analysis of trabecular microstructure derived from DEXA data is the trabecular bone score. In patients with primary hyperparathyroidism, the trabecular bone score shows decreased connectivity of the trabecular spinal microstructure, even though the T-score on the DEXA may not be significantly lower. Primary hyperparathyroidism is characterized by fewer, thinner, and more widely spaced trabeculae on high-resolution peripheral quantitative CT scans of the tibia and distal radius. The comparatively high incidence of vertebral fractures in primary hyperparathyroidism may be attributed to trabecular microstructural defects, even in cases where lumbar spine bone mineral density appears to have been preserved. These fractures might not always cause any symptoms (Young and Stanson, 2009).

10.5.4. Management

Surgical intervention, medication, and watchful waiting are available treatment options for primary hyperparathyroidism.

10.5.4.1. Management Approach

The only effective treatment for primary hyperparathyroidism is still surgery. For certain patients, particularly those who are elderly and have mild hypercalcemia without significant complications, nonoperative surveillance may be the best course of action. For certain patients, medical treatment with bisphosphonates or cinacalcet can be very beneficial. Age, the severity of the hypercalcemia, the existence or nonexistence of hyperparathyroidism complications, patient comorbidities, and the risk of anesthesia and surgery are taken into consideration when deciding whether to recommend surgery.

For patients who are not candidates for surgery, medical treatment of primary hyperparathyroidism may be beneficial. Calcium is frequently supplemented in the setting of bone disease, so limiting calcium intake could further stimulate PTH production. There is strong evidence that hyperparathyroidism is predisposed to by long-term vitamin D deficiency. It is advised by experts that individuals suffering from hyperparathyroidism and with low vitamin D levels take supplements to raise their 25-hydroxyvitamin D level above 30 ng/mL. Patients with hyperparathyroidism who are followed for up to 15 years have been found to have favorable long-term outcomes without surgery. In general, their chemistries appear to be fairly stable. During nonoperative surveillance, there is a decrease in bone mineral density that starts at 8 to 9 years and gets more noticeable after year 10. After 15 years, a small number of patients had lost more than 10% of their measured bone mineral density. Nephrolithiasis risk is elevated because hypercalciuria continues while renal function is stable.

The following is advised by current guidelines for the monitoring of patients receiving medical treatment for primary hyperparathyroidism:

- Annual measurement of serum calcium, 25-hydroxyvitamin D, and creatinine clearance;
- PTH levels can be repeated as clinically indicated;
- Repeat 24-hour urine calcium excretion, abdominal imaging for calcifications, and vertebral X-rays can be repeated if clinically indicated;

- Three-site DEXA scans are recommended either annually or biannually.

10.5.4.2. Medical Management

The goal of medical treatment for individuals with primary hyperparathyroidism is to manage hypercalcemia or osteoporosis. While antiresorptive drugs can increase bone density but are less successful in lowering serum calcium, cinacalcet can lower serum calcium but usually not increase bone mineral density. It is advised to use combination therapy if both issues need to be treated.

The following medications can be used to treat primary hyperparathyroidism medically:

- Patients with osteoporosis or osteopenia who are hyperparathyroid may benefit from oral bisphosphonates and denosumab, two antiresorptive medications, which can promote bone mineral density. While intravenous bisphosphonates have been shown to effectively treat severe hypercalcemia, they are not a practical long-term treatment. Reports have indicated that denosumab can control refractory hypercalcemia.
- Patients with hyperparathyroidism will typically see a significant decrease in serum PTH and calcium when taking medications that activate the calcium-sensing receptor, such as cinacalcet, but their bone density will not usually increase. With these drugs, more than 70% of patients' blood calcium levels will return to normal. Even after serum calcium levels return to normal, PTH levels often decline by 35 to 50% and may never fully recover. Cinacalcet can normalize serum calcium even in cases of inoperable parathyroid carcinoma and is quite effective in treating patients with hyperparathyroidism that would otherwise be unmanageable. Urinary calcium levels and vitamin D levels do not vary much. Patients with chronic kidney disease can also receive treatment for secondary hyperparathyroidism with cinacalcet.
- Although estrogen therapy does not alter serum PTH or calcium levels, it has been shown to be beneficial in increasing bone mineral density, especially in the lumbar spine, in postmenopausal women with primary hyperparathyroidism. For the medical treatment of primary hyperparathyroidism, estrogen is not usually advised due to concerns about long-term, chronic use.
- Serum calcium levels can be decreased by up to 1 mg/dL with oral phosphates. They decrease vitamin D levels, lessen bone resorption, and inhibit intestinal calcium absorption through calcium binding. Phosphates used to be commonly used in the long-term medical management of primary hyperparathyroidism are no longer do so because they raise PTH levels and increase the risk of soft tissue calcification.

10.5.4.3. Surgical Therapy

For patients with symptomatic disease, such as those with overt bone disease or recurrent kidney stones, surgery is the preferred course of treatment. A successful parathyroidectomy leads to a significant improvement in bone mineral density across the board and a permanent normalization of serum calcium and PTH levels (Young and Stanson, 2009). Bone mineral density, microstructure, and strength all increase after a successful parathyroid procedure, and patients also have a lower chance of fractures and kidney stones. Following a successful parathyroidectomy, Rubin et al. reported an improvement in bone mineral density of about 10% at all sites, a benefit that lasted for at least 15 years. All patients who had parathyroidectomies, regardless of whether they fulfilled the requirements for surgery, experienced these advantages. On the other hand, there is inconsistent evidence regarding the improvement of cardiovascular events or neurocognitive function following successful parathyroid surgery. Although there are reports that patients with cognitive impairment who are hyperparathyroid may experience improvements in their mental functioning as soon as two weeks after parathyroid surgery, the 5th International Workshop task force found insufficient evidence to recommend parathyroidectomy for improving cardiovascular indices, neurocognitive function, or quality of life.

If both the patient and the doctor approve and there are no contraindications, surgery is a possibility for every patient with primary hyperparathyroidism. The best people to perform the surgery should be skilled parathyroid surgeons who have performed these procedures often and are familiar with preoperative localization. In these hands, success rates are higher than 95%. According to current guidelines, the gold standard of care for all patients with symptomatic primary hyperparathyroidism is surgery. Patients with asymptomatic primary hyperparathyroidism may benefit from surgery in the following situations like:

- Age younger than 50 years;
- GFR or creatinine clearance is <60 mL/min;
- Evidence of renal calcifications, nephrocalcinosis, or urinary stones;
- Hypercalciuria (>300 mg/24 hours in men or 250 mg 24 hours in women);
- Osteoporosis on DEXA scan (T-score <-2.5 at any site);
- Serum calcium >1 mg/dL above the upper limit of normal;
- Vertebral compression fracture on imaging.

Patients undergoing surgery should have preoperative localization studies performed, particularly if a minimally invasive procedure is being used. With a false-positive rate of up to 25% and low sensitivity and specificity, imaging studies are not advised for use in diagnosis alone. For hyperparathyroidism, minimally invasive parathyroidectomy is currently the procedure of choice in the majority of centers. The precise site of the previously discovered aberrant parathyroid gland is the focus of this surgery. Furthermore, it is advised to use intraoperative PTH measurements to confirm the surgery's effectiveness. Since PTH has a short half-life (3–4 minutes), following a successful excision, the PTH level should decrease by at least 50% from its preoperative level in 10–20 minutes and return to normal in 30 minutes. The thyroid gland is the site of about 2% of abnormal parathyroid tissue sources, which include an adenoma in 88% of cases and hyperplastic tissue in 12%. The abnormally functioning tissue can typically be located and successfully imaged using sestamibi scanning and ultrasonography. In most cases, thyroid lobe excise or local excision can result in surgical recovery. In small series, radiofrequency ablation of isolated parathyroid adenomas has been reported to be successful with few complications. For patients who would not otherwise be candidates for surgery, this could be a suitable substitute (Young et al., 2017).

Many patients with primary hyperparathyroidism experience progressive loss of cortical bone if they are left untreated. On the other hand, a successful procedure results in a significant increase in bone mineral density, which can last for up to 15 years. After surgery, patients with nephrolithiasis typically have fewer stones. It is still recommended to do a 24-hour urine kidney stone risk profile analysis because there are still potential chemical promoters of kidney stones. If patients experience symptoms, complications, worsening hypercalcemia, or any of the following during the nonoperative surveillance period, surgery is advised which includes:

- Low trauma fracture;
- Nephrolithiasis or nephrocalcinosis;
- Serum calcium consistently >1 mg/dL above the upper limit of normal;
- Significant reduction in BMD to a T-score <2.5 at any site;
- Significant decrease in creatinine clearance.

10.5.4.4. Hungry Bone Syndrome

Hungry bone syndrome is the term used to describe the period of profound, severe, and prolonged hypocalcemia that may occur immediately after the surgical correction of primary or secondary hyperparathyroidism. The majority of sources characterize hungry bone syndrome as a persistently low serum calcium level of less than 8.4 mg/dL for more than 4 days following definitive parathyroid surgery, though there is no universal agreement on this. Following surgery, there is an abrupt decrease in PTH levels, which leads to unopposed accelerated osteoblastic activity. This rapid incorporation of serum calcium into new bone causes significant hypocalcemia. Hypophosphatemia, hypomagnesemia, and elevated alkaline phosphatase are frequently present in conjunction with this.

It is possible for hypophosphatemia and hypocalcemia to last for months or even years. Following parathyroid surgery, hypocalcemia can also result from hypoparathyroidism and hypomagnesemia. Those with hypoparathyroidism should have higher serum phosphorus levels than those with hungry bone syndrome. The likelihood of developing hungry bone syndrome rises as hyperparathyroidism worsens and lasts longer. This syndrome may also develop following treatment for malignant tumors that impair calcium metabolism, such as prostate cancer, thyrotoxicosis, vitamin D supplementation in calcitriol-deficient patients, or correction of secondary hyperparathyroidism. Patients with chronic dialysis and renal failure who have secondary hyperparathyroidism are more likely to experience hungry bone syndrome than those with primary parathyroid disease.

High oral calcium supplementation—calcium citrate is preferred—and vitamin D are the usual forms of treatment. However, intravenous calcium supplementation is necessary if the serum calcium level is less than 7.6 mg/dL, symptoms of hypocalcemia are present, or there are associated EKG abnormalities (such as prolonged QT). For intravenous calcium supplementation, calcium gluconate is typically preferred over calcium chloride because it is simpler to administer, doesn't require a central line, and has a lower risk of causing tissue necrosis if the IV infiltrates (Young et al., 2017).

10.5.4.5. Differential Diagnosis

Although there are many possible diagnoses for primary hyperthyroidism, laboratory tests can frequently be used to make distinctions. Secondary hyperparathyroidism, normocalcemic primary hyperparathyroidism, familial hypocalciuric hypercalcemia, malignancy-related hypercalcemia, granulomatous diseases, hyperthyroidism, lithium therapy, thiazide therapy, milk-alkali syndrome, vitamin A intoxication, and vitamin D intoxication are some conditions that present with hypercalcemia or other similar presentations.

10.6. DIAGNOSIS AND MANAGEMENT OF RENAL ARTERY STENOSIS AND OTHER RARE FORMS OF RENIN DRIVEN HYPERTENSION

The narrowing of one or both renal arteries is known as renal artery stenosis. It is the primary cause of hypertension and, based on some reports, the reason behind hypertension in 1% to 5% of the 50 million Americans living with the condition. It is primarily caused by fibromuscular dysplasia or atherosclerosis. End-stage renal disease and chronic kidney disease are two more complications linked to renal artery stenosis.

10.6.1. Pathophysiology

10.6.1.1. Pathogenesis of Hypertension

Although the exact cause of endothelial injury in atherosclerosis is unknown, it may be caused by dyslipidemia, smoking, viruses, immunological damage, or elevated homocysteine levels. Permeability to low-density lipoprotein (LDL) and macrophage migration rise at the lesion site, leading to the eventual formation of atherosclerotic plaque and the proliferation of smooth muscle and endothelial cells. One of the key factors influencing the glomerular filtration rate (GFR) is the renal blood flow, which is much higher than the perfusion to other organs. The other factor is the hydrostatic pressure of the glomerular capillaries. Renal artery stenosis patients experience chronic ischemia due to renal blood flow obstruction, which causes adaptive changes in the kidney. These changes include the formation of collateral blood vessels and renin secretion by the juxtaglomerular apparatus. Because it changes angiotensinogen into angiotensin I, the renin enzyme plays a crucial part in preserving homeostasis. The lungs' angiotensin-converting enzyme (ACE) then helps to convert angiotensin I into angiotensin II. Angiotensin II is in charge of vasoconstriction and aldosterone release, which lead to water and salt retention and secondary hypertension, also known as renovascular hypertension.

10.6.1.2. Pathogenesis of Chronic Renal Insufficiency

Between the afferent and efferent arteries, angiotensin II and other modulators auto-regulate the glomerular filtration rate (GFR). When renal perfusion pressure drops below 70 mmHg to -85 mmHg, the maintenance of GFR is no longer possible. Therefore, until arterial luminal narrowing surpasses 50%, significant functional impairment of autoregulation, resulting in a decrease in the GFR, is unlikely to be observed. Research indicates that glomerular filtration can be reduced by up to 40% when renal perfusion pressure and renal blood flow are moderately reduced (mean 30%). Nevertheless, tissue oxygenation in the kidney cortex and medulla can adjust to these changes without leading to severe hypoxia. As a result, early-stage patients can often receive medical therapy without experiencing a progressive loss of function or irreversible fibrosis—sometimes for years at a time.

More advanced stenosis, which corresponds to 70–80% vascular occlusion, is reported to cause demonstrable cortical hypoxia. It is hypothesized that this hypoxia causes rarefaction of microvessels and activates oxidative and inflammatory pathways that result in interstitial fibrosis. Thus, in addition to being a generally reversible side effect of antihypertensive medication, loss of renal function in renovascular disease may also be a sign of progressive intrinsic renal disease or a narrowing of the renal arteries. Long-term parenchymal injury eventually turns into an irreversible process. Restoring renal blood flow does not currently result in a return of renal function or any therapeutic advantages (Palermo et al., 2004).

10.6.2. Epidemiology

Renal artery stenosis is probably less than 1% common in patients with mild hypertension but can reach 10–40% in patients with acute, severe, or refractory hypertension (even if it is imposed on top of an already-existing blood pressure elevation). According to many studies, the prevalence of unilateral stenosis ranges from roughly 53% to 80% when compared to bilateral stenosis.

Research shows that among patients over the age of 50, ischemic nephropathy may be responsible for 5% to 22% of cases of advanced renal disease. In those with fibromuscular dysplasia, the renal arteries are affected in approximately 75% to 80% of cases, with around two-thirds of patients having multiple arteries involved. This condition is more prevalent in females than in males.

10.6.3. Diagnosis

Your doctor may begin by diagnosing renal artery stenosis by doing the following:

- A physical examination during which your doctor listens for noises that could indicate a narrowed kidney artery with a stethoscope over the kidney regions.
- An analysis of your past medical records.
- Tests on your blood and urine to assess kidney function. tests on the blood and urine to determine the hormone levels that control blood pressure.

Renal artery stenosis is frequently diagnosed with imaging tests such as these:

- **Ultrasound Doppler:** Your doctor can see and examine your kidneys and arteries with the use of high-frequency sound waves. This process also aids in the identification and assessment of blood vessel blockages by your physician.
- **CT Scan:** An X-ray machine connected to a computer produces a detailed image during a CT scan that displays cross-sectional views of the renal arteries. To demonstrate blood flow, you might be given an injection of dye.
- **MRA stands for Magnetic Resonance Imaging:** MRA creates precise three-dimensional (3D) images of the kidneys and renal arteries using radio waves and powerful magnetic fields. During imaging, blood vessels are outlined by an injection of dye into the arteries.
- **Renal Artery Mapping:** This particular kind of X-ray examination aids in the diagnosis of renal artery blockage by your physician, who may use a balloon or stent to open the narrowed portion. Your

doctor uses a long, thin tube called a catheter to inject a dye into the renal arteries before taking an X-ray to better define the arteries and demonstrate blood flow. This test is primarily performed if it is also likely that you will require the implantation of a small tube, or stent, to widen your blood vessel.

10.6.4. Management

Renal artery stenosis treatment options include medication, lifestyle modifications, and kidney blood flow restoration surgery. Sometimes the best course of action is to combine several treatments. Your overall health and symptoms may determine whether you require any special treatment or not.

10.6.4.1. Lifestyle Changes

A healthy lifestyle that includes eating a diet low in salt, exercising frequently, and getting regular physical activity can help control blood pressure if it is moderately or severely elevated.

10.6.4.2. Medication

Even when the primary cause of high blood pressure is renal artery stenosis, medication is frequently an effective treatment. It might take some time and patience to find the right medication or combination of medications.

Some drugs that are frequently prescribed to treat high blood pressure brought on by renal artery stenosis are as follows:

- Angiotensin II receptor blockers (ARBs) and angiotensin-converting enzyme (ACE) inhibitors help relax blood vessels and prevent the body's natural production of the blood vessel-narrowing chemical angiotensin II.
- Diuretics, commonly referred to as water pills, aid the body in getting rid of extra water and salt.
- Depending on the medication you take, beta blockers and alpha-beta blockers may cause your heart to beat more slowly and gently or they may cause your blood vessels to dilate.
- Calcium channel blockers: they aid in blood vessel relaxation.

If renal artery stenosis is caused by atherosclerosis, your doctor might also suggest aspirin and a cholesterol-lowering drug. The right drugs for you will depend on your unique circumstances.

10.6.4.3. Procedures

To enhance blood flow to the kidney, a procedure to reopen the renal artery may be advised for some individuals. Findings from clinical trials comparing medication with renal angioplasty and stenting for patients with moderate renal artery stenosis did not demonstrate any distinction between the two treatment modalities in terms of lowering hypertension and enhancing renal function. Those who are not well treated with medicine alone, have medication intolerance issues, frequently retain fluids, or have treatment-resistant heart failure should think about having the vessel opened (Young et al., 2017).

Procedures to treat renal artery stenosis may include:

- **Stent Placement and Renal Angioplasty:** During this procedure, a device called a stent is inserted into your blood vessel to hold its walls open and improve blood flow, while also widening the narrowed renal artery.
- **Surgery for Renal Artery Bypass:** To create a new path for blood to get to your

kidneys, doctors graft a replacement blood vessel to the renal artery during a bypass procedure. This may occasionally entail joining the renal artery to a vessel from another organ, like the spleen or liver. These procedures are typically carried out in cases where angioplasty proves unsuccessful or when additional surgical procedures become necessary.

10.6.4.4. Lifestyle and Home Remedies

As a part of your treatment plan for renal artery stenosis, your doctor may recommend making certain lifestyle changes:

- **Sustain a Healthy Weight:** Your blood pressure rises as you gain weight. Reducing your weight could assist in lowering your blood pressure if you are overweight.
- **Limit the Amount of Salt You Eat:** Your body retains fluid when exposed to salt and salty foods. Your blood pressure may rise as a result of this increasing blood volume.
- **Engage in Physical Activity:** Regular physical activity has been shown to help people reduce their blood pressure, cholesterol, risk of heart disease, and weight. Before starting an exercise program, especially if you have high blood pressure and haven't been active in the past, consult your doctor.
- **Lessen Your Tension:** Your blood pressure may drop if you reduce your stress levels.
- **Avoid Alcohol:** If you use alcohol at all, do so in moderation. Your blood pressure may rise if you drink too much alcohol.
- **Avoid Smoking:** Smoking damages the walls of blood vessels and hastens the artery-hardening process. Ask your doctor for assistance in quitting if you smoke.

A Closer Look

Pseudo-Cushing's Syndrome

Non-neoplastic hypercortisolism, also known as pseudo-Cushing's syndrome, is a medical condition where patients exhibit the symptoms, signs, and abnormal cortisol levels typically seen in Cushing's syndrome. Unlike Cushing's, pseudo-Cushing's is not caused by issues with the hypothalamic-pituitary-adrenal axis but rather is often idiopathic in nature. However, a Cushingoid appearance can sometimes be linked to excessive alcohol consumption. In addition, elevated total cortisol levels can be attributed to estrogen present in certain oral contraceptive pills containing both estrogen and progesterone. This is because estrogen can lead to an increase in cortisol-binding globulin, ultimately resulting in higher total cortisol levels.

Summary

- Primary aldosteronism (PA) is the most common form of secondary hypertension (HTN), with an estimated prevalence of 4% of hypertensive patients in primary care and around 10% of referred patients. Primary aldosteronism is screened for by measuring plasma aldosterone (PA) and plasma renin activity (PRA) or direct renin concentration.
- Cushing syndrome is caused by prolonged exposure to high circulating levels of cortisol. The most common cause of cushingoid features is iatrogenic corticosteroid use, while some herbal preparations can also increase circulating corticosteroid levels leading to Cushing syndrome.
- The prevalence of hypertension in patients with growth hormone excess is approximately 46% and more frequent than in the general population. Growth hormone has anti natriuretic actions and may lead to sodium retention and volume expansion.
- Thyroid disease is a general term for a medical condition that keeps your thyroid from making the right amount of hormones. It can affect people of all ages. Your thyroid is a small, butterfly-shaped gland located at the front of your neck under your skin. The symptoms of hypothyroidism can be different from person to person. And they often look like symptoms of other health problems. Because of that, a diagnosis of hypothyroidism doesn't rely on symptoms alone. It is usually based on the results of blood tests.
- Parathyroid hormone levels in hypertensive patients usually are in the normal range and appropriate for the serum calcium concentration. However, patients with essential hypertension excrete more calcium compared to normotensive people, suggesting an enhanced parathyroid gland function.
- Renal artery stenosis is narrowing of the one or both of renal arteries. It is the major cause of hypertension and according to some reports is the cause of hypertension in 1% to 10% of the 50 million people in the United States. Atherosclerosis or fibromuscular dysplasia most often cause it. Other associated complications of renal artery stenosis are chronic kidney disease and end-stage renal disease.

References

1. Arnaldi, G., Angeli, A., Atkinson, A. B., et al. (2003). Diagnosis and complications of Cushing's syndrome: A consensus statement. *Journal of Clinical Endocrinology & Metabolism, 88*(12), 5593–5602. https://doi.org/10.1210/jc.2003-030871.
2. Bakris, G. L., Agarwal, R., Anker, S. D., et al. (2020). Effect of finerenone on chronic kidney disease outcomes in type 2 diabetes. *New England Journal of Medicine, 383*(23), 2219–2229. https://doi.org/10.1056/NEJMoa2025845.
3. Chiang, W. F., Cheng, C. J., Wu, S. T., et al. (2013). Incidence and factors of post-adrenalectomy hyperkalemia in patients with aldosterone-producing adenoma. *Clinica Chimica Acta, 424*, 114–118. https://doi.org/10.1016/j.cca.2013.05.009.
4. Colao, A., Ferone, D., Marzullo, P., & Lombardi, G. (2004). Systemic complications of acromegaly: Epidemiology, pathogenesis, and management. *Endocrine Reviews, 25*(1), 102–152. https://doi.org/10.1210/er.2002-0022.

5. Freeman, M. W., Halvorsen, Y. D., Marshall, W., et al. (2023). Phase 2 trial of baxdrostat for treatment-resistant hypertension. *New England Journal of Medicine, 388*(5), 395–405. https://doi.org/10.1056/NEJMoa2210718.

6. Funder, J. W., Carey, R. M., Mantero, F., et al. (2016). The management of primary aldosteronism: Case detection, diagnosis, and treatment: An Endocrine Society Clinical Practice Guideline. *Journal of Clinical Endocrinology & Metabolism, 101*(5), 1889–1916. https://doi.org/10.1210/jc.2015-4061.

7. Giraldi, F. P., Ambrogio, A. G., De Martin, M., et al. (2007). Specificity of first-line tests for the diagnosis of Cushing's syndrome: Assessment in a large series. *Journal of Clinical Endocrinology & Metabolism, 92*(11), 4123–4129. https://doi.org/10.1210/jc.2007-0892.

8. Kelly, W. (2009). Cushing's syndrome: A review of diagnosis and treatments. *Sudan Medical Journal, 45*(3), 3–7.

9. Kempers, M. J., Lenders, J. W., van Outheusden, L., et al. (2009). Systematic review: Diagnostic procedures to differentiate unilateral from bilateral adrenal abnormality in primary aldosteronism. *Annals of Internal Medicine, 151*(5), 329–337. https://doi.org/10.7326/0003-4819-151-5-200909010-00007.

10. Lentini, S., Heinig, R., Kimmeskamp-Kirschbaum, N., & Wensing, G. (2016). Pharmacokinetics, safety, and tolerability of the novel, selective mineralocorticoid receptor antagonist finerenone: Results from first-in-man and relative bioavailability studies. *Fundamental & Clinical Pharmacology, 30*(2), 172–184. https://doi.org/10.1111/fcp.12194.

11. Orth, D. N. (1995). Cushing's syndrome. *New England Journal of Medicine, 332*(12), 791–803. https://doi.org/10.1056/NEJM199503233321207.

12. Pagana, K., & Pagana, T. (2009). *Mosby's Diagnostic and Laboratory Reference* (9th ed., p. 303). St. Louis, MO: Mosby.

13. Palermo, M., Quinkler, M., & Stewart, P. M. (2004). Apparent mineralocorticoid excess syndrome: An overview. *Arquivos Brasileiros de Endocrinologia & Metabologia, 48*(5), 687–696. https://doi.org/10.1590/s0004-27302004000500003.

14. Parthasarathy, H. K., Menard, J., White, W. B., et al. (2011). A double-blind, randomized study comparing the antihypertensive effect of eplerenone and spironolactone in patients with hypertension and evidence of primary aldosteronism. *Journal of Hypertension, 29*(5), 980–990. https://doi.org/10.1097/HJH.0b013e328344da92.

15. Rakugi, H., Ito, S., Itoh, H., Okuda, Y., & Yamakawa, S. (2019). Long-term phase 3 study of esaxerenone as mono or combination therapy with other antihypertensive drugs in patients with essential hypertension. *Hypertension Research, 42*(12), 1932–1941. https://doi.org/10.1038/s41440-019-0315-4.

16. Rubin, M. R., Bilezikian, J. P., McMahon, D. J., Jacobs, T., Shane, E., Siris, E., Udesky, J., & Silverberg, S. J. (2008). The natural history of primary hyperparathyroidism with or without parathyroid surgery after 15 years. *Journal of Clinical Endocrinology & Metabolism, 93*(9), 3462–3470. https://doi.org/10.1210/jc.2007-1215.

17. Schirpenbach, C., Seiler, L., Maser-Gluth, C., Beuschlein, F., Reincke, M., & Bidlingmaier, M. (2006). Automated chemiluminescence-immunoassay for aldosterone during dynamic testing: Comparison to radioimmunoassay's with and without extraction steps. *Clinical Chemistry, 52*(9), 1749–1755. https://doi.org/10.1373/clinchem.2006.070532.

18. Seiler, L., Rump, L. C., Schulte-Mönting, J., Slawik, M., Borm, K., Pavenstädt, H., Beuschlein, F., & Reincke, M. (2004). Diagnosis of primary aldosteronism: Value of different screening parameters and influence of antihypertensive medication. *European Journal of Endocrinology, 150*(3), 329–337. https://doi.org/10.1530/eje.0.1500329.

19. Stowasser, M., & Gordon, R. D. (2006). Aldosterone assays: An urgent need for improvement. *Clinical Chemistry, 52*(9), 1640–1642. https://doi.org/10.1373/clinchem.2006.075713.

20. Streeten, D. H. P., Tomycz, N., & Anderson, G. H. (1979). Reliability of screening methods for the diagnosis of primary aldosteronism. *American Journal of Medicine, 67*(3), 403–413. https://doi.org/10.1016/0002-9343(79)90418-6.

21. Tsiavos, V., Markou, A., Papanastasiou, L., et al. (2016). A new highly sensitive and specific overnight combined screening and diagnostic test for primary aldosteronism. *European Journal of Endocrinology, 175*(1), 21–28. https://doi.org/10.1530/EJE-16-0146.

22. Vaidya, A., & Dluhy, R. (2000). Hyperaldosteronism. *MDText.com, Inc.*

23. Yoneda, T., Karashima, S., Kometani, M., et al. (2016). Impact of new quick gold nanoparticle-based cortisol assay during adrenal vein sampling for primary aldosteronism. *Journal of Clinical Endocrinology & Metabolism, 101*(7), 2554–2561. https://doi.org/10.1210/jc.2015-4139.

24. Young, W. F., & Stanson, A. W. (2009). What are the keys to successful adrenal venous sampling (AVS) in patients with primary aldosteronism? *Clinical Endocrinology, 70*(1), 14–17. https://doi.org/10.1111/j.1365-2265.2008.03301.x.

25. Young, W. F., Calhoun, D. A., Lenders, J. W. M., Stowasser, M., & Textor, S. C. (2017). Screening for endocrine hypertension: An Endocrine Society scientific statement. *Endocrine Reviews, 38*(2), 103–122. https://doi.org/10.1210/er.2017-00054.

INDEX

B

C

H

I

K

L

M

N

O

P

R

S

T

U

V

W

Z

FSC
www.fsc.org
MIX
Papier | Fördert gute Waldnutzung
FSC® C083411

Kolibri 360 GmbH
Ferdinand-Jühlke-Straße 7
99095 Erfurt, Deutschland
produktsicherheit@kolibri360.de